Online Resources

Included with your purchase are multiple online resources. This includes the practice tests in an interactive format and a convenient study timer to help you manage your time.

Instructions for accessing these resources can be found on the last page of this book.

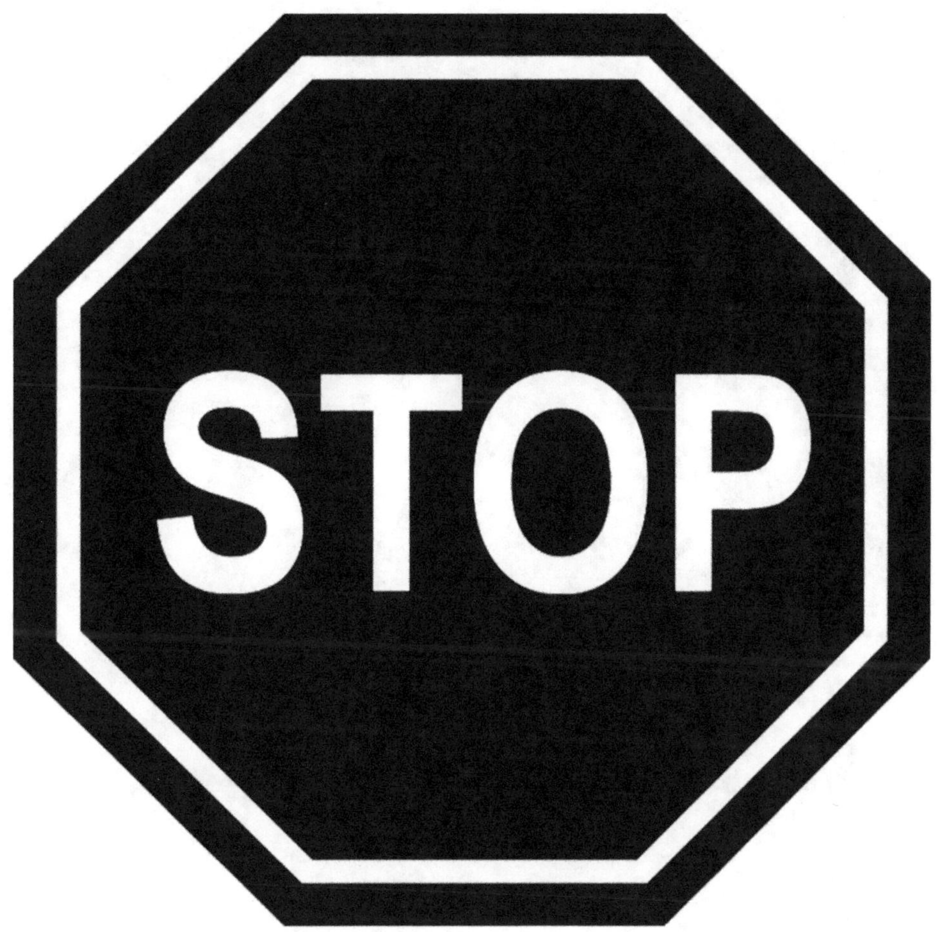

Women's Health Nurse Practitioner Study Guide

WHNP Review Book with Full-Length Practice Tests (375+ Questions) for the NCC® Exam [Includes Detailed Answer Explanations]

Lydia Morrison

Written and edited by TPB Publishing.

ISBN 13: 9781637757383

Table of Contents

Welcome

Dear Reader,

Welcome to your new Test Prep Books study guide! We are pleased that you chose us to help you prepare for your exam. There are many study options to choose from, and we appreciate you choosing us. Studying can be a daunting task, but we have designed a smart, effective study guide to help prepare you for what lies ahead.

Whether you're a parent helping your child learn and grow, a high school student working hard to get into your dream college, or a nursing student studying for a complex exam, we want to help give you the tools you need to succeed. We hope this study guide gives you the skills and the confidence to thrive, and we can't thank you enough for allowing us to be part of your journey.

In an effort to continue to improve our products, we welcome feedback from our customers. We look forward to hearing from you. Suggestions, success stories, and criticisms can all be communicated by emailing us at support@testprepbooks.com.

Sincerely,

Test Prep Books Team

Quick Overview

As you draw closer to taking your exam, effective preparation becomes more and more important. Thankfully, you have this study guide to help you get ready. Use this guide to help keep your studying on track and refer to it often.

This study guide contains several key sections that will help you be successful on your exam. The guide contains tips for what you should do the night before and the day of the test. Also included are test-taking tips. Knowing the right information is not always enough. Many well-prepared test takers struggle with exams. These tips will help equip you to accurately read, assess, and answer test questions.

A large part of the guide is devoted to showing you what content to expect on the exam and to helping you better understand that content. In this guide are practice test questions so that you can see how well you have grasped the content. Then, answer explanations are provided so that you can understand why you missed certain questions.

Don't try to cram the night before you take your exam. This is not a wise strategy for a few reasons. First, your retention of the information will be low. Your time would be better used by reviewing information you already know rather than trying to learn a lot of new information. Second, you will likely become stressed as you try to gain a large amount of knowledge in a short amount of time. Third, you will be depriving yourself of sleep. So be sure to go to bed at a reasonable time the night before. Being well-rested helps you focus and remain calm.

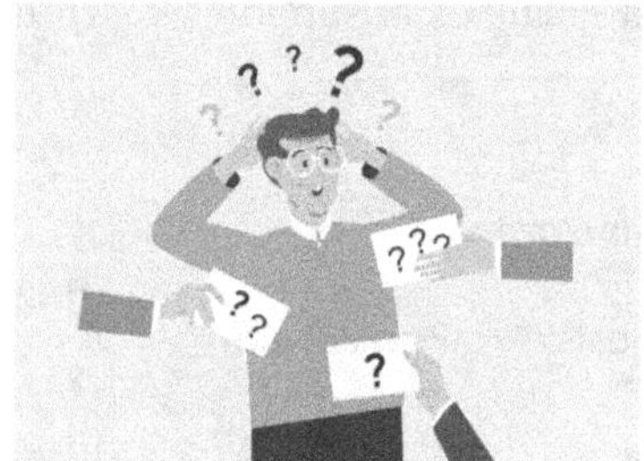

Be sure to eat a substantial breakfast the morning of the exam. If you are taking the exam in the afternoon, be sure to have a good lunch as well. Being hungry is distracting and can make it difficult to focus. You have hopefully spent lots of time preparing for the exam. Don't let an empty stomach get in the way of success!

When travelling to the testing center, leave earlier than needed. That way, you have a buffer in case you experience any delays. This will help you remain calm and will keep you from missing your appointment time at the testing center.

Be sure to pace yourself during the exam. Don't try to rush through the exam. There is no need to risk performing poorly on the exam just so you can leave the testing center early. Allow yourself to use all of the allotted time if needed.

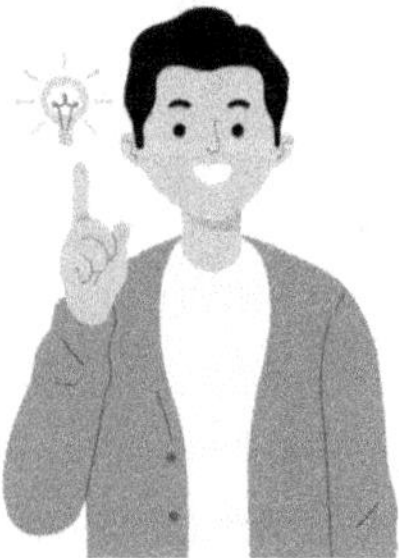

Remain positive while taking the exam even if you feel like you are performing poorly. Thinking about the content you should have mastered will not help you perform better on the exam.

Once the exam is complete, take some time to relax. Even if you feel that you need to take the exam again, you will be well served by some down time before you begin studying again. It's often easier to convince yourself to study if you know that it will come with a reward!

Test-Taking Strategies

1. Predicting the Answer

When you feel confident in your preparation for a multiple-choice test, try predicting the answer before reading the answer choices. This is especially useful on questions that test objective factual knowledge. By predicting the answer before reading the available choices, you eliminate the possibility that you will be distracted or led astray by an incorrect answer choice. You will feel more confident in your selection if you read the question, predict the answer, and then find your prediction among the answer choices. After using this strategy, be sure to still read all of the answer choices carefully and completely. If you feel unprepared, you should not attempt to predict the answers. This would be a waste of time and an opportunity for your mind to wander in the wrong direction.

2. Reading the Whole Question

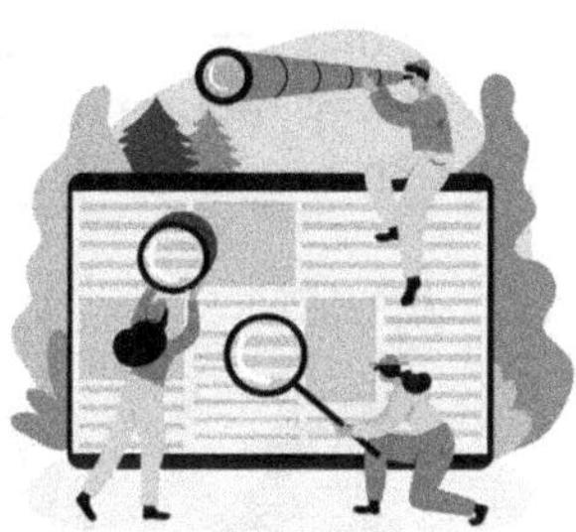

Too often, test takers scan a multiple-choice question, recognize a few familiar words, and immediately jump to the answer choices. Test authors are aware of this common impatience, and they will sometimes prey upon it. For instance, a test author might subtly turn the question into a negative, or he or she might redirect the focus of the question right at the end. The only way to avoid falling into these traps is to read the entirety of the question carefully before reading the answer choices.

3. Looking for Wrong Answers

Long and complicated multiple-choice questions can be intimidating. One way to simplify a difficult multiple-choice question is to eliminate all of the answer choices that are clearly wrong. In most sets of answers, there will be at least one selection that can be dismissed right away. If the test is administered on paper, the test taker could draw a line through it to indicate that it may be ignored; otherwise, the test taker will have to perform this operation mentally or on scratch paper. In either case, once the obviously incorrect answers have been eliminated, the remaining choices may be considered. Sometimes identifying the clearly wrong answers will give the test taker some information about the correct answer. For instance, if one of the remaining answer choices is a direct opposite of one of the eliminated answer choices, it may well be the correct answer. The opposite of obviously wrong is obviously right! Of course, this is not always the case. Some answers are obviously incorrect simply because they are irrelevant to the question being asked. Still, identifying and eliminating some incorrect answer choices is a good way to simplify a multiple-choice question.

4. Don't Overanalyze

Anxious test takers often overanalyze questions. When you are nervous, your brain will often run wild, causing you to make associations and discover clues that don't actually exist. If you feel that this may be a problem for you, do whatever you can to slow down during the test. Try taking a deep breath or counting to ten. As you read and consider the question, restrict yourself to the particular words used by the author. Avoid thought tangents about what the author *really* meant, or what he or she was *trying* to say. The only things that matter on a multiple-choice test are the words that are actually in the question. You must avoid reading too much into a multiple-choice question, or supposing that the writer meant something other than what he or she wrote.

5. No Need for Panic

It is wise to learn as many strategies as possible before taking a multiple-choice test, but it is likely that you will come across a few questions for which you simply don't know the answer. In this situation, avoid panicking. Because most multiple-choice tests include dozens of questions, the relative value of a single wrong answer is small. As much as possible, you should compartmentalize each question on a multiple-choice test. In other words, you should not allow your feelings about one question to affect your success on the others. When you find a question that you either don't understand or don't know how to answer, just take a deep breath and do your best. Read the entire question slowly and carefully. Try rephrasing the question a couple of different ways. Then, read all of the answer choices carefully. After eliminating obviously wrong answers, make a selection and move on to the next question.

6. Confusing Answer Choices

When working on a difficult multiple-choice question, there may be a tendency to focus on the answer choices that are the easiest to understand. Many people, whether consciously or not, gravitate to the answer choices that require the least concentration, knowledge, and memory. This is a mistake. When you come across an answer choice that is confusing, you should give it extra attention. A question might be confusing because you do not know the subject matter to which it refers. If this is the case, don't eliminate the answer before you have affirmatively settled on another. When you come across an answer choice of this type, set it aside as you look at the remaining choices. If you can confidently assert that one of the other choices is correct, you can leave the confusing answer aside. Otherwise, you will need to take a moment to try to better understand the confusing answer choice. Rephrasing is one way to tease out the sense of a confusing answer choice.

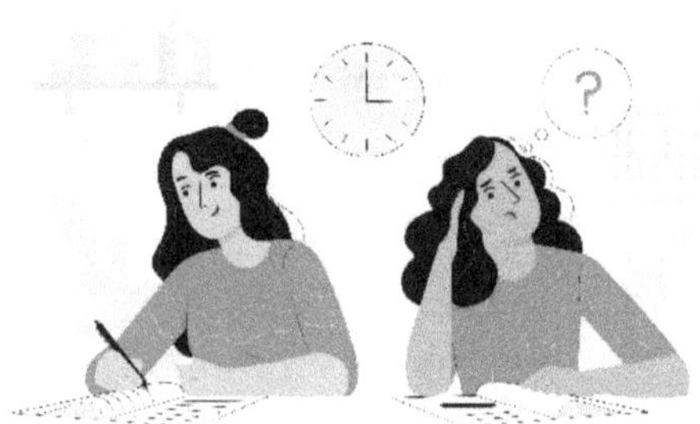

7. Your First Instinct

Many people struggle with multiple-choice tests because they overthink the questions. If you have studied sufficiently for the test, you should be prepared to trust your first instinct once you have carefully and completely read the question and all of the answer choices. There is a great deal of research suggesting that the mind can come to the correct conclusion very quickly once it has obtained all of the relevant information. At times, it may seem to you as if your intuition is working faster even than your reasoning mind. This may in fact be true. The knowledge you obtain while studying may be retrieved from your subconscious before you have a chance to work out the associations that support it. Verify your instinct by working out the reasons that it should be trusted.

8. Key Words

Many test takers struggle with multiple-choice questions because they have poor reading comprehension skills. Quickly reading and understanding a multiple-choice question requires a mixture of skill and experience. To help with this, try jotting down a few key words and phrases on a piece of scrap paper. Doing this concentrates the process of reading and forces the mind to weigh the relative importance of the question's parts. In selecting words and phrases to write down, the test taker thinks about the question more deeply and carefully. This is especially true for multiple-choice questions that are preceded by a long prompt.

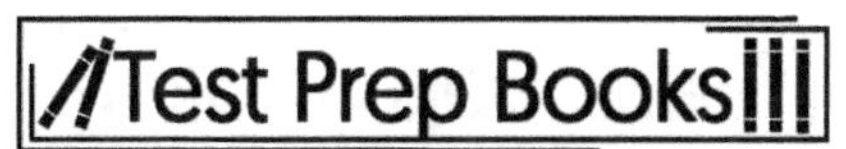

9. Subtle Negatives

One of the oldest tricks in the multiple-choice test writer's book is to subtly reverse the meaning of a question with a word like *not* or *except*. If you are not paying attention to each word in the question, you can easily be led astray by this trick. For instance, a common question format is, "Which of the following is...?" Obviously, if the question instead is, "Which of the following is not...?," then the answer will be quite different. Even worse, the test makers are aware of the potential for this mistake and will include one answer choice that would be correct if the question were not negated or reversed. A test taker who misses the reversal will find what he or she believes to be a correct answer and will be so confident that he or she will fail to reread the question and discover the original error. The only way to avoid this is to practice a wide variety of multiple-choice questions and to pay close attention to each and every word.

10. Reading Every Answer Choice

It may seem obvious, but you should always read every one of the answer choices! Too many test takers fall into the habit of scanning the question and assuming that they understand the question because they recognize a few key words. From there, they pick the first answer choice that answers the question they believe they have read. Test takers who read all of the answer choices might discover that one of the latter answer choices is actually *more* correct. Moreover, reading all of the answer choices can remind you of facts related to the question that can help you arrive at the correct answer. Sometimes, a misstatement or incorrect detail in one of the latter answer choices will trigger your memory of the subject and will enable you to find the right answer. Failing to read all of the answer choices is like not reading all of the items on a restaurant menu: you might miss out on the perfect choice.

11. Spot the Hedges

One of the keys to success on multiple-choice tests is paying close attention to every word. This is never truer than with words like *almost*, *most*, *some*, and *sometimes*. These words are called "hedges" because they indicate that a statement is not totally true or not true in every place and time. An absolute statement will contain no hedges, but in many subjects, the answers are not always straightforward or absolute. There are always exceptions to the rules in these subjects. For this reason, you should favor those multiple-choice questions that contain hedging language. The presence of qualifying words indicates that the author is taking special care with his or her words, which is certainly important when composing the right answer. After all, there are many ways to be wrong, but there is only one way to be right! For this reason, it is wise to avoid answers that are absolute when taking a multiple-choice test. An absolute answer is one that says things are either all one way or all another. They often include words like *every*, *always*, *best*, and *never*. If you are taking a multiple-choice test in a subject that doesn't lend itself to absolute answers, be on your guard if you see any of these words.

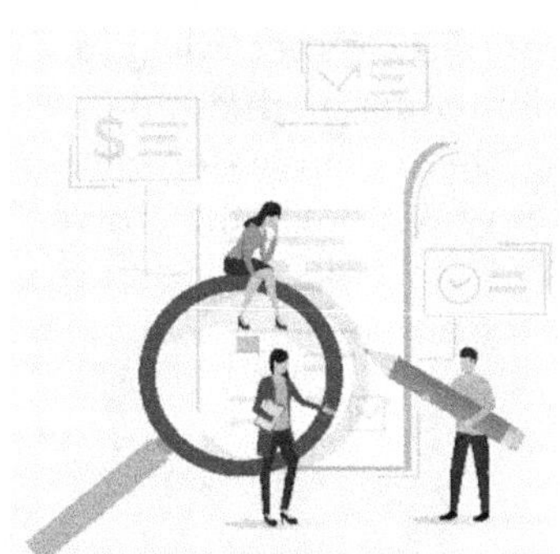

12. Long Answers

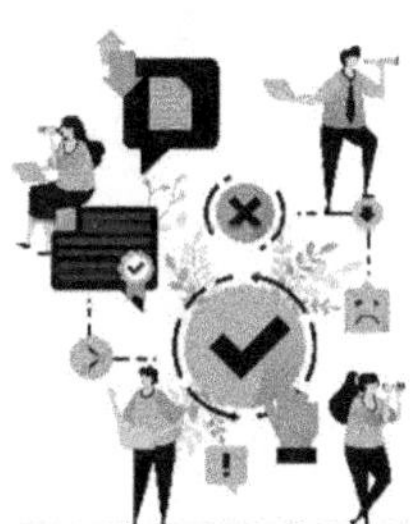

In many subject areas, the answers are not simple. As already mentioned, the right answer often requires hedges. Another common feature of the answers to a complex or subjective question are qualifying clauses, which are groups of words that subtly modify the meaning of the sentence. If the question or answer choice describes a rule to which there are exceptions or the subject matter is complicated, ambiguous, or confusing, the correct answer will require many words in order to be expressed clearly and accurately.

In essence, you should not be deterred by answer choices that seem excessively long. Oftentimes, the author of the text will not be able to write the correct answer without offering some qualifications and modifications. Your job is to read the answer choices thoroughly and completely and to select the one that most accurately and precisely answers the question.

13. Restating to Understand

Sometimes, a question on a multiple-choice test is difficult not because of what it asks but because of how it is written. If this is the case, restate the question or answer choice in different words. This process serves a couple of important purposes. First, it forces you to concentrate on the core of the question. In order to rephrase the question accurately, you have to understand it well. Rephrasing the question will concentrate your mind on the key words and ideas. Second, it will present the information to your mind in a fresh way. This process may trigger your memory and render some useful scrap of information picked up while studying.

14. True Statements

Sometimes an answer choice will be true in itself, but it does not answer the question. This is one of the main reasons why it is essential to read the question carefully and completely before proceeding to the answer choices. Too often, test takers skip ahead to the answer choices and look for true statements. Having found one of these, they are content to select it without reference to the question above. The savvy test taker will always read the entire question before turning to the answer choices. Then, having settled on a correct answer choice, he or she will refer to the original question and ensure that the selected answer is relevant. The mistake of choosing a correct-but-irrelevant answer choice is especially common on questions related to specific pieces of objective knowledge.

15. No Patterns

One of the more dangerous ideas that circulates about multiple-choice tests is that the correct answers tend to fall into patterns. These erroneous ideas range from a belief that B and C are the most common right answers, to the idea that an unprepared test-taker should answer "A-B-A-C-A-D-A-B-A." It cannot be emphasized enough that pattern-seeking of this type is exactly the WRONG way to approach a multiple-choice test. To begin with, it is highly unlikely that the test maker will plot the correct answers according to some predetermined pattern. The questions are scrambled and delivered in a random order. Furthermore, even if the test maker was following a pattern in the assignation of correct answers, there is no reason why the test taker would know which pattern he or she was using. Any attempt to discern a pattern in the answer choices is a waste of time and a distraction from the real work of taking the test. A test taker would be much better served by extra preparation before the test than by reliance on a pattern in the answers.

Introduction

Function of the Test

The Women's Health Care Nurse Practitioner Board Certification Examination (WHNP-BC) is one of many specialty certification exams administered by the American Nurses Credentialing Center (ANCC). This exam is designed for registered nurses who are graduates of an accredited Women's Health Care Nurse Practitioner degree program and seek to demonstrate competency in their field prior to obtaining state licensure. The exam is accredited by the National Commission for Certifying Agencies (NCCA). After receiving a passing score, the advanced practice nurse will be awarded the WHNP-BC credential, which is valid for three years.

The first step in taking the Women's Health Care Nurse Practitioner Board Certification Examination begins with an online application. Eligibility requirements for the exam include the following:

- Active Registered Nurse (RN) or advanced practice nursing licensure
- Graduate of a Women's Health Care Nurse Practitioner Master's, Doctorate, or Post-Master's degree program within the last eight years
- Submission of diploma and official transcript from degree program

The content of the exam is developed by a panel of nurse practitioners and experts in the specialty area who serve as writers and reviewers. Based on the recommendations of the content team, the exam focuses on six areas of competency: Assessment, Diagnostic Testing, and Interpretation; Primary Care; Gynecologic and Reproductive Health; Obstetrics; Pharmacology; and Professional Issues. This supports the goal of accurately validating the candidate's knowledge and skillset in the women's health care nurse practitioner field.

Test Administration

Candidates who meet eligibility requirements will receive approval to schedule their exam within a 90-day testing window. The exam is delivered in a computer-based format at a testing center or via live remote proctoring. For special testing accommodations, a signed document from the candidate's physician or healthcare professional must be submitted prior to scheduling the exam. Appointments may be rescheduled or canceled at least two days prior to the testing date to avoid loss of exam fees. If needed, extensions to the testing window may be requested for an additional cost. To provide proof of identity on the day of the exam, candidates must bring two forms of identification (e.g., driver's license or passport and student ID or credit card). Prohibited items in the testing area include items such as cell phones, books, study notes, and food/drink. Candidates should plan to arrive at least fifteen minutes prior to their appointment time to allow adequate time for check-in and preparation for the exam.

Test Format

The Women's Health Care Nurse Practitioner Board Certification Examination (WHNP-BC) consists of 175 questions. Of these questions, 150 are scored and the remaining 25 are unscored questions. While the unscored questions do not affect the candidate's results, all test questions must be answered since the difference between the two is not distinguished on the exam. Candidates will have three hours in which to complete the exam. The following table represents a breakdown of exam topics by percentage:

Competency Area	Percentage
Assessment, Diagnostic Testing, and Interpretation	12%
Primary Care	13%
Gynecologic and Reproductive Health	33%
Obstetrics	29%
Pharmacology	10%
Professional Issues	3%
Total	**100%**

Scoring

Test results are determined based on the established minimum passing score for the exam. Upon completion of the exam, candidates will receive a score of pass or fail. For those who do not pass the exam, a detailed report of performance in each content area will be provided to aid in studying for a future attempt. Following a 45-day time period and submission of a new application, retesting can be scheduled. Candidates can retest a maximum of two times within a 12-month time period.

Study Prep Plan

1 **Schedule -** Use one of our study schedules below or come up with one of your own.

2 **Relax -** Test anxiety can hurt even the best students. There are many ways to reduce stress. Find the one that works best for you.

3 **Execute -** Once you have a good plan in place, be sure to stick to it.

One Week Study Schedule

Day	Topic
Day 1	Assessment, Diagnostic Testing...
Day 2	Primary Care
Day 3	Obstetrics
Day 4	Pharmacology
Day 5	Practice Test #1
Day 6	Practice Test #2
Day 7	Take Your Exam!

Two Week Study Schedule

Day	Topic	Day	Topic
Day 1	Assessment, Diagnostic Testing...	Day 8	Postpartum Care and Complications
Day 2	Imaging Studies (common indications)	Day 9	Pharmacology
Day 3	Primary Care	Day 10	Practice Quiz
Day 4	Practice Quiz	Day 11	Ethical Principles
Day 5	Fertility Awareness and Contraception	Day 12	Quality Improvement
Day 6	Practice Quiz	Day 13	Practice Test #2
Day 7	Prenatal Care	Day 14	Take Your Exam!

One Month Study Schedule

Day	Topic	Day	Topic	Day	Topic
Day 1	Assessment, Diagnostic Testing...	Day 11	Menstrual Disorders	Day 21	Pharmacotherapeutics
Day 2	Blood Typing and Antibody Screening	Day 12	Adnexal Masses	Day 22	Professional Practice Issues
Day 3	Comprehensive Metabolic Panel (CMP)	Day 13	Pelvic Organ Relaxation & Prolapse	Day 23	Bioethics
Day 4	Testing and Cultures for Vaginal Discharge...	Day 14	Infertility	Day 24	PDCA Cycle
Day 5	Hepatitis Panel	Day 15	Male Reproductive System Disorders	Day 25	Research Utilization
Day 6	Primary Care	Day 16	Practice Quiz	Day 26	Pharmacology
Day 7	Genitourinary Conditions	Day 17	Gestational Age Determination	Day 27	Professional Issues
Day 8	Age-Appropriate Primary, Secondary	Day 18	Common Discomforts of Pregnancy	Day 28	Pharmacology
Day 9	Healthy Lifestyles	Day 19	Ultrasound	Day 29	Professional Issues
Day 10	Preconception Counseling	Day 20	Postpartum Complications	Day 30	Take Your Exam!

Build your own prep plan by visiting the Online Resources page.

Instructions and a QR code can be found on the last page of this guide.

As you study for your test, we'd like to take the opportunity to remind you that you are capable of great things! With the right tools and dedication, you truly can do anything you set your mind to. The fact that you are holding this book right now shows how committed you are. In case no one has told you lately, you've got this! Our intention behind including this coloring page is to give you the chance to take some time to engage your creative side when you need a little brain-break from studying. As a company, we want to encourage people like you to achieve their dreams by providing good quality study materials for the tests and certifications that improve careers and change lives. As individuals, many of us have taken such tests in our careers, and we know how challenging this process can be. While we can't come alongside you and cheer you on personally, we can offer you the space to recall your purpose, reconnect with your passion, and refresh your brain through an artistic practice. We wish you every success, and happy studying!

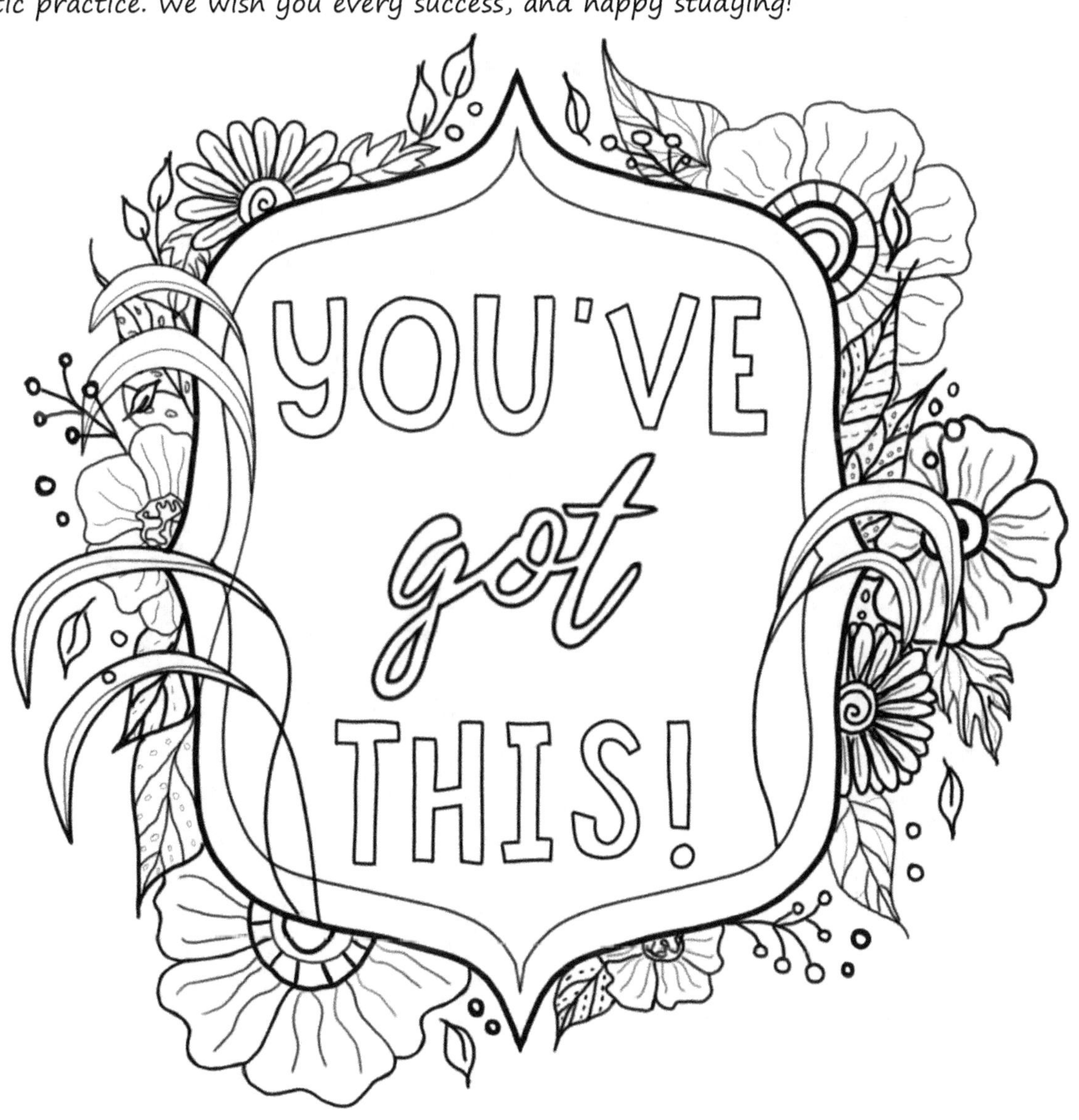

Assessment, Diagnostic Testing, and Interpretation

Health History and Physical Exam

Health History

Comprehensive Health History

The comprehensive history and a physical assessment are essential first steps in establishing a therapeutic patient-provider relationship for a hospitalized patient or a patient who is new to a primary practice. The WHNP has the opportunity to collect baseline data and to identify or eliminate physical assessment data that relate to the information provided by the patient in the interview portion of the assessment. As the WHNP becomes familiar with the patient's condition, they can use this teachable moment to provide health promotion information. The WHNP will develop and maintain expertise in conducting all phases of the history and physical assessment.

The seven elements of the **comprehensive health history** are as follows:

- Patient's identifying information
- Chief complaint
- History of the present illness
- Past history
- Family history
- Personal and social history
- Review of systems (ROS)

The patient's identifying information includes the date of the examination and the patient's name, gender, age, marital status, and occupation. This element also contains the identity and the reliability of the informant, who may be the patient, a family member, or an interpreter. The WHNP will assess and document the veracity of the information that is provided. If the patient has been referred to the care of the WHNP, any information recorded in the electronic health record (EHR) referencing the reason for the referral should be reviewed and documented in the comprehensive health history.

Focused Health History

The **focused history** is appropriate for follow-up visits for established patients. This form of the patient's history addresses specific symptoms or areas of concern, and the physical examination is targeted on these symptoms as well. The details of the focused history are built on the results of the initial health history. The patient's symptoms may be physical or somatic, which are either acute, such as pain that requires intervention, or self-limiting, which most often resolve without treatment within six weeks. Up to 30 percent of the patient's symptoms may have no medical explanation, whereas other symptoms that occur in groups may be identified as a functional syndrome such as irritable bowel syndrome or chronic fatigue syndrome.

Chief Complaint and History of Present Illness

The **chief complaint** is the patient's description of the problem or issue that prompted the visit. The patient's narrative may only vaguely describe the details of the current complaint, or the patient may prove to be an excellent historian. In either event, the WHNP will document the information received from the patient using the patient's exact words whenever possible.

The **history of the present illness** is a chronological narrative that identifies the events from the onset of symptoms to the point at which the patient decides to access care for the problem. The WHNP will also question the context in which the problem developed, all manifestations associated with the problem, and any treatments that have been used to address the problem.

The **seven cardinal elements** of each of the manifestations that are associated with the present illness must be identified and documented. The seven elements are location; quality; quantity or severity; the element of time, which includes, onset, duration, and frequency; context; factors that alleviate or exacerbate the manifestations; and associated manifestations. This section will also identify the patient's assessment of how the current complaint has affected their ability to carry out activities of daily living (ADLs) and other activities. This section will also include the identification of "pertinent positives" or "pertinent negatives" among the manifestations associated with the present illness, which are signs that are either present or absent and may be associated with one of the conditions to be considered in the differential diagnosis for the present illness.

Allergies, Substance Use, and Medication Reconciliation

The WHNP will also include the assessment of the patient's drugs, allergies, tobacco, alcohol, and recreational drug use. The review of the patient's drugs should include all prescription and nonprescription drugs as well as oral contraceptives and herbal supplements. Patients are often instructed to bring all of their drugs with the containers for review by the WHNP. Specific details of any reaction to drugs, foods, insect bites, or environmental allergens must be reviewed and recorded. The patient's **smoking history** should be documented in the form of packs per day; for instance, a person who smoked 1.5 packs per day for ten years has a smoking history documented as a fifteen-pack-year history. If the patient has quit smoking, the length of time will be recorded. The use of and amounts of alcohol and recreational drugs is documented.

Medical, Surgical, and OB/GYN History

The patient's past history begins with the documentation of infectious childhood illnesses, chronic illnesses, and surgeries. There are four elements of the adult history, including the following:

- Medical
- Surgical
- Obstetric/Gynecologic
- Psychiatric

Medical issues should include documentation of chronic diseases including human immunodeficiency virus (HIV) status, sexual preference, and identification of high-risk sexual behaviors. Each surgical procedure should be documented with the identification of the purpose, recovery course, and surgical outcome. The obstetric/gynecologic history will document all pregnancies, induced and naturally occurring abortions, contraceptive use, and menstrual history. The psychiatric history includes specific disorders, hospitalizations, and treatments. This section should also include an assessment of the patient's age-specific immunization status and any screening tests that have been completed. WHNPs should understand that many patients will not be able to identify each of these details; however, the information from the EHR or referral documentation can be used to prompt the patient's answers.

The **family history** is a comprehensive assessment of all members of the patient's family for the presence or absence of chronic and genetically linked conditions such as renal disease, hypertension (HTN), cardiovascular disease, arthritis, suicide, seizure disorders, breast cancer, ovarian cancer, and prostate cancer. The WHNP will construct a chart that identifies the health status and age or the age and health status at the time of death for the patient's parents, grandparents, siblings, and grandchildren. The personal and social history identifies the patient's support structure, ways of coping, educational level, risk behaviors, and safety measures. The **review of systems** (**ROS**) can be completed during the physical examination; however, WHNPs should understand that the review of systems should be included with the comprehensive health history if there are multiple symptoms identified in the current complaint.

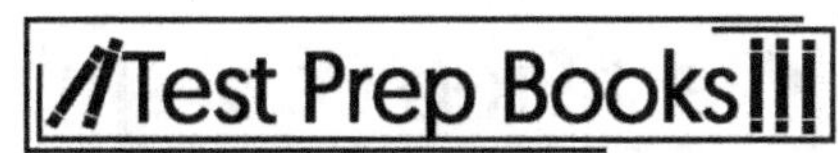

Health Risk Assessment

Advanced practice nurses provide various types of counseling to patients. Counseling arises from the need to educate patients on certain risks that can affect their health decisions. After performing a health history, a genetic risk assessment, which includes questions about health conditions in their family history, can be obtained. Parents and siblings are considered immediate family. Grandparents, aunts, and uncles are part of the extended family and are important to include in the assessment. Genetic conditions include HTN, cancer, diabetes, high cholesterol, obesity, drug addiction, alcoholism, and mental illness. Bringing awareness to the probability of disease in patients is a method of health promotion and risk reduction. Behavioral and mental health are an important part of a psychosocial risk assessment.

Patients need to be interviewed regarding their life stressors and coping mechanisms. **Life stressors** can include losing a job, losing a loved one, divorce, chronic illnesses, and increased family obligations. The goal of risk reduction is keeping the patient safe and helping them avoid self-harm. A **suicide risk assessment** should be performed when patients verbalize suicide ideation or poor coping skills. The patient should be asked if they have a suicide plan and the means to carry it out. The SAD PERSONAS suicide risk assessment can be used to assess a patient's suicide risk. Eleven major areas (sex, age, depression, previous attempt, ethanol abuse, rational thinking loss, social supports lacking, organized plan, no spouse, availability of lethal means, sickness) are assessed and scored. The higher the score, the higher the risk. Lifestyle risk factors can contribute to disease and chronic illness. Establishing patterns during the health interview allows for education and counseling. Exercise habits determine a patient's activity level and the potential for the development of sedentary lifestyle–related illnesses, such as obesity and high blood pressure. Patients should be counseled on exercise plans that meet their physical needs. Poor nutrition can lead to heart-related conditions. WHNPs should assess their patients' dietary habits and provide counseling on meals that meet their dietary requirements.

Genetic Risk Factors

A **genetic risk assessment** estimates an individual's risk for the development of chronic and rare diseases that are genetically linked. This assessment only identifies a statistical probability, not cause and effect, because diseases that result from variants in multiple genes as opposed to a single gene increase the complexity of estimating the risk. There is a wide variation in the degree to which the genetically linked diseases contribute to the possibility of expression of the disease in the offspring. For instance, the genetic risk associated with the development of melanoma is 21 percent whereas the risk associated with type 1 diabetes is 88 percent. There are two categories of risk: absolute risk and relative risk. **Absolute risk** means that if the patient has a one in ten chance of developing a disease in their lifetime, that person has a 10 percent risk for that disease. **Relative risk** compares the risk for two groups for the same disease. For instance, the risk of breast cancer is higher for descendants of Ashkenazi Jews who emigrated from Eastern Europe than for the average female population in the United States.

There are family patterns that increase the risk for the development of diseases including having multiple first-degree relatives with the same condition, having a relative diagnosed with the condition before the age of 55, having a relative with a disease that is more common in the opposite gender, and having more than one genetically linked disease in the family. The genetic pedigree, which is a visual representation of the patient's family tree, may be used to assess the patient's genetic risk factors. Providers must also support patients and families as they decide whether or not to access formal genetic testing. The **Genetic Information Nondiscrimination Act** (**GINA**) and the **Health Insurance Portability and Accountability Act** (**HIPAA**) of 1996 provide some protection against discrimination due to the findings of the testing. There also can be ethical questions related to reproductive planning and family dynamics. The patient should be encouraged to seek professional counseling when considering genetic testing. The patient should also understand that direct-to-consumer genetic tests may or may not provide reliable information for the patient's unique circumstances and that none of the commercial products provides counseling.

Behavior and Lifestyle Risk Factors

The Centers for Disease Control (CDC) identifies and tracks four **lifestyle risk factors**: poor exercise habits, inadequate nutrition, smoking, and excessive alcohol intake. Each of these lifestyle behaviors increases the risk of chronic diseases such as HTN, stroke, and respiratory disease. The research clearly implicates smoking as a factor in the development of all of these conditions; yet, adults and young people continue to smoke. The government has enacted age restrictions on the sale of tobacco in addition to imposing a significant tariff that is included in the price of cigarettes, and commercial companies market a wide array of prescription and nonprescription smoking cessation products. There are commercial and medical weight loss programs that provide one-on-one and peer support and twelve-step programs for all forms of addiction. The WHNP is responsible for supporting patients' plans to change by providing the necessary information prior to the change in behavior and then to support patients as they initiate and maintain the changed behavior.

The patient should understand that persistent change requires effort continued over time and that even modest reductions in lifestyle risks will have some effect on the progression of chronic diseases. In other words, the patient does not have to run a marathon to gain some benefit from regular, light exercise. Modest dietary improvement and increased activity can lower blood pressure and lipids; however, smoking cessation requires total abstinence to be effective in reducing the development or progression of chronic illness. The WHNP will monitor the patient's medication needs as these risk factors are addressed to be sure that medication doses are reduced as necessary. It is not uncommon for patients who eliminate smoking, increase exercise, and improve their nutritional status to be able to discontinue or limit their use of antihypertensive drugs, oral hypoglycemic drugs, or antilipidemic drugs. A patient who has accurate health-promoting information, contacts for needed community resources, and the support of the provider will have the greatest chance for successful change.

Host Risk Factors

Host risk factors, or host factors, are terms that refer to a patient's susceptibility to certain diseases. Several factors can affect the probability that someone will develop an acute or chronic illness. Assessing these factors via a health history interview followed by a physical assessment can direct the advanced practice nurse to develop a treatment plan that will prevent possible complications. Microorganisms thrive when they invade the body and overpower the immune response. The first line of defense in the body is the skin. When the skin is broken, it opens up a pathway for microorganisms to enter the body and cause illness. Assessing the patient's skin integrity is an important component of a physical assessment. Patients who have skin integrity issues are more at risk of developing infections. To survive, the body must maintain an acid-base balance. The pH levels vary throughout the body. The stomach is highly acidic, whereas the large intestine is more basic. In females, vaginal pH is moderately acidic. When pH levels in these areas change, microorganisms can grow.

For example, when the vaginal pH turns alkaline, there is an increased risk of developing bacterial vaginosis (BV), which can cause itchiness, discharge, and discomfort. The immune response is activated when a microorganism enters the body. Cell mediators alert the body that there is a potentially harmful organism present. White blood cells (WBCs) help fight off infection in the body. When patients have decreased levels of WBCs, they are more susceptible to infection due to a delayed or weakened immune response. Medications can alter a patient's immune response. Corticosteroids, a class of anti-inflammatory drugs, suppress the immune system. They are helpful in autoimmune illnesses in which the body attacks its own immune system. However, a practitioner should always balance the risks and benefits of suppressing immunity. Age is an important host factor for susceptibility. Older adults go through age-related changes, such as loss of skin elasticity, a decrease in sphincter control of the bladder, and a decreased cough reflex. These changes can increase the risk of skin, urinary tract, and pulmonary infections.

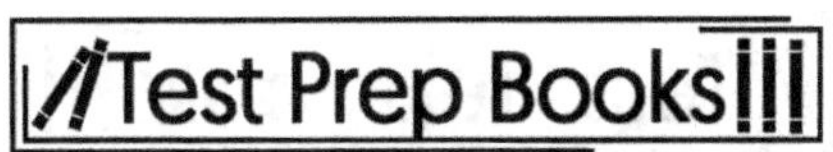

Communicable Disease Risk Factors

An infectious disease that has the risk of transmission from one person to another is known as a **communicable disease**. Because these diseases are a risk to the public, some are reportable to the county or state health department. A large number of these diseases are also reported nationally. Among these communicable diseases are STIs. WHNPs should perform a health history regarding the patient's sexual health to determine if further testing is required. The provider should question the patient on number of sexual partners, history of STIs, use of protection, and frequency of screening. Respiratory infections, such as tuberculosis, pertussis, diphtheria, and severe acute respiratory syndrome, are all reportable at a national level. The patient's respiratory history and possible risk factors should be assessed. Screening patients for a history of respiratory disease should include the exposure time, onset of symptoms, treatment, and outcome.

Occupational and environmental factors should also be assessed. Patients should be asked about travel outside of their immediate area in order to verify places that have a high risk of acquiring respiratory infections. Hepatitis A, B, and C are reportable. Hepatitis A is transmitted via the fecal-oral route or contaminated food and water. Providers should ask questions related to safe food handling, handwashing practices, and sexual practices. Hepatitis B is transmitted via blood or bodily fluids. The patient should be asked about any occupational hazards or close contact with an infected person. Hepatitis C is transmitted primarily through blood. Patients should be asked about any needle exposure, such as tattoos or drug usage. Healthcare workers and those in occupations with exposure to needles are at a higher risk of transmission. Many communicable diseases are preventable with vaccinations.

Immunization records can alert the provider of the potential risk of infection. Poliomyelitis, rubella, mumps, and measles are among the vaccine-preventable diseases. Providers should reference the vaccination schedules provided by entities such as the CDC when reviewing immunization records.

Demographic Risk Factors

It is important for the WHNP to know which diseases or conditions ethnic and racial groups are prone to. The white population is more prone to atrial fibrillation than people of other races. The Hispanic population has high rates of obesity and diabetes; in individuals from Puerto Rico, there is an increased incidence of HIV infection and AIDS.

Obesity and type 2 diabetes are common in African Americans, and the death rate from HTN, stroke, HIV infection, and AIDS is higher than the rate in the non-Hispanic white population. Asian Americans have an increased incidence of tuberculosis, and hepatitis B infection occurs more commonly in recent immigrants to the United States. Asian Americans also have an increased rate of chronic obstructive pulmonary disease (COPD), in spite of the fact that smoking rates among Chinese and Japanese Americans are lower than average. Native Americans have a high incidence of alcoholism; recent pharmacologic research indicates that altered metabolic pathways may contribute to this finding. As with the Asian American population, the nurse will be aware of the frequent use of herbal preparations in the Native American population as well.

Social History

Prevention of disease and promotion of health requires exploration of social factors that may affect the patient's compliance with the medical plan of care. Assessing the patient's financial means allows a practitioner to determine what treatment options are viable. If a patient cannot purchase the prescribed medications or supplies, the likelihood that they will remain compliant with the treatment plan will be decreased. In conjunction with case managers and social workers, the patient's housing and utilities, such as a running water and electricity, are important to assess. Patients may prioritize obtaining these resources over their treatment plans. Transportation is also crucial to patient compliance. Attending health appointments may be an obstacle if patients do not have reliable transportation. Patients who are required to attend rehabilitation services, dialysis treatments, or infusion therapy may need to rely on public transportation that may not always be available.

Support systems are required for patients who cannot perform their own care. Patients who develop acute injuries or progressive chronic illnesses may need daily assistance in the home setting. Ensuring that these patients have available resources is important. Collaborative planning with case management and social workers is needed. In the elderly population, assessing home safety is a preventive strategy to avoid injuries. The removal of clutter and ensuring good lighting and level flooring can help prevent falls. Falls are a frequent occurrence among geriatric patients and can be prevented with adequate assessment and intervention. Providing patient education is a main role of the advanced practice nurse.

The patient's education level is an important factor to determine before the delivery of the treatment plan. Patients must be able to understand their health instructions to increase compliance. The patient's culture should be established during the health interview to ensure that the treatment plan respects their traditions and practices. Practitioners should always strive to promote culturally competent care. When a patient's culture is different from the practitioner's, every effort should be made to understand the patient's perception of illness and therapeutic preferences. Tools such as the Ecosystemic Structural Family Therapy (ESFT) Model, which addresses the patient's conception of illness, social and environmental factors, fears, concerns, and therapeutic understanding, are essential to providing culturally competent care. The patient's perception of their health status will alert the practitioner to their potential coping skills. Minimizing stress and safe handling of emotions will allow the patient to adhere to the treatment plan.

Social Determinants of Health

Social determinants of health can be an overwhelmingly complex concept for the WHNP who cares for a diverse patient population. Each nurse should understand the general social determinants of health, representing the nonmedical factors that directly or indirectly affect the patient's healthcare experience. Several general talking points fall under social determinants of health: economic stability, level of education, access to quality healthcare, community resources, and environmental status—essentially, each patient's socioeconomic status.

Economic stability refers to the patient's level of consistent income. Poor economic stability can affect the foods a patient eats, the medications the patient can take, the resources the patient can utilize, and access to certain forms of healthcare. Level of education includes the highest level of education achieved, along with general access to education. Access to healthcare relates to the patient's ability to physically get to anything healthcare related (e.g., a patient without a car in a rural area would have a harder time getting to routine doctor's appointments) as well as the quality of healthcare provided. Lastly, the community factor includes the safety of the neighborhood/housing as well as community resources available. Considering that all these points are related and each one can impact the others (e.g., economic stability could affect the level of education), social determinants of health will vary from patient to patient and will require the nurse to closely assess for gaps in healthcare needs.

Regarding the WHNP's understanding of social determinants of health, the main goal is to ensure safe, consistent patient care with appropriate referrals in place. Low-income patients with a low level of education are at a higher risk of poor care coordination, noncompliance, and gaps in healthcare. The WHNP can provide patient-appropriate education (i.e., education resources that are appropriate for the patient's education and understanding level), ensure follow-up appointments, and assist in referrals to community resources.

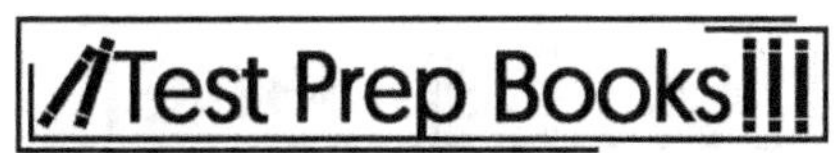

Sexual History

Assessing a patient's sexuality is an important part of a comprehensive assessment by a practitioner. **Sexuality** includes biological sex, gender identity and roles, and sexual activity and orientation. Several factors affect sexuality, and they must be explored. Cultural considerations regarding gender preference during intimacy, acceptable sexual positions and stimulation, and role behaviors are important questions to ask patients during a health history. Asking adolescents about sexuality is a challenging task. Teenagers require a sense of belonging and understanding. Communication gaps occur when practitioners do not understand adolescents' needs. Practitioners should be confident about asking sexuality questions and ask them objectively. Medical terminology should be explained in lay terms to make it relatable to patients. Patients should be asked about their gender identities so that the appropriate pronoun is used during the assessment. Many patients struggling with acceptance of their gender or sexual identity can benefit from community-based programs that address their healthcare requirements. Organizations such as the Gay and Lesbian Alliance Against Defamation (GLAAD) aim to promote equality.

Physical Examination

Comprehensive Physical Examination

Once each element of the health history has been addressed, the WHNP will complete the **comprehensive physical assessment** in the following order:

- General assessment of appearance and weight change
- Skin
- Head and neck
- Breasts

The following systems are then assessed:

- Respiratory
- Cardiovascular
- Gastrointestinal
- Peripheral vascular
- Urinary
- Genital
- Musculoskeletal
- Psychiatric
- Neurologic
- Hematologic
- Endocrine

The WHNP is aware that the goal of the physical examination is to gather relevant data in an efficient manner that maintains the patient's maximum comfort and privacy. Proficiency in moving from one area of assessment to another requires practice, and the WHNP will develop a consistent pattern that is followed with each assessment. There are four cardinal techniques associated with physical assessment: inspection, palpation, percussion, and auscultation. With the exception of the abdominal assessment, these techniques are used in sequence as appropriate for each body system.

Inspection is the process of visually assessing the body surface area of irregularities such as petechiae or bruises, peripheral edema, or alterations of skin color. In addition, inspection also includes the assessment of the patient's general appearance and body habitus. **Palpation** is the process of applying tactile pressure to assess the body part for abnormal contours, tenderness, or temperature. The technique can also be used to assess the presence of crepitus in the joints. **Percussion** is defined as the creation of a sound wave to assess resonance or dullness in the chest cavity or the abdomen. **Auscultation** with the diaphragm or bell of the stethoscope allows the assessment of the location, timing, intensity, and pitch of the sounds for the heart, lungs, and abdomen. This technique is also used to detect heart murmurs and bruits over the peripheral arterial vessels. The diaphragm of the stethoscope is used to assess high-pitched sounds such as lung sounds, whereas the bell is used to assess low-pitched sounds such as heart murmurs.

Universal precautions must be maintained, with proper disposal of all materials. Environmental factors that affect the quality of the assessment include lighting, room temperature, and the height of the patient's bed or examining table. For some assessments, such as the identification of jugular vein distension, direct lighting can obscure the result, whereas tangential or indirect lighting significantly improves the accuracy of the assessment. The room temperature should be maintained at a level that is comfortable for the patient and the examiner. The height of the bed or examining table should be adjusted to accommodate the height of the examiner. The novice WHNP often requires time to process the information gained from the focused assessment before sharing the findings with the patient. With experience, the WHNP will be able to appreciate the "gestalt" of the patient's condition without making the clinical decisions in a step-by-step process.

Focused Physical Examination

All providers determine their own best sequence for the **focused physical assessment**; however, the WHNP is encouraged to consider the frequent position changes required for optimum assessment of the different body systems in terms of the patient's functional abilities and to modify that sequence as necessary. The generally recommended assessment sequence proceeds from head to toe, and the focused assessment will address only the specific systems that are relevant to the current complaint. For instance, a full neurological assessment is not generally required for a complaint of constipation. The focused assessment may also address specific patient conditions that are not directly linked to a body system such as depression or addiction.

The cardinal elements of each symptom or issue are frequently addressed by the PQRSTU assessment pneumonic. The P refers to provocation, which identifies the patient's perceptions of conditions that provoke or decrease the symptom, and it places the occurrence of the symptom in the context of the patient's activities. The Q identifies the quality or amount of the symptom, and the R refers to the radiation of the symptom to an area some distance from the point of origin. The S refers to the score on a rating system for the severity of the symptom. In addition, severity also identifies the patient's perception of whether the symptom is getting worse, better, or remaining the same. The T refers to the timing of the symptom, such as when did it first appear and how long does it last. The U refers to an assessment of the patient's understanding of the significance of the symptom.

Body Positions/Draping

The provider will use proper draping to maximize the patient's privacy and to facilitate the planned procedures.

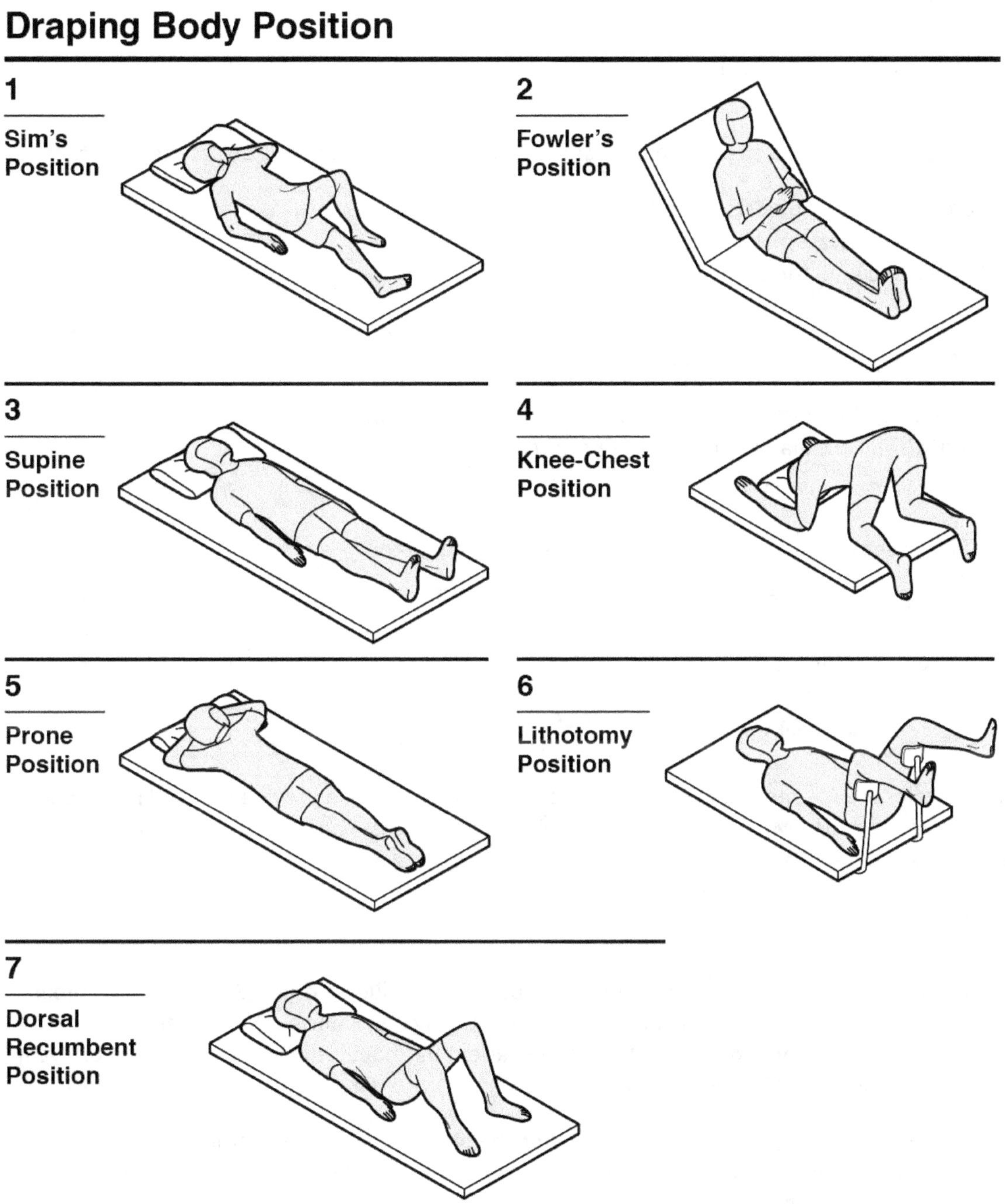

Draping Body Position

1 Sim's Position

2 Fowler's Position

3 Supine Position

4 Knee-Chest Position

5 Prone Position

6 Lithotomy Position

7 Dorsal Recumbent Position

Anthropometric Measurements

Height

To record an accurate height, the provider must instruct the patient to:

- Remove all footwear.
- Stand straight with the back against the wall.
- Remain still until the height is recorded.

Weight

To record an accurate weight, the provider must first zero the scale and then instruct the patient to:

- Remove all heavy objects from the pockets.
- Stand on the scale facing forward.
- Remain still until the weight is recorded.

BMI

The **BMI** (**body mass index**) is equal to:

- Imperial English BMI Formula: $weight\ (\text{lbs}) \times 703 \div height\ (\text{in}^2)$
- Metric BMI Formula: $weight\ (\text{kg}) \div height(\text{m}^2)$

For example:

The BMI of a patient who weighs 150 pounds and is 5'6" is equal to:

$$150 \times 703 = 105{,}450$$

$$66 \times 66 = 4{,}356$$

$$\frac{105{,}450}{4{,}356} = 24.2 \text{ or } 24.0$$

Bodyweight scales may be mechanical or digital. Some digital scales also provide detailed metabolic information including the BMI in addition to the weight. Other scales can accommodate patients who are confined to bed.

Vital Signs

Body Temperature

There are five possible assessment sites for body temperature, including oral, axillary, rectal, tympanic, and temporal. The route will depend on the patient's age and the agency policies. Assessment of oral temperatures requires the provider to verify that the patient has had nothing to eat or drink for five minutes before testing in order to avoid inaccurate readings.

Thermometers may be digital with disposal covers for the probe, wand-like structures that use infrared technology and are moved across the forehead to the temporal area, or handles with disposable cones that measure the tympanic temperature.

Blood Pressure

To obtain an accurate measurement, the provider will:

- Assist the patient to a seated position.
- Expose the upper arm at the level of the heart.

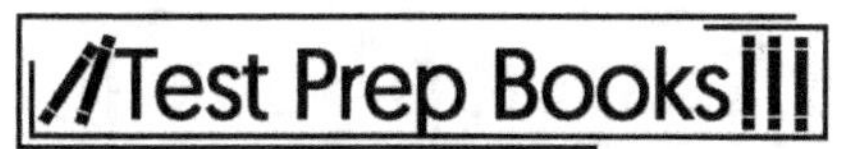

- Apply the appropriately sized cuff.
- Palpate the antecubital space to identify the strongest pulsation point.
- Position the head of the stethoscope over the pulsation point.
- Slowly inflate the cuff to between 30 and 40 mm Hg above the patient's recorded blood pressure (BP). If this information is unavailable, the cuff may be inflated to between 160 and 180 mm Hg.
- Note the point at which the pulse is initially audible, which represents the systolic BP.
- Slowly deflate the cuff and record the point at which the pulse is initially audible as the systolic BP.
- Record the point at which the sounds are no longer audible as the diastolic BP.

Pulse

To assess the pulse the provider will:

- Expose the intended pulse point.
- Palpate the area for the strongest pulsation.
- Position the middle three fingers of the hand on the point.
- Count the pulse for one full minute.

The provider will identify the pulse points that include the radial artery in the wrist, the brachial artery in the elbow, the carotid artery in the neck, the femoral artery in the groin, the popliteal artery behind the knee, and the dorsalis pedis and the posterior tibialis arteries in the foot.

The provider will assess the pulse rate by counting the number of pulsations per sixty seconds. In addition to the pulse rate, the provider will document the regularity or irregularity and strength of the pulsations.

Oxygen Saturation

When every hemoglobin molecule in the circulating blood volume is carrying the maximum number of four oxygen molecules, the oxygen saturation rate is 100 percent. The normal oxygen saturation level is 95 percent to 100 percent, and levels below 90 percent must be treated.

The provider measures oxygen saturation noninvasively by the application of a pulse oximetry device, which the provider will attach to the patient's finger. The device may be used for continuous or intermittent monitoring of the saturation rate.

The pulse oximeter is a foam-lined clip that attaches to the patient's finger and uses infrared technology to assess the oxygen saturation level, which is expressed as a percentage.

Respiration Rate

The respiratory rate is counted, and the breathing pattern is assessed. The provider should ensure that the patient is unaware that the breathing rate is being counted by leaving the fingers resting on the radial pulse site while the respiratory rate is assessed.

Age-Specific Normal and Abnormal Vital Signs

Age	**Temperature** Degrees Fahrenheit	**Pulse** Range	**Respiratory Rate** Range	**Blood Pressure** mmHg
Newborns	98.2 axillary	100-160	30-50	75-100/50-70
0 - 5 years	99.9 rectal	80-120	20-30	80-110/50-80
6 - 10 years	98.6 oral	70-100	15-30	85-120/55-80
11 - 14 years	98.6 oral	60-105	12-20	95-140/60-90
15 - 20 years	98.6 oral	60-100	12-30	95-140/60-90
Adults	98.6 oral	50-80	16-20	120/80

Pain

Pain has been called the fifth vital sign. This is because along with heart rate, blood pressure, temperature, and rate of breathing, pain as reported by the patient is an important clue as to how well the patient is doing.

Pain is almost completely subjective data. Pain is as the patient reports it and is very difficult to measure otherwise. Whereas the heart rate can easily and accurately be counted in beats per minute, assessing pain requires the WHNP to use clinical judgement by applying a patient-by-patient assessment.

The most common measure of pain is the **Numerical Rating Pain Scale**, rated zero to ten, with zero being no pain at all and ten being the worst pain imaginable to the patient.

The WHNP will assess pain by asking the patient what exacerbates the pain and what alleviates the pain. The provider should ask about the location of the pain, the quality, and the onset. The provider should ask about when exacerbations occur and what signs and symptoms accompany an exacerbation. Finally, the provider should assess how the pain affects the patient's overall functioning ability, how intense it becomes, and its temporal characteristics.

Grimacing, sweating, clutching, and guarding are all examples of non-verbal signs that pain is being experienced. Additional pain scales for the WHNP include the **Wong-Baker Faces Pain Scale**, FLACC Pain Scale, and COMFORT Pain Scale. These pain scales are used predominantly for pediatric patients or those who cannot adequately communicate their pain level.

Pain can also be acute or chronic. **Acute pain** is pain that is generally related to an injury and slowly gets better over time as the injury heals. Acute pain usually lasts for less than three months. **Chronic pain** continues for at least three months and is often caused by underlying disease. Patients who come to the hospital setting may be experiencing acute on top of chronic pain, and their pain may be more difficult to manage, as they may have developed a tolerance to pain medications.

HEENT Assessment

Eyes

The eyes are sensory organs responsible for vision. Vision is possible when the cornea, iris, and retina are intact. The **cornea** allows light rays to enter the eye. The **iris** regulates the amount of light, and the **retina** transmits visual stimuli to the brain. Vision loss is a symptom that gets reported to primary care providers often. A practitioner should ask direct questions to assess whether the patient is experiencing blurring of vision, the inability to focus, or total vision loss. Patients should be asked when the vision loss started and if it is occurring in both eyes. Laterality is important in determining whether the vision loss is due to a lesion, trauma, or a progressive chronic illness. Sudden loss of vision may indicate **retinal detachment**. Patients

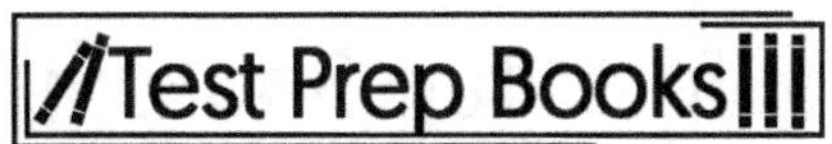

should be asked about accompanying symptoms, such as a flash of light shortly before vision loss, because this may indicate the retina has detached.

Assessment of the visual fields is important to assess the center of the retina. Peripheral vision should be tested by bringing an object from behind the patient's ear toward the center of their face. The patient should be able to detect the object at the same distance bilaterally. Blurry vision may be caused by conditions such as cataracts or glaucoma. **Cataracts** are caused by changes in the tissue of the eye that leads to cloudiness of the lens. This is a common finding in the older population. Assessing the eyes using an ophthalmoscope will provide a more in-depth look at the internal structures of the eye. The **red light reflex** is checked with an ophthalmoscope and can reveal opacities in the back of the eye. Absence of a red reflex can be caused by cataracts.

Glaucoma can occur when increased pressure is being exerted onto the optic nerve. Glaucoma can be a progressive condition that leads to loss of vision. Glaucoma will make the optic disc appear enlarged. To further assess for glaucoma, a practitioner can refer a patient to an eye specialist. A **tonometer** is a tool used to assess for intraocular pressure. The inability of the eye to focus can be caused by trauma, neurological conditions, or medication intoxication. Repetitive and uncontrolled movements of the eye is termed **nystagmus**. Several tests can be performed to assess for vision loss. Visual acuity can be tested by tools such as the Snellen chart or Rosembaum card. The **Snellen chart** is used to assess distance vision. Normal findings are 20/20. A result of 20/70 indicates visual impairment, and 20/200 is considered legal blindness. The **Rosembaum card** is held 15 inches from the eyes and is used to assess near vision. Practitioners should be prepared to make a referral if a child's vision is 20/50 at the age of 5 and 20/40 if they are 6 years or older.

Ears

The ears are sensory organs responsible for the sense of hearing and equilibrium. Three portions inside the ear provide for auditory function. The **external ear** guides sound waves into the auditory canal. The **middle ear** conducts sound waves to the **inner ear**, which translates sound with the assistance of the auditory nerve. **Otalgia** is the medical term for ear pain. A practitioner should perform various assessments and ask health questions to determine the root cause of otalgia. Inflammation of the middle ear, which is common in children, is known as **acute otitis media (AOM)**. **Referred pain** is when the primary pain site originates somewhere else.

Many patients with AOM experience referred pain from dental, mouth, or facial disorders. One of the first questions to ask patients is whether fever is present. In children, AOM will be accompanied by fever in up to 60 percent of cases. Smoking can have an impact on the frequency of otitis media cases. Smoking can causes blockage of the **eustachian tube**, which connects the middle ear to the back area of the nose and throat. Ear wax, or **cerumen**, protects the ear canal from foreign bodies. Prolonged water exposure can decrease cerumen and cause irritation. This may lead to a condition known as **swimmer's ear**, or **otitis externa**. The practitioner should inspect the external ears for pain, lesions, or swelling in the opening of the ear canal. These may be indicative of a bacterial infection. Practitioners should also palpate the ears and pre-auricular lymph nodes. Tenderness may be felt when otitis is present.

Nose/Throat

The nose and throat are part of the upper respiratory tract and help to warm, filter, humidify, and transport air to the lower respiratory tract.

The throat is known as the **oropharynx** and includes the tonsils, which are part of the lymphatic system. One of the most common complaints in primary care is sore throat, or **pharyngitis**. Infections are usually the cause for inflammation of the oropharynx mucosa. The most common cause of bacterial pharyngitis is **B-hemolytic streptococcus**, or **group A streptococcus** (**GAS**). Prompt treatment of GAS is necessary to avoid complications, such as an abscess, rheumatic fever, or glomerulonephritis. Fever is a key symptom in patients with GAS. Practitioners should inspect the oral cavity for any exudate, lesions, or enlarged papillae. The tonsils, if present, should be observed and graded accordingly. A grade of 4 on the tonsillar scale requires rapid attention because they can obstruct the airway. Yellow tonsillar exudate may be present in GAS. If GAS is suspected, a throat swab should be obtained and sent for analysis of streptococcal antigens. A **throat culture** will provide the gold standard for diagnosis. Exudate and crusting should be removed from lesions prior to swabbing.

Cardiovascular Assessment

Cardiovascular issues can be life threatening. Any condition that impedes circulation has the potential to damage the myocardium, or heart muscle. A damaged myocardium may be unable to meet the oxygen demands of the body. It is important to quickly identify any patient exhibiting symptoms indicative of such emergencies so that they can receive prompt treatment to prevent further cardiovascular injury or death. Every patient presenting with possible cardiovascular symptoms should immediately be given a focused assessment followed by a history and physical. The triage, assessment, diagnostics, and treatment of such patients must be prioritized to preserve cardiac function and, ultimately, life.

Upon completion of a focused health history, the WHNP should examine the patient for signs and symptoms of cardiovascular compromise, including chest pain, palpitations, paresthesia, cold extremities, and edema. In general, the nurse should note overall appearance (e.g., demeanor, posture, and gait); examine skin tone (e.g., pink, pallor, red, or cyanotic); look for skin abnormalities (e.g., rashes and lesions); and assess nail beds (e.g., color and capillary refill). A through assessment of the patient's pain should be completed, including exacerbating and relieving factors. If edema is noted, the WHNP should use the assessment scale for pitting edema to note specifics, which ranges from 1+ for slight pitting to 4+ for very deep pits lasting 2–5 minutes.

The WHNP should palpate carotid pulses and assess range of motion in the neck. Using a pulse scale rated from 0-4+, with 0 meaning absent and 4+ meaning strong and bounding, the WHNP should assess the following pulse points: temporal, apical, brachial, radial, ulnar, femoral, popliteal, posterior tibial, and dorsal pedis. The WHNP should auscultate the aortic area, which is found at the second right intercostal space and right sternal border; the pulmonic area, which is found second to the left intercostal space and left sternal border; the tricuspid area, which is located at the fourth left intercostal space and the left sternal border; and finally, the mitral area, which spans the fifth left intercostal space and the midclavicular line.

Cardiac Monitoring

The **electrocardiogram** (**ECG**) captures a graphic record of the depolarization and repolarization of the atria and ventricles to understand the direction and magnitude of the electrical activity and determine a diagnosis. The results will help to reveal if the patient has experienced a STEMI (ST-elevation myocardial infarction), which is one of the most serious types of myocardial infarction (MI). When working with a 12-lead cardiac monitoring system, the WHNP should review changes to determine the affected area of the heart. If changes are noted in leads I, aVL, V5, and V6, the patient is suffering from lateral wall ischemia, injury, or infarction. If changes are noted in leads II, III, and aVF, the patient is suffering from inferior wall ischemia, injury, or infarction. If changes are noted in leads V1 and V2, the patient is suffering from septal wall ischemia, injury, or infarction. Finally, if changes are noted in leads V3 and V4, the patient is suffering from anterior wall ischemia, injury, or infarction.

In addition to cardiac monitoring, the WHNP should review the homeostatic state of the patient to include primary diagnosis, comorbidities, and lifestyle. Hemodynamic parameters to monitor include blood pressure, heart rate, respiratory rate, cardiac output, mean arterial perfusion, systemic vascular resistance, systolic time intervals, and lung congestion. When electing to use noninvasive monitoring systems, the WHNP should detect cardiovascular homeostasis via external applications of automated or manual detection devices

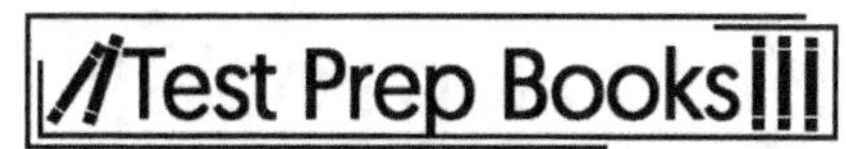

including the following: manual blood pressure cuff, stethoscope, automated blood pressure cuff with pulse detection, and pulse oximetry. The WHNP should also assess capillary refill for color and timing, skin temperature through a thermometer and via physical assessment, and quality of pulse.

Invasive hemodynamic monitoring may be necessary if the care team deems that a highly accurate and reliable reading is necessary for the severity of the patient's vulnerable condition. Invasive monitoring typically takes place in critical care environments and includes devices such as pulmonary artery catheter and arterial line. The need to monitor via invasive devices typically centers on obtaining precisely accurate measurements of blood pressure and cardiac function when early intervention is crucial to avoid devastating outcomes. Some examples of conditions that may warrant invasive monitoring include myocardial injury, ischemic stroke, renal injury, and myocardial infarction, along with the postoperative period following cardiac surgeries such as coronary bypass. The WHNP implements care plans with evolving interventions that follow unique changes to hemodynamic status.

Respiratory Assessment

Working in tandem with the cardiovascular system is the respiratory (also referred to as pulmonary) system, composed of the two lungs and the airway. Airway and breathing are part of the airway, breathing, circulation (ABC) mnemonic representing the patient's most vital functions. While each bodily system serves a unique and vital function, the respiratory system represents two of the three priority assessments in an emergent situation—following the ABC mnemonic.

The assessment of the respiratory system is multifaceted and includes an in-depth review of the patient's overall pulmonary status. First, the WHNP should assess the depth of respirations and note if breaths are shallow or deep, and then assess the rhythm and note whether it is even or uneven. Next, the WHNP should assess the level of effort needed to breathe. Continuing on, the WHNP should note chest expansion (including symmetry), along with any presence of a cough (productive or nonproductive). Finally, the WHNP should auscultate the lungs to assess air exchange throughout and determine the presence of adventitious, absent, lowered, diminished, or distant sounds.

Various patterns of respiration exist; therefore, the WHNP must closely examine the patient to ensure accuracy in the assessment. Normal respirations for a resting adult are regular, comfortable, and at a rate of 12-20 breaths per minute. If the rate is lower than 12 breaths per minute, the patient is displaying **bradypnea**; if the rate is higher than 20 breaths per minute, the patient is displaying **tachypnea**. **Hyperventilation** is when the rate is higher than 20 breaths per minute, accompanied by deep breathing. Similar to hyperventilation, **hyperpnea** also encompasses deep, rapid breathing, but is typically in response to an increase in oxygen demand—therefore not altering blood gases. **Cheyne-Stokes respiration** involves varying periods of increased depth, alternating with periods of apnea, which is breathlessness. **Kussmaul respirations** involve rapid, deep, and labored breaths. **Biot respirations** (also referred to as cluster breathing) are irregular and disorganized respirations with random periods of apnea.

In order to measure the oxygen level of the blood, the nurse should place a pulse oximeter on the patient's finger; this device provides an indirect reading that displays how well oxygen is reaching peripheral areas of the body, noted as SpO_2. The pulse oximetry must be interpreted, and then appropriate action must take place, including determining the patient's need for continuous or intermittent monitoring. When additional information is warranted, such as during periods of alterations from normal (e.g., outside of either the reference range or the patient's usual baseline), an invasive measurement can be obtained via laboratory blood work. This method is used to gather direct **arterial oxygen saturation levels** (**SaO2**). While both laboratory analysis and pulse oximetry display the arterial oxygen saturation level, noting the finding through the use of SpO_2 terminology simply denotes that the level was obtained via pulse oximetry rather than via arterial blood gas sampling. **End-tidal carbon dioxide** (**ETCO2**) monitoring, also called **capnography**, is a noninvasive technique used to measure the amount of CO2 at the end of exhalation, which is displayed as a plateau waveform in terms of mmHg. Measured with a nasal prong device equipped with sensors, the normal range value for capnography is 5–6 percent CO_2, or 35-45 mmHg. These values are important for understanding cardiac output and pulmonary blood flow. While capnography can adequately measure ventilation, there is no indication of oxygenation status. Capnography can provide an earlier detection of hypoventilation, including the impending poor oxygenation, sooner than pulse oximetry.

Arterial Blood Gas Interpretation

A two-step system should be used when assessing **arterial blood gases** (**ABGs**). First, the care team should check the pH level to determine if an imbalance exists; however, it is important to note that even if the pH is normal, the patient may still be suffering from a disturbance, as the system attempts to compensate to maintain homeostasis. Review of various levels, including pH, $PaCO_2$, PaO_2, HCO_3-, and O_2 saturation, helps the care team to understand a complete clinical picture of acid-base manifestations.

If **acidosis** is present, the pH will be below 7.35; alternatively, a pH above 7.45 is indicative of **alkalosis**, as normal blood pH is around 7.4. If an imbalance is detected, the care team must determine the primary cause of the disturbance. The WHNP should look to the primary abnormal lab value to determine the cause of the acid-base imbalance. For a respiratory imbalance, the $PaCO_2$ or serum CO_2 will be abnormal. For a metabolic imbalance, the HCO_3- will be abnormal. The body can respond with either partial or full compensation. If a metabolic disturbance is occurring, the respiratory system will likely compensate; if a respiratory imbalance is occurring, the renal system will likely compensate.

Arterial blood gases are drawn using a heparinized syringe. The blood should not come into contact with room air and should be transported to the lab immediately. In the event of a delay in the transfer or inability of the lab to process the blood sample immediately, the sample should be placed on ice. Simple hypoxia may be seen in acute respiratory distress and pneumonia. Acidosis is seen in chronic obstructive pulmonary disease (COPD), lung edema, shock, and diabetes mellitus. Alkalosis is seen in anxiety disorders, vomiting, and diuretic use. The WHNP must understand that hypoventilation may lead to respiratory acidosis, while hyperventilation may lead to respiratory alkalosis. Alterations in acid-base status are closely monitored and fluctuations in ABGs are reported to the care team and the patient.

Normal ABG values:

- pH: 7.35-7.45
- $PaCO_2$: 35-45 mm Hg
- PaO_2: 75-100 mm Hg
- HCO_3-: 22-26 mEq/L
- O_2 sat: 95%-100%

Pulmonary Function Tests

Pulmonary function tests evaluate the two main functions of the pulmonary system: air exchange and oxygen transport. The specific tests measure the volume of the lungs, the amount of air that can be inhaled or exhaled at one time, and the rate at which that volume is exhaled. The tests are used to monitor the progression of chronic pulmonary disorders, including asthma, emphysema, chronic obstructive lung disease, and sarcoidosis.

Spirometry

Spirometry is one of the two methods used to measure pulmonary function. The provider attaches the mouthpiece to the spirometer and instructs the patient to form a tight seal around its edge. The provider will

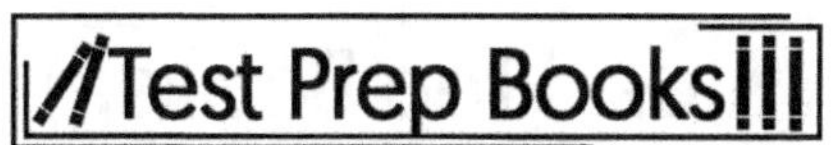

then demonstrate the breathing patterns that are necessary for successful evaluation of each of the pulmonary measurements. The spirometry device calculates each of the values based on the patient's efforts.

Peak Flow Rate

Peak flow rate is defined as the speed at which the patient can exhale. This measure is commonly used to evaluate pulmonary function in patients with asthma.

Breast Assessment

The **breast examination** is one of the most crucial defenses against breast cancer. It should be performed slowly and meticulously, taking at least three minutes per side. Crucially, always ensure a staff chaperone is present for this examination. First, visually inspect the breasts, assessing their color, contour, and symmetry to each other. Look for visible lumps, areas of thickness, or dimpling. Note the size and shape of the nipples, and assess for any ulceration, retraction, or discharge. Perform this inspection with the patient's hands on her hips, with her arms raised overhead, and with the patient leaning forward, as these maneuvers may reveal retraction or dimpling that may otherwise be hidden. Next, have the patient lie supine, as this is the best position for palpation. Beginning with the posterior axillary line at the level of the clavicle, use the vertical strip pattern to palpate in a serpentine fashion down to the inframammary fold (that is, the bra line). Move 2 centimeters medially, and palpate superiorly until reaching the clavicle. Continue this pattern until reaching the sternum. Palpation should be performed with the pads of the middle three digits in small concentric circles. Palpate first with light pressure and then with deeper pressure, especially with larger breasts. While palpating, note the consistency of the tissues, the presence and mobility of any lumps or masses, and any nipple discharge. Additionally, palpate high into the axilla to assess for lymphadenopathy. Prior to this portion of the exam, advise the patient that she may experience mild discomfort. Other than when comparing symmetry, ensure the contralateral breast remains covered to maintain as much modesty as possible.

Abdominal Assessment

The gastrointestinal (GI) tract is composed of three main structures. The **stomach** is responsible for digestion of food that is ingested via the esophagus. The **small intestine** absorbs nutrients that are passed from the stomach. Elimination of waste and absorption of excess water occurs in the **large intestine** and the rectum. When stool does not get properly eliminated or is hard to pass, patients will present with constipation. Constipation is a common symptom that can have many etiologies. The practitioner should establish the patient's bowel habits, asking about frequency and characteristics of stool. Questions about diet preferences can be a factor in diagnosing constipation. **Acute constipation** is a sudden change from the patient's normal bowel habits. **Persistent constipation** can last weeks and increases in frequency. **Chronic constipation** is a long-term dysfunction in bowel elimination.

An abdominal assessment should be performed when a patient presents with symptoms of constipation. Abdominal contour should be assessed for distention. Bowel sounds will determine if smooth muscle within the intestine is contracting and passing along the stool. Absent bowel sounds may signal an **obstruction**. Light and deep palpation of the abdomen may elicit tenderness when an obstruction is present. An **intestinal obstruction** results from the inability of waste to pass through the bowel. Obstructions that are not relieved can perforate and cause immediate sepsis. Several conditions may cause an intestinal obstruction. Decreased peristalsis can lead to paralytic ileus. Muscle contractions that slow significantly will cause a backup of feces.

Peritonitis, pancreatitis, and appendicitis may cause a non-mechanical obstruction. Scar tissue within the intestines is a form of mechanical obstruction. An abdominal x-ray and CT scan can detect the obstruction. Management is geared toward preventing fluid imbalance and relieving pressure. Ingestion of fiber can help bulk up the stool and make it easier to pass through the bowel. Lack of fiber in the diet can lead to irritation of the intestinal mucosa. Outpouching of the mucosa is known as **diverticula**. When diverticula become inflamed, the condition is known as **diverticulitis**. Diverticula that are not inflamed is termed **diverticulosis**. Risk factors for diverticulosis and diverticulitis include a diet high in refined carbohydrates and low in fiber, increased age, and obesity. Patients will present with pain that is localized around the affected area of the colon. Change in bowel habits may also be reported. Bowel sounds should be auscultated and the abdomen palpated for tenderness. To rule out rectal bleeding, a fecal occult test should be ordered. An ultrasound and CT scan with contrast can confirm the diagnosis. Treatment is aimed at increasing dietary fiber and promoting physical activity and weight loss if applicable.

Reproductive Assessment

Female Reproductive System

The female reproductive system consists of several structures. The **vagina** contains three layers of muscular tissue that increase in flexibility, especially during childbirth. The **uterus** is lined with endometrial tissue and serves as a womb when an ovum is implanted. The **cervix** is the posterior portion of the uterus that visibly protrudes into the vagina. The **fallopian tubes** are used to transport ova to the uterus. The **ovaries** are structures that contain ova that may be fertilized by sperm during ovulation.

The **pelvic exam** is done to assess the organs of the female reproductive system. The ovaries and the uterus are assessed by palpation, and the cervix is assessed by inspection. The PAP smear sample is a screening test for cervical cancer. The sample, obtained from the opening of the cervix, is transferred to glass slides for processing.

Male Reproductive System

The male reproductive organs include the penis, scrotum, testicles, vas deferens, seminal vesicles, and the prostate gland. In addition to the urethra, the penis contains three sections of erectile tissue. The **scrotum** is a fibromuscular pouch that contains the testes, the spermatic cord, and the epididymis. The pair of **testes** is suspended in the scrotum and each one is approximately 2 inches by 1 inch long. The **vas deferens** is a tubular pathway between the testes and the penis, and the **seminal vesicles** are small organs located between the bladder and the bowel. The **prostate gland** surrounds the proximal end of the urethra within the pelvic cavity.

The main function of the male reproductive system is the production of **sperm**. Unlike the female, beginning at puberty, several million immature sperm are produced every day in the testes. The sperm are transported through the vas deferens to the penis, and the prostate gland and seminal vesicles contribute fluids that support the activity of the sperm after ejaculation.

At **puberty**, egg maturation, menses, and sperm production begin, and the secondary sex characteristics appear. Female fertility declines at thirty years of age, and the maturation of eggs in the ovaries ceases at menopause, which occurs at fifty years of age. Sperm production continues from puberty until death; however, after sixty years of age the ability of the sperm to travel to the fallopian tube to fertilize an egg is decreased.

Colorectal Assessment

The **colorectal exam** may be performed in a similar fashion for a female patient as for a male patient. Always ensure a staff chaperone is present before beginning. Typically, the patient is positioned on her left side. Visually inspect the perianal and sacrococcygeal regions for rashes, ulcers, masses, or evidence of bleeding. Next, lubricate a gloved index finger, inform the patient of the next step in the exam, and explain that she should feel pressure but not pain. Position the finger on the outside of the anus, and insert it as the anal sphincter gradually relaxes. Palpate circumferentially to assess for tenderness, lesions, or masses. Additionally, have the patient tighten the external anal sphincter, allowing for assessment of muscle tone. A retroverted uterus or the cervix itself may be palpable through the rectal wall and should not be confused for

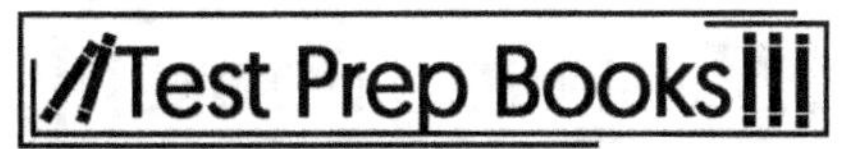

a mass. This exam may also be performed in the lithotomy position after a pelvic exam, allowing for bimanual palpation and evaluation for any pelvic or adnexal masses.

Extremity Assessment

Peripheral Pulses

Knowledge of **peripheral pulse assessment** is necessary to evaluate the patient's circulatory status. Strong pulses at a normal rhythm are good; faint pulses that are either too fast or too slow are worrisome and need further evaluation. Pulses are graded on a scale of 0 to 4, 0 being absent, 1 being weak, 2 being normal, 3 being increased volume, and 4 being a bounding pulse. The pulse is assessed and documented with further action being taken if necessary.

Edema

Another way to evaluate the health of the circulatory system is to assess for and grade edema. **Edema**, a fluid accumulation in the peripheral tissues of the body, can get to a point where, when pushed down upon with a finger, the impression stays in the skin. These impressions can be graded by their depth, ranging from +1 to +4 as shown in the diagram below.

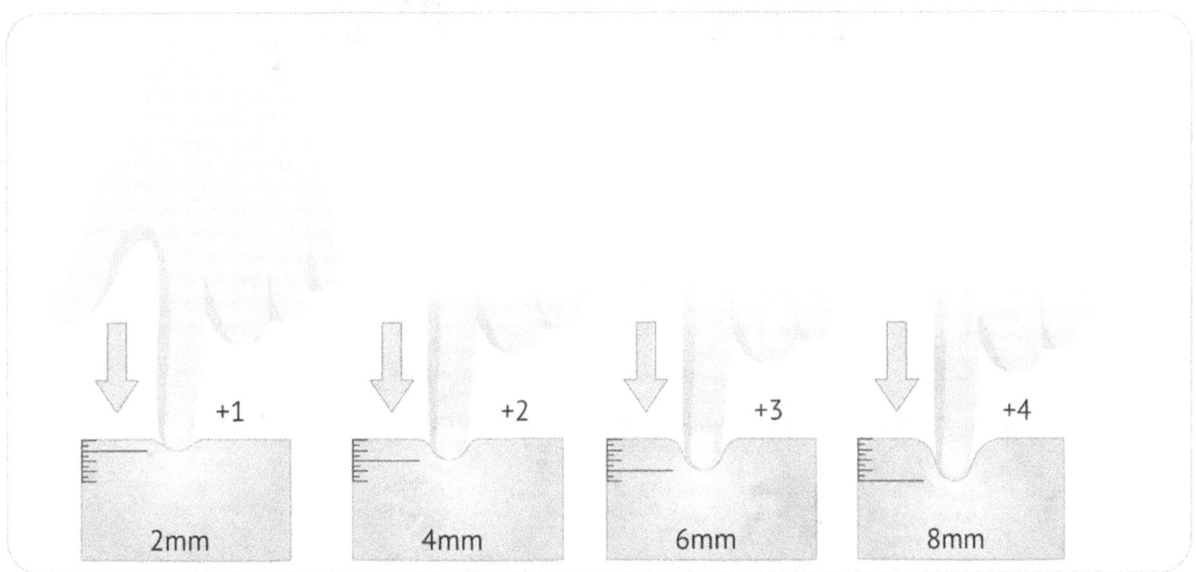

Musculoskeletal Assessment

The WHNP can assess the client's musculoskeletal system by testing for bilateral strength and equality of movement. **Muscular strength** can be graded on a 0 to 5 scale. A patient with no visible muscle contraction is graded as a 0, a patient who has visible contraction but still no movement is graded as a 1, a patient that is contracting and trying to move but cannot overcome gravity is graded as a 2, the same without the ability to push against resistance is a 3, the same with only a limited effect of resistance on their effort is a 4, and finally, a full contraction with movement that can overcome elevated levels of resistance is a 5.

Range of Motion Techniques

Range of motion exercises involve moving the body's limbs in particular ways to keep the joints healthy and flexible. Active range of motion exercises are performed by the patient independently. Passive range of motion exercises are done for patients who are unable to perform active ones. When performing passive

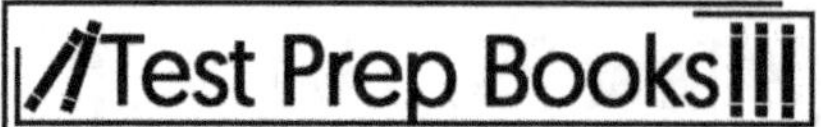

range of motion exercises, gently guide the patient's limbs through their range of motion. Never force the limbs, as this can harm the patient.

With the patient resting in the supine position, take each joint through its range of motion. **Adduction** is the movement of a limb toward the midline of the body. **Abduction**, the opposite of adduction, is the movement of a limb away from the midline of the body.

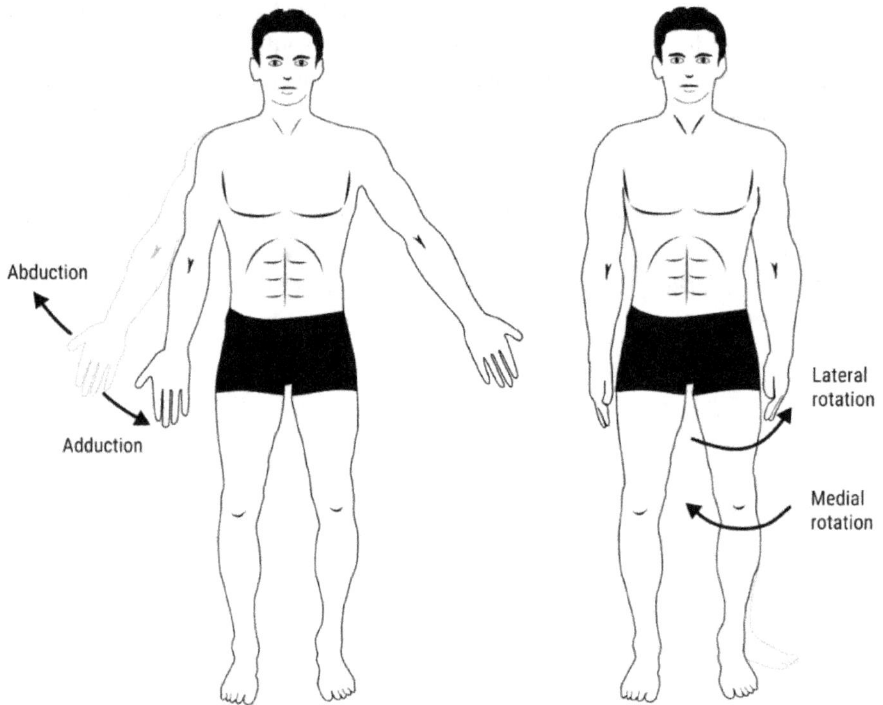

Flexion is the bending of a limb at the joint, while **extension** is the straightening of a limb at the joint.

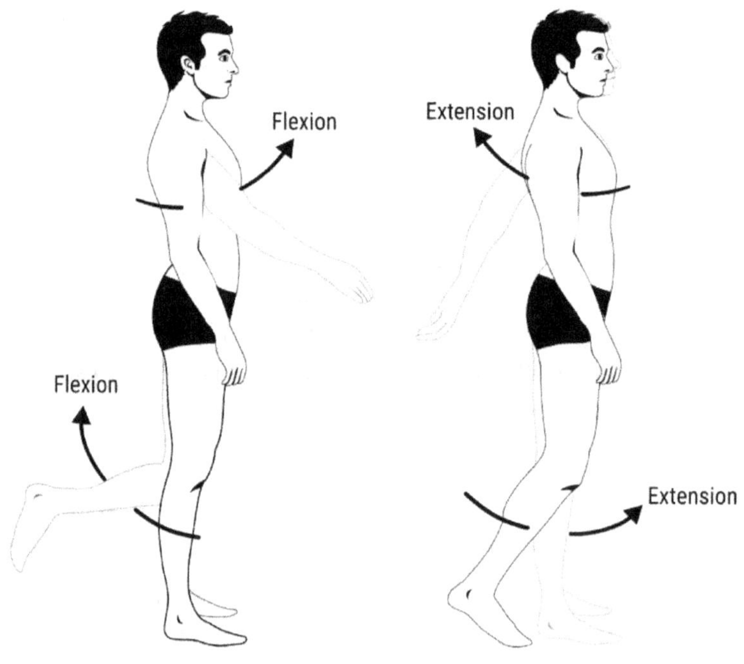

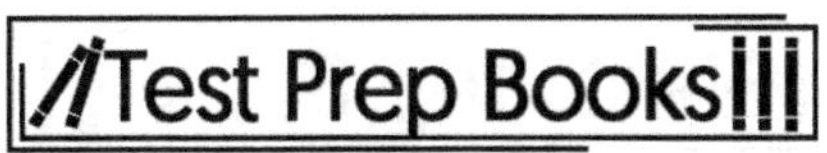

Neurological Assessment

The neurological system may need specific evaluation requiring the provider's keen assessment skills. The WHNP will start by evaluating the client's **level of consciousness**, which is measured by interviewing the client and their knowledge of who they are, where they are, and the time. A client oriented to all three of these components is said to be oriented times three, while a client who only knows their name, for example, is only oriented times one. Commonly, this is noted in the nurse's notes as "A&OX3" or something similar. The "A" stands for "alert," as opposed to obtunded, drowsy, sleepy, difficult to arouse, and other altered levels of consciousness.

Other components of the neurological assessment include assessment of the cranial nerves, usually used on stroke assessments, motor and sensory function, pupillary response, reflexes, cerebellar function, and vital signs.

Endocrine Assessment

The endocrine system is made up of multiple glands throughout the body. Glands secrete hormones that help regulate the function of organs. Hormones are responsible for growth and development and differentiation of the male and female reproductive systems. Hormones also maintain a neutral environment inside the body and will operate when changes occur. Abnormal levels of hormones within the body result in endocrine disorders. The **pancreas** is a glandular organ that sits behind the stomach in the abdominal cavity. It is the producer of insulin. **Insulin** is a hormone that helps regulate the metabolism of protein, fats, and carbohydrates. It also maintains a normal level of glucose in the body. Alterations in insulin production can lead to abnormally high or low levels of glucose in the body.

The hormones of the body play a key role in metabolism and the regulation of body processes. Each hormone, produced in various glands throughout the body, has a specific target tissue that it acts upon, producing a specific result. Dysfunction of hormonal regulation can lead to disease states.

The endocrine system is maintained through homeostatic balance of a variety of hormones. To ensure proper maintenance and detection of disease, laboratory values are monitored via individualized, patient-centered treatment plans regarding frequency and response to results. If medication management is initiated in response to laboratory and clinical findings, repeat laboratory values should be assessed on an individualized basis to provide follow-up response to treatment.

Major Human Endocrine Glands and Some of Their Hormones

Gland		Hormone	Chemical Class	Representative Actions	Regulated By
Hypothalamus		Hormones released from the posterior pituitary and hormones that regulate the anterior pituitary *see below*			
Posterior pituitary gland *Releases neurohormones made in hypothalamus*		Oxytocin	Peptide	Stimulates contraction of uterus and mammary gland cells	Nervous system
		Antidiuretic hormone **ADH**	Peptide	Promotes retention of water by kidneys	Water/salt balance
Anterior pituitary gland		Growth hormone **GH**	Protein	Stimulates growth (especially bones) and metabolic functions	Hypothalamic hormones
		Prolactin **PRL**	Protein	Stimulates milk production and secretion	Hypothalamic hormones
		Follicle-stimulating hormone **FSH**	Glycoprotein	Stimulates production of ova and sperm	Hypothalamic hormones
		Luteinizing hormone **LH**	Glycoprotein	Stimulates ovaries and testes	Hypothalamic hormones
		Thyroid-stimulating hormone **TSH**	Glycoprotein	Stimulates thyroid gland	Hypothalamic hormones
		Adrenocorticotropic hormone **ACTH**	Peptide	Stimulates adrenal cortex to secrete glucocorticoids	Hypothalamic hormones
Thyroid gland		Triiodothyrocine T_3 Thyroxine T_4	Amine	Stimulate and maintain metabolic processes	TSH
		Calcitonin	Peptide	Lowers blood calcium level	Calcium in blood
Parathyroid glands		Parathyroid hormone **PTH**	Peptide	Raises blood calcium level	Calcium in blood
Pancreas		Insulin	Protein	Lowers blood calcium level	Glucose in blood
		Glucagon	Protein	Raises blood calcium level	Glucose in blood
Adrenal glands	*Adrenal medulla*	Epinephrine Norepinephrine	Amines	Raises blood glucose level; Increases metabolic activities; Constrict certain blood vessels	Nervous system
	Adrenal cortex	Glucocorticoids	Steroid	Raises blood glucose level	ACTH
		Mineralocorticoids	Steroid	Promote reabsorbtion of Na^+ and excretion of K^+ in kidneys	K^+ in blood; angiotensin II
Gonads	*Testes*	Androgens	Steroid	Support sperm formation; Promote development and maintenance of male secondary sex characteristics	FSH LH
	Ovaries	Estrogens	Steroid	Stimulate uterine lining growth; Promote development and maintenance of female secondary sex characteristics	FSH LH
		Progestins	Steroid	Promote uterine lining growth	FSH and LH
Pineal gland		Melatonin	Amine	Involved in biological rhythms	Light/dark cycles

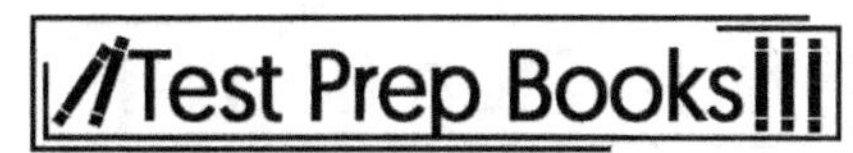

Skin Assessment

The skin or integumentary body system is the largest organ of the body in surface area and weight. It is composed of three layers, which include the outermost layer or epidermis, the dermis, and the hypodermis. The thickness of the epidermis varies according to the specific body area. For example, the skin is thicker on the palms and the soles of the feet than on the eyelids. The dermis contains the hair follicles, sebaceous glands and sweat glands. Melanin is the pigment that is responsible for skin color.

The main function of the skin is the protection of the body from the outside environment. The skin regulates body temperature, using the insulation provided by body fat and the secretion of sweat, which acts as a coolant for the body. Sebum lubricates and protects the hair and the skin, and melanin absorbs harmful ultraviolet radiation. Special cells that lie on the surface of the skin also provide a barrier to bacterial infection. Nerves in the skin are responsible for sensations of pain, pressure, and temperature. In addition, the synthesis of Vitamin D, which is essential for the absorption of calcium from ingested food, begins in the skin.

Vernix caseosa is a thick, protein-based substance that protects the skin of the fetus against infection and irritation from the amniotic fluid from the third trimester until it dissipates after birth. Several childhood illnesses, such as measles and chicken pox, are associated with specific skin alterations. Acne related to hormonal changes is common in adolescents, and the effects of sunburn are observed across the life span. In the elderly, some of the protections provided by the skin become less effective; decreases in body fat and altered sweat production affect cold tolerance, loss of collagen support results in wrinkling of the skin, and decreased sebum secretions lead to changes in hair growth and skin moisture content.

Diagnostic Studies

The WHNP is responsible for selecting diagnostic tests that are accurate, necessary, and whenever possible, cost-effective. There is a large selection of evaluation measures, and they can be divided into screening tests and diagnostic tests. **Screening tests** are used to identify risk factors for a disease or the presence of early manifestations of the disease in asymptomatic individuals. **Diagnostic tests** are used to confirm the presence of the disease in a symptomatic patient or in an asymptomatic patient who has tested positive for the disease. Screening tests are used to identify common diseases in large numbers of people; therefore, the tests need to be inexpensive, generally less invasive than diagnostic tests, easy to administer, and highly sensitive.

The WHNP will select those diagnostic tests that are most likely to provide the relevant information needed to support all clinical decisions. The appropriate selection of a diagnostic test also relies on the provider's intuitive assessment skills. For instance, the context of the likelihood ratio is dependent on the identification of the pretest probability by the provider, and the pretest probability is derived from the physical assessment. The WHNP also must remain current with recommendations related to the use of new assessment measures that might replace older measures that are more expensive, invasive, or less reliable. That being said, every new test should not automatically replace an existing test without careful consideration. The WHNP will consider the possible benefits of the new versus the old before changing the diagnostic plan.

The patient's preferences should be reviewed by the WHNP because the patient may have cultural concerns with invasive testing. Other common diagnostic tests such as magnetic resonance imaging (MRI) are not tolerated well by many patients, and if the MRI or any diagnostic test that is essential for appropriate patient care is refused by the patient, the WHNP works with the patient to be certain that the needed information is collected. Anxious patients might need mild sedation in order to tolerate a procedure. However, if the patient does refuse to complete the test, the refusal should be well documented.

The WHNP will use best practices to select the appropriate diagnostic tests to develop the patient's care plan. In making these choices, the WHNP will consider the metrics of each test, the patient's preferences, and the cost effectiveness.

Differential Diagnosis

Patients present to primary care clinics with one symptom or a cluster of manifestations. To reach a final diagnosis, WHNPs must first create a list of differential diagnoses. A **differential diagnosis** is a list of possible etiologies for the presenting symptoms. Obtaining a thorough medical history and asking clarifying questions will guide the provider down a pathway to reach a final diagnosis.

For example, a common symptom is shortness of breath. Labored breathing may cause the patient anxiety and will produce a number of physical findings. Providers must first rule out emergency diagnoses, such as a PE, pneumothorax, or foreign body aspiration. A physical assessment will assist in eliminating potential diagnoses. Auscultation of the lung sounds can reveal adequate airflow. The absence of lung sounds or audible wheezing can point to ineffective airflow in the airways. Essential vital signs, such as heart rate, respiratory rate, and blood pressure, can reveal changes in cardiac output and lung effort. Examination of the skin may reveal color changes. Blue discoloration may indicate inadequate gas exchange at the base of the lungs. Obtaining the oxygen saturation level via a pulse oximeter can aid the provider in determining whether the patient is oxygenating adequately.

A chest x-ray is essential in visualizing opacities in the chest cavity. A physical assessment and diagnostic studies can determine if shortness of breath is caused by an acute condition such as pneumonia or a chronic condition such as COPD. Chest pain is a symptom that should be addressed promptly. Pain characteristics and accompanying symptoms will help determine if the chest pain is due to a life-threatening condition. The chest cavity incases the heart and lungs. Radiating pain away from the chest cavity toward the shoulders may indicate a respiratory condition. Concurrent vital signs and lung auscultation can rule out respiratory disorders. Crushing chest pain with concurrent numbness to the left arm may be indicative of a cardiac event. An ECG can assist with ruling out ischemia or infarction. Laboratory data such as cardiac enzymes can assist with measuring cardiac tissue injury. Investigation of risk factors and onset of symptoms can help determine if the chest pain is cardiac in nature or due to a non-emergent condition such as esophagitis and peptic ulcer disease.

Hematologic Studies

Complete Blood Count (CBC) and Differential

The **complete blood count** (**CBC**) is a type of diagnostic test that requires a small vial of blood to be drawn from the patient. The blood is sent to the lab, and the components of the blood are measured. The CBC measures red blood cells (RBCs), white blood cells (WBCs), hemoglobin, hematocrit, and platelets. This simple test can give the clinician a quick look at the body's oxygen-carrying capacity, immune function, and clotting capability all in one go.

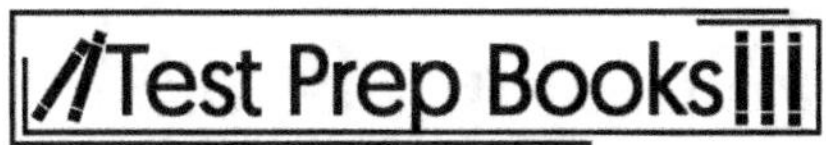

Normal Laboratory Values

Blood Count	Normal Range (Adult Male)	Normal Range (Adult Female)
Red blood cell	5 to 6 million cells/mcL	4 to 5 million cells/mcL
White blood cell	4,500 to 10,000 cells/mcL	
Platelets	140,000 to 450,000 cells/mcL	
Hemoglobin	14 to 17 gm/dL	12 to 15 gm/dL
Hematocrit	41% to 50 %	36% to 44%
Mean corpuscular volume	0 to 95 fl	

Information from the National Heart, Lung, and Blood Institute (NIH)

Blood Typing and Antibody Screening

Blood typing and **antibody screening** is a cornerstone of routine prenatal care and should occur in the first trimester. This testing identifies the ABO and RhD (that is, "positive" or "negative") blood types of both mother and baby. This testing identifies patients who need **Rh immune globulin** (**RhoGAM®**) to prevent Rh alloimmunization. It also screens for maternal antibodies such as anti-Fy, anti-Jk, anti-C, anti-E, and anti-Kell, among others. Though rare, if these antibodies are present and not identified in the mother's blood, they can cross the placenta and cause hemolytic disease of the newborn (HDN) or suppression of myeloid progenitor cells in fetal bone marrow. If such antibodies are detected, their presence and concentration should be monitored at least every four weeks with a low threshold for referral to maternal-fetal medicine or other high-risk pregnancy specialists for treatment to ensure the health of the fetus.

Hemoglobin Electrophoresis

Hemoglobin electrophoresis is the process of separating and quantifying hemoglobin proteins based on their ionic characteristics, such as their electric charge. This testing can aid in diagnosis of certain hemoglobinopathies, the most significant of which include sickle cell disease (SCD) and thalassemia syndromes. Originally, gel electrophoresis was the most established such method, but over time, other methods for identification of abnormal hemoglobin have emerged, including capillary zone electrophoresis, isoelectric focusing, and high-pressure liquid chromatography. All neonates should undergo screening for hemoglobinopathy shortly after birth. Pregnant women should also undergo this testing if there is reason for suspicion of a hemoglobinopathy, such as if red blood cell testing demonstrates microcytosis and/or if the patient is of an ethnicity that is predisposed to hemoglobinopathies. These include patients of Mediterranean, African, Middle Eastern, and Southeast Asian descent. The earlier a potential hemoglobinopathy is identified, the more rapidly the appropriate resources can be arranged to ensure the best possible outcome for both mother and baby.

Diabetic Testing

Diabetes mellitus is a disease characterized by chronic hyperglycemia. There are three main types of diabetes.

Type 1 diabetes is primarily an autoimmune disorder in which pancreatic beta cells are destroyed. Insulin production is decreased, and glucose levels in the body are unregulated. Type 1 diabetes is commonly diagnosed during childhood. **Type 2 diabetes** results from insulin resistance and decreased production of insulin from beta cells. Type 2 diabetes is preventable by initiating lifestyle modifications. Practitioners should assess for dietary and exercise habits. Obesity is a main risk factor for the development of type 2 diabetes. **Gestational diabetes** can occur in pregnant females and is characterized by glucose intolerance.

Gestational diabetes increases the risk of developing type 2 diabetes later in life. Characteristic signs of diabetes development include increased thirst, urination, hunger, and unintentional weight loss. Several tests can be performed to diagnose diabetes. The **hemoglobin A1C** test measures the level of sugar in the blood for the previous 60 to 120 days. Normal findings are A1C levels below 5.7 percent. Levels of 6.5 percent or higher indicate diabetes. A **fasting blood sugar** test measures the blood sugar levels after not eating overnight. Patients should not eat for a period of at least 8 hours before a fasting blood test. Normal levels are 99 mg/dL or lower. Blood sugar levels of 126 mg/dL or higher are indicative of diabetes.

Protein/Creatinine (PC) Ratio

The **PC ratio** has multiple diagnostic uses. Most broadly, an elevated ratio may suggest kidney disease, particularly in patients with diabetes. In obstetrics, an increased PC ratio is concerning for preeclampsia, a serious condition that can threaten both mother and baby if untreated. Specifically, a PC ratio greater than 0.3 is highly suggestive of preeclampsia and relates directly to the pathophysiology of the condition. Preeclampsia involves microvascular damage across multiple organs resulting from abnormal interactions between maternal and placental tissue. In the kidneys, this microvascular damage leads to renal insufficiency, which is manifested by proteinuria and evidenced by a urine dipstick with 2+ protein, a 24-hour urine collection with more than 300 milligrams of protein, or an elevated PC ratio. Expectant mothers with preeclampsia must undergo more frequent monitoring and aggressive treatment of hypertension. Delivery should occur by 37 weeks of gestation, but in some high-risk patients, it may be necessary as early as 34 weeks.

Blood Clotting Studies

PT/INR

PT/INR and **PTT** are two common tests that assess the rapidity at which a patient's blood clots. PT stands for *prothrombin time* and measures the extrinsic and common pathways of the coagulation cascade. It is performed by adding thromboplastin to a plasma sample and measuring the time to clot formation. This test in particular is subject to high variability due to different thromboplastin formulations. For this reason, the international normalized ratio (INR) was developed. The INR conveys PT results in a standardized format, with less than 1.1 considered a normal value. This is highly useful in patients who take warfarin, which inhibits the extrinsic and common pathways via vitamin K antagonism.

PTT

Partial thromboplastin time (PTT) focuses more on the intrinsic pathway of the coagulation cascade, which involves factors XII, XI, IX, and VIII. Generally, 25 to 35 seconds is considered a normal PTT. Elevated values may occur with hemophilia or von Willebrand disease, but they may be appropriately elevated in a patient receiving heparin. Indeed, PTT is the test of choice for monitoring a patient's response to anticoagulation with heparin.

D-Dimer

The **D-dimer** test differs from the above in that it indicates the presence of a clot somewhere in the body. It is a product of fibrin degradation; its elevation suggests ongoing coagulation and fibrinolysis but does not indicate where this is occurring. In other words, D-dimer is a highly sensitive test that, when negative, effectively rules out blood clots in a patient. This is particularly useful in screening patients for deep vein thrombosis or pulmonary embolism. However, a positive D-dimer does not rule in such a diagnosis, as it is not specific to any organ or region of the body. In such cases, further testing is required.

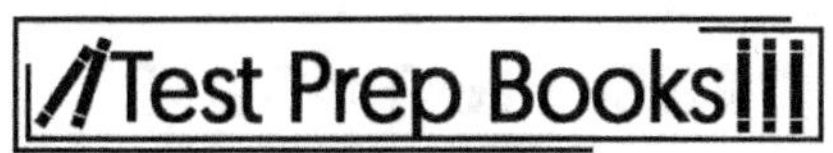

Serologic Screening

RPR

Rapid plasma reagin (**RPR**) is a common serological screening test for *Treponema pallidum*, better known as syphilis. Screening appropriate patients is vital because, if undetected and untreated, syphilis can produce chronic cardiovascular and neurologic disease as well as fetal anomalies in congenital syphilis. The RPR test assesses for the presence of antibodies to antigens associated with—but not specific for—syphilis. If found, the antibodies are diluted in solution, and results are expressed in a ratio that quantifies the maximum dilution at which antibody agglutination is visible. Negative results are generally reassuring against syphilis infection, while positive results require confirmation with a more specific test, such as fluorescent treponemal antibody (FTA) or *T. pallidum* enzyme immunoassay (TP-EIA).

CMV

Cytomegalovirus (**CMV**) is also known as human herpesvirus 5 (HHV 5) and, though often asymptomatic or mild with flu-like symptoms, can cause serious disease in immunosuppressed patients and in utero via congenital CMV infection. CMV is a double-stranded DNA virus that is present worldwide. Fortunately, infection is not particularly common in pregnancy, and routine immunoglobulin M (IgM) antibody screening before or during pregnancy is not recommended due to high rates of false positive results related to cross-reactivity with non-CMV antibodies. It may be considered in immunosuppressed patients or those with known exposure to a CMV-positive patient. In such cases, quantitative CMV DNA polymerase chain reaction (PCR) studies are considered the most sensitive screening tests.

HSV

Herpes simplex virus 2 (**HSV-2**) is classically associated with genital herpes and can cause neonatal illness if vertical transmission occurs. However, in most patients, the best screening test for HSV is a history and physical exam. Ask patients about history of HSV or contact with an infected partner, the presence of vesicular lesions, or a sensation of tingling or burning in the genital region. They should also be examined for such lesions at the onset of labor. Though the gold standard for diagnosis, routine serologic screening in asymptomatic patients is not currently recommended. If necessary, suppressive antiviral therapy may generally be initiated based on history and physical findings suggestive of active or recurrent HSV infection.

Toxoplasmosis

Congenital **toxoplasmosis** can cause severe fetal illness, including blindness and neurological anomalies. Fortunately, however, congenital infection is uncommon, occurring in as few as 1 in 10,000 pregnancies. Thus, indications for testing are generally limited to immunosuppressed mothers with a history of infection, exposure to cats or undercooked meat, or findings of cerebral ventriculomegaly or intracranial calcifications on imaging. When indicated, toxoplasmosis is identified via toxoplasmosis IgM, IgG, or IgA or positive PCR for toxoplasma DNA. The PCR test may identify toxoplasma in urine, blood, or cerebrospinal fluid. Though routine prenatal testing is not recommended, regular prenatal visits are essential to ensure the ongoing health of both mother and baby.

HIV

The **human immunodeficiency virus** (**HIV**) is a sphere-shaped virus that is a fraction of the size of a red blood cell. There are primarily two types of HIV: HIV-1 and HIV-2. HIV-2 is not highly transmissible and is poorly understood. It has mainly affected people in West Africa. HIV-1 is more severe and more highly transmissible. It is the dominant strain among global HIV cases, and when literature and media refer to HIV, this is usually the type that is being referred to.

HIV is highly contagious. It is found in human bodily fluids and can be transmitted through infected breast milk, blood, mucus, and sexual fluids. The most common forms of transmission are through anal or vaginal sex, but transmission can also occur through contaminated syringe use, blood transfusions, or any other method where membranes are compromised. Once in the body, HIV attacks and destroys CD4/T cells. These cells are responsible for attacking foreign bodies (e.g., bacteria, infections, other viruses). As the body's CD4/T-cell count diminishes, the patient is left immunocompromised.

The HIV-1 type can be broken further into four groups: M, N, O, and P. M is the most commonly seen group globally. Within group M, there are nine different subtypes of HIV. These are noted as A, B, C, D, E, F, G, H, J, and K. Subtype B is prevalent in the Western world, and most research has been conducted on this subtype. This research has led to the manufacturing of antiretroviral (ARV) drugs. Antiretroviral therapy (ART) has been a major breakthrough in the management of HIV and in the quality of life for patients with HIV. In conjunction with medical care, many patients with HIV are able to have completely normal, healthy, active lives. It is important to treat HIV as early as possible. The better a patient's HIV is managed, the lower their viral load. Viral load refers to how much HIV is present in a patient's blood; when a viral load is low, transmission of the disease is far less likely to occur. With ART, many patients with HIV are viral-suppressed, and some even have an undetectable viral load. Viral load in other transmitting fluids, such as semen, cannot be detected but the virus is still present. Therefore, transmission is still possible, and all precautions should be taken.

Globally, most HIV patients have subtype C, but subtypes are mixing as travel and migration become more widespread. Most subtypes can be treated with ART, though these drugs were researched and manufactured to treat subtype B. However, ART is not always physically available or financially accessible in countries that need it most.

Without early intervention or adequate managed care of HIV, the virus can deteriorate the host body's immune system to a point where it cannot be rehabilitated. This stage is marked by extremely low levels of CD4/T cells (less than two hundred cells per cubic millimeter of blood) and is referred to as **acquired immunodeficiency syndrome** (**AIDS**). When a patient's HIV diagnosis progresses to AIDS, he or she often succumbs to serious chronic diseases, such as cancer. Mild illnesses, such as a cold or flu, can also be fatal to someone with AIDS. Not everyone who is diagnosed with HIV will also be diagnosed with AIDS. Once diagnosed with AIDS, the patient has approximately one to three years to live unless he or she receives adequate treatment.

Hormone Studies

Many different hormones are involved in the reproductive system, and their levels individually and in relation to each other can help identify the causes of conditions such as anovulation and infertility, oligo- or amenorrhea, galactorrhea, and a host of other nonspecific symptoms. In patients struggling with infertility, in addition to sperm studies for the male partner, **follicle-stimulating hormone** (**FSH**) and **luteinizing hormone** (**LH**) are evaluated to distinguish ovarian versus hypothalamic insufficiency. **Progesterone** is also drawn halfway through the luteal phase of the menstrual cycle to determine whether ovulation is occurring. Of note, increased FSH levels may also indicate menopause in women of the appropriate age who are experiencing such symptoms. In patients with menstrual irregularities, FSH and LH are useful, and thyroid studies (TSH and free T4) should be obtained as well. Elevated **prolactin** levels cause galactorrhea, or milky breast discharge that is usually bilateral. Hyperprolactinemia may also cause oligo- or amenorrhea. Crucially, clinicians must check the β-subunit of **human chorionic gonadotropin** (**β-hCG**) in any patient of childbearing age reporting amenorrhea, as pregnancy is the most common cause of secondary amenorrhea.

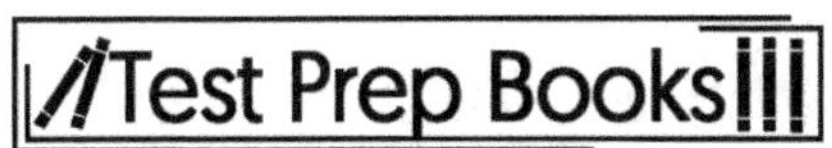

Comprehensive Metabolic Panel (CMP)

The **comprehensive metabolic panel** (**CMP**) is a group of lab values that are often taken together that measure how well the kidneys and liver are functioning and levels of blood sugar, cholesterol, calcium, and protein levels in the body. The electrolytes may be measured using the CMP or as part of a smaller lab test called a **basic metabolic panel** (**BMP**). Though it varies based on facility, the CMP generally consists of fourteen separate lab tests, while a BMP may only contain eight separate lab tests. The practitioner will determine which of these tests to perform.

Normal Laboratory Values

Comprehensive Metabolic Panel	Normal Range
Albumin	3.4 to 5.4 g/dL
Alkaline phosphatase	20 to 130 U/L
ALT (alanine aminotransferase)	4 to 36 U/L
AST (aspartate aminotransferase)	8 to 33 U/L
BUN (blood urea nitrogen)	6 to 20 mg/dL
Calcium	8.5 to 10.2 mg/dL
Chloride	96 to 106 mEq/L
CO2 (carbon dioxide)	23 to 29 mEq/L
Creatinine	0.6 to 1.3 mg/dL
Glucose	70 to 100 mg/dL
Potassium	3.7 to 5.2 mEq/L
Sodium	135 to 145 mEq/L
Total bilirubin	0.1 to 1.2 mg/dL
Total protein	6.0 to 8.3 g/dL

Information from the National Library of Medicine (NLM)

Lipid Profile

Total cholesterol is determined from two components: **high-density lipoproteins** (**HDL**) cholesterol, considered the "good" cholesterol, and **low-density lipoproteins** (**LDL**) cholesterol, considered the "bad" cholesterol. Although it is helpful to keep a lower total cholesterol level for health and reduced disease risk, it is more critical to keep the ratio of HDL to LDL elevated.

Cholesterol levels can be obtained from a **lipid panel**. High levels of total cholesterol can increase the risk of heart disease. Total cholesterol levels should be below 200 mg/dL. High levels of low-density lipoprotein (LDL) cause plaque buildup in the artery walls. A level less than 100 mg/dL is ideal. Patients who have a high risk of heart attacks should aim for a level less than 70 mg/dL. High triglyceride levels can increase the risk of heart disease. **Triglyceride** levels should be below 150 mg/dL.

Normal Laboratory Values

Lipid Panel	Normal Range
Cholesterol	Less than 200 mg/dL
HDL	40 to 60 mg/dL
LDL	Less than 100 mg/dL
VLDL	2 to 30 mg/dL
Triglycerides	Less than 150 mg/dL

Information from the National Library of Medicine (NLM)

Urinalysis/Urine Cultures

Urinalysis

The provider can collect a random **urinalysis** any time the patient voids.

To obtain a midstream/clean catch urine sample, the provider will instruct the patient to first clean the urinary meatus with the appropriate antiseptic solution, void without collecting the initial volume, and then deposit the remaining output into the container.

Before beginning the collection of a timed twenty-four-hour collection, the provider must obtain a storage container containing any necessary preservative from the laboratory and confirm the accommodations for refrigeration of the sample if required. The first time the patient voids, the provider will discard the specimen and record the time. All urine collected in the following twenty-four-hour period will be collected by the provider and stored in the prepared container at the prescribed temperature.

Catheterization may be used to obtain a sterile specimen. The provider will pass the sterile catheter into the bladder to drain the urine into a sterile container, which must then be labeled and transported to the lab according to agency policy.

The **pediatric urine collector** is a plastic pouch attached to a foam adhesive backed base. The provider will verify that the skin around the urinary meatus is clean, dry, and free of powder or lotions. The provider will adhere the adhesive section of the collection device over the urinary meatus and replace the patient's diaper.

Urine Cultures

Urine cultures allow for the identification of a specific causative organism in conditions such as urinary tract infections (UTIs) and pyelonephritis. This allows for the tailoring of antibiotic therapy to the specific organism, preventing ineffective or unnecessarily broad coverage. Many institutions now perform "reflex" cultures, in which the urine sample of any patient whose urinalysis suggests UTI is automatically sent for culture, and empiric antibiotic coverage is initiated in the meantime. Accurate cultures require a clean-catch specimen and aseptic technique in handling. Importantly, cultures are only considered positive if they demonstrate more than 100,000 colony-forming units (CFUs). Furthermore, antibiotics are not indicated unless the patient is experiencing irritative voiding symptoms and/or systemic symptoms, regardless of culture results. Pregnant women represent the exception to this rule: Asymptomatic bacteriuria, defined by the same urine culture results, should be treated during pregnancy. If a patient's culture results demonstrate a pathogen not covered by the previously initiated empiric antibiotic, the patient should be contacted and a new prescription sent.

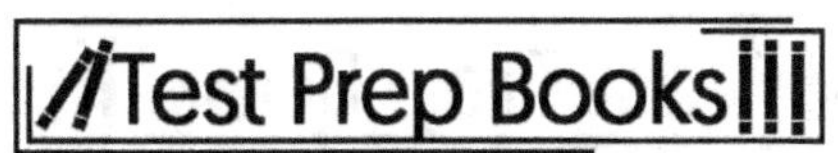

Fecal Occult Blood Testing

Occult bleeding is not visibly apparent, which means that detection methods rely on the chemical reaction between the blood and the testing reagents for identification of blood in a sample. For home sample collection with guaiac testing, the provider will instruct the patient to collect three samples on three different days to optimize results. The patient will secure the test card and submit it to the provider for testing. The provider will apply a guaiac solution to the sample to identify a bluish tinge in the test area, which is considered positive for the presence of occult blood.

Vaginal Microscopy

Vaginal microscopy is typically indicated for women complaining of irritative vaginal symptoms, including itching, burning, erythema, odor, and/or discharge. Microscopy is an inexpensive and widely available method of testing that helps differentiate the common causes of vulvovaginitis, including candidiasis, trichomoniasis, and bacterial vaginosis (BV). The provider first obtains a sample of vaginal tissue or discharge with a swab or brush; then, he or she spreads it on a microscope slide and applies saline or potassium hydroxide to prepare a wet mount. A **wet mount** revealing budding hyphae and yeast (often compared to spaghetti and meatballs) indicates candidiasis. The presence of motile, flagellated trichomonads is diagnostic for trichomoniasis. Additionally, the microscopic finding of clue cells (that is, squamous cells studded with bacteria) combined with other findings in Amsel's criteria suggests BV. As always, accurate diagnosis is essential for proper treatment.

Cervical and Vaginal Cultures

Cervical and vaginal cultures are primarily used for the evaluation of vaginitis and cervicitis, which are caused by **sexually transmitted infections (STIs)**. The most frequent causative organisms are *Neisseria gonorrhoeae* and *Chlamydia trachomatis*. However, with these infections, cultures are not the most commonly used method of testing. Rather, **nucleic acid amplification testing (NAAT)** is preferred due to higher sensitivity and specificity. However, cultures are an appropriate option in certain circumstances, such as when NAAT is unavailable, when antibiotic resistance is suspected, or when symptoms recur or persist despite treatment. In most patients, vaginal swabs, performed by either the patient herself or the clinician, are often sufficient for obtaining an accurate culture. Similar to blood or urine cultures, cervical and vaginal cultures typically take 48 to 72 hours for definitive results. Empiric antibiotics should be initiated based upon history and exam findings and any other previous test results. Therapy should then be narrowed to the causative pathogen when results are reported.

Testing and Cultures for Vaginal Discharge and STIs

Many conditions can cause abnormal **vaginal discharge**, including candidiasis, BV, trichomoniasis, and vaginitis or cervicitis caused by bacteria such as chlamydia and gonorrhea. Each of these may be diagnosed with relatively fast and inexpensive testing. Importantly, ensure that patients complaining of vaginal discharge are not pregnant, as this may impact both diagnosis and treatment. Utilize microscopy with wet mount for candidiasis, BV, and trichomoniasis. For vaginitis or cervicitis, cultures are no longer considered first-line, as NAAT boasts high accuracy and, increasingly often, rapid results. The best initial diagnostic workup for vaginal discharge is a history and physical. Ask about the color, volume, and consistency of discharge and any associated symptoms, such as fever, chills, pelvic or back pain, itching, burning, tingling, rashes, or lesions. Ask about their own sexual history and that of their partner(s). Furthermore, remember that multiple causes can coexist, so maintain a low threshold to perform both microscopy and NAAT or culture.

Throat and Skin Cultures

Throat Swab

After assisting the patient to a seated position in a chair or bed, the provider will use sterile swabs to remove the sample from the back of the throat while avoiding contact with the uvula and tongue. The provider will then break the tips of the swabs and secure them in the labeled collection sleeve, transport the sample to the lab according to agency policy, and document the sample collection time and site.

Wound Swab

The provider will position the patient according to the site being sampled. The provider will remove and discard the existing dressing, use sterile swabs to obtain the sample from the center of the wound, then break the tips of the swabs and secure them in the labeled collection sleeve. Once the swabs are secured, the provider will dress the wound, ensure that the sample is delivered to the laboratory, and document the wound assessment and the sample collection time and site.

Cervical Cytology and HPV Testing

Cervical intraepithelial neoplasia (CIN) involves a spectrum of abnormal cell growth ranging from benign to cancerous; dysplasia is screened for by **Papanicolaou tests**, or **pap smears**. The leading risk factor for CIN is **human papillomavirus** (**HPV**)—specifically, HPV types 16 and 18. More than 75 percent of Americans are estimated to have some type of HPV, though the highest-risk types are much less common. Risk factors for HPV include early sexual activity, multiple partners, immunosuppression, and low socioeconomic status. Current guidelines advise screening for CIN from ages twenty-one to sixty-five. This usually involves cervical cytology via pap smear every three years, but screenings can be extended to every five years if HPV co-testing is performed. Testing is essential because a physical exam cannot identify dysplasia.

Abnormal pap smear results include ASCUS (atypical squamous cells of undetermined significance), LSIL (low-grade squamous intraepithelial lesions), HSIL (high-grade squamous intraepithelial lesions), and atypical glandular cells. LSIL refers to mild dysplasia (CIN1), while HSIL involves moderate or severe dysplasia (CIN2-3). Colposcopy with biopsy is indicated for HSIL. For limited dysplasia, the lesion can be excised via conization or trachelectomy (cervical removal), which can preserve fertility. Advanced dysplasia and cancer may require hysterectomy and possible oophorectomy with or without chemotherapy and radiation.

Test for Ruptured Membranes

Classically, patients with **rupture of membranes** (**ROM**) report leakage of fluid from the vagina and often describe it as clear and watery. Importantly, ask about gestational age, prior pregnancies and any complications, history of prenatal care, and other medical history. Inquire also about any associated symptoms (e.g., blood, contractions, recent trauma or physical activity) and the color, consistency, and volume of the fluid. Workup should begin with a physical exam, wherein direct visualization of fluid leaking from the cervical os is diagnostic of ROM. If in doubt, ROM may be confirmed in several ways. On microscopy, dried amniotic fluid crystallizes resemblant of a fern tree. An elevated fluid pH relative to that of normal vaginal secretions (approximately 4) also suggests ROM. If ROM is confirmed, ensure fetal stability with ultrasound and/or tocometry, and monitor for signs of spontaneous labor. Expectant management is typically appropriate, and antenatal corticosteroids should be strongly considered if gestational age is less than 37 weeks.

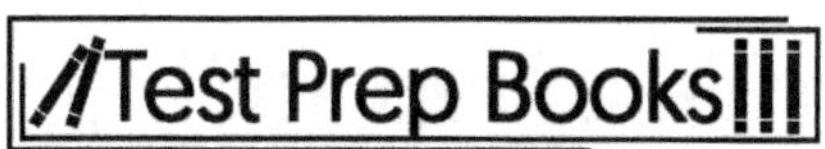

Fetal Fibronectin

Fetal fibronectin (FF) is an extracellular matrix glycoprotein that is present throughout gestation and useful in stratifying the risk of preterm birth in women with symptoms of preterm (that is, prior to 37 weeks) labor. Testing is performed by placement of a swab into the posterior vaginal fornix for collection of secretions. A low value (often <10 ng/mL) on quantitative testing or a negative value on qualitative testing predicts a low likelihood of delivery in the next 1 to 2 weeks. These negative results can help prevent unnecessary hospitalization, tocolytics, and corticosteroids. The test is most useful in women with symptoms of preterm labor with minimal cervical dilation and intact amniotic membranes. Of note, positive results are less reliable. Therefore, use of FF for routine screening tests in preterm patients is not recommended because false positive testing may lead to overutilization of resources, hindering those who truly need hospitalization.

Biopsies

Depending on the location and form of the cancer, ultrasonography, CT scans, bone scans, MRI, nuclear imaging studies, and blood and body fluid analyses will be considered. In some instances, the definitive diagnosis can only be established by a **biopsy** of the malignant cells, which can identify the characteristics of the cells. Biopsy samples can be collected by shaving a thin layer of skin, by punching a core of tissue from the skin, by aspirating fluid and tissue from a superficial tumor with a fine needle or a coring needle, by an incisional or excisional biopsy, or by removing lymph nodes that are proximal to the malignancy.

Endometrium

The most crucial indication for **endometrial biopsy** is that of abnormal uterine bleeding and particularly postmenopausal bleeding, which is highly suspicious for endometrial cancer. This cancer is the fourth most common affecting women. Endometrial biopsy can be performed in-office, and patients without contraindications may benefit from a pre-procedure nonsteroidal anti-inflammatory drug (NSAID) to alleviate post-biopsy cramping. It is also advisable to have a chaperone present, as with any exams or procedures requiring undressing. Absolute contraindications to this procedure include pregnancy, cervical cancer, and active vaginal, cervical, or pelvic infection. Otherwise, prompt biopsy is essential for timely diagnosis and treatment of suspected endometrial cancer.

Cervix

Cervical cancer remains a highly prevalent cancer worldwide, though in the US, vaccines against human papillomavirus (HPV) have directly caused a 90 percent decrease in cervical cancer rates. Cervical biopsy is indicated in patients with specific abnormal Pap smear findings, including, but not limited to: confirmed high-grade squamous intraepithelial lesion (HSIL); low-grade squamous intraepithelial lesion (LSIL) plus a positive HPV test; and a calculated HSIL risk over 4 percent. Additional indications include postcoital or postmenopausal bleeding despite normal Pap results; unexplained vaginal bleeding; or evaluation of persistent pruritus. Active vaginal or cervical infection represents the only contraindication to cervical biopsy. The procedure begins with direct visualization via colposcopy and application of 5 percent acetic acid. The presence of acetowhitening is concerning for neoplasia; every visible lesion requires its own biopsy.

Vulva

Vulvar cancer is not particularly common, but the prevalence of risk factors such as HPV infection, smoking, and immunosuppression means many patients face some degree of risk for vulvar cancer. Some patients may describe itching, irritation, or pain, but many lack symptoms. Though squamous cell carcinoma (SCC) occurs most often, patients with vulvar melanoma may experience bleeding, ulceration, and discoloration. Any suspicious lesion, including those that are asymmetric, irregular, growing, or of various colors, must be biopsied. Depending on proximity to the urethra or rectum, cystoscopy or proctoscopy should also be considered, as well as advanced imaging, to assess for possible spread.

Breast

Breast biopsy is indicated in any patient with exam and/or imaging findings concerning for breast cancer. Potential findings include a fixed, irregular mass, nipple inversion, unilateral discharge, orange-peel discoloration, and rash or other skin irritation. Clinicians should correlate suspicious findings with ultrasound or mammogram. Mammogram findings are expressed on the **Breast Imaging-Reporting and Data System** (**BI-RADS**) scale, which runs from 0 to 6. A score of 0 indicates inconclusive findings requiring further imaging; a 6 represents previous biopsy-proven malignancy. Importantly, scores of 4 or 5 depict highly suspicious lesions requiring urgent biopsy. Options for biopsy include ultrasound-guided core needle biopsy, open surgical biopsy, and stereotactic biopsy utilizing multiple mammograms. The preference for each biopsy depends on the size, location, and nature of the suspected tumor.

Genetic Testing

Screening Tests for Obstetrical Patients

Routine prenatal visits should begin with a comprehensive history and physical encompassing the patient's medical and surgical history, medications and substance use, family history, social history, including screening for **intimate partner violence**. Obtain β-hCG early to confirm pregnancy. Additional initial testing should include complete blood count, ABO and RhD type, antibody screen, and serology for syphilis, hepatitis B, rubella, and HIV. All patients should also undergo initial screening for gonorrhea and chlamydia. Obtain urine cultures at an early visit for detection of asymptomatic bacteriuria. Furthermore, check blood pressure (BP) at every visit. If the patient's BP is greater than 140/90 millimeters of mercury, screen for proteinuria using a urinalysis, as these findings are concerning for preeclampsia, especially after 20 weeks' gestation.

Monitoring for fetal development is also crucial. Screen for **fetal aneuploidy** (such as trisomy 13, 18, and 21) with cell-free DNA as early as 10 weeks or with quad screening in the second trimester. Maternal alpha-fetoprotein is included in the quad screen and is effective in detecting **neural tube defects**, such as spina bifida or anencephaly. The fetal anatomic scan should be performed between 18 and 22 weeks. Finally, screen for gestational diabetes between 24 and 28 weeks, or earlier if the patient's BMI is over 30 kg/m^2 or if other risk factors are present.

Ethnic-Specific Genetic Testing

Genetic testing has historically been performed on members of specific ethnic groups to identify parents who are asymptomatic carriers of abnormal genes associated with particular diseases. However, most guidelines and organizations now recommend standardized carrier testing rather than ethnic-based testing given the increasing diversity in many patient populations. Still, certain ethnic groups face higher risk for certain heritable diseases. In those of African, Mediterranean, and Southeast Asian descent, cystic fibrosis and hemoglobinopathies like sickle cell disease and thalassemia are more prevalent than in the general population. Patients of Ashkenazi Jewish descent are, unfortunately, predisposed to a host of genetic disorders, including the above two as well as Tay-Sachs disease, familial dysautonomia, Niemann-Pick type A, and several others. While carrier testing is available and encouraged for all patients both pre-conception and throughout the antepartum period, it is of particular importance in those communities described above. Should an anomaly be detected, clinicians should refer parents to a genetic counselor who can provide guidance regarding expectations and specific care the child may need after birth.

Cancer Genetic Screening

Inherited mutations in an individual's chromosomes, genes, or proteins may be harmful, beneficial, or have no effect on the individual's health. Harmful mutations increase the risk of diseases such as cancer, and research indicates that 5 to 10 percent of all cancers are genetically linked. Cancer-specific mutations have

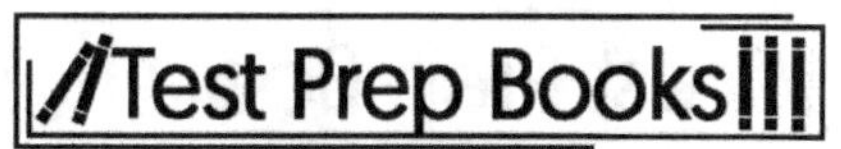

been identified, and the presence or absence of these defects in an individual can be confirmed with **genetic testing**.

Gene TP53, which produces a protein that suppresses tumor growth, is the most commonly mutated gene in all forms of cancer. Mutations of this gene cause Li-Fraumeni, a rare inherited disorder that is associated with an increased risk for several cancers. Hereditary breast and ovarian cancer syndromes, which result from mutations of the BRCA1 and BRCA2 genes, are associated with an increased lifetime risk for the development of breast and ovarian cancer. These two genes are thought to be responsible for 5 to 10 percent of all breast cancers in women and 100 percent of breast cancers in men. This inherited mutation is also associated with an increased risk for pancreatic cancer and prostate cancer. Mutations of gene PTEN, which also produces a protein that suppresses tumor growth, may result in an inherited disorder identified as Cowden syndrome, which is associated with an increased risk of breast, thyroid, and endometrial cancers. The most common inherited cancer is Lynch syndrome—or hereditary nonpolyposis colon cancer—, which occurs as the result of mutations in a group of five different genes.

Patient characteristics that are associated with inherited cancer syndromes include a history of cancer that was diagnosed at a very early age, simultaneous evidence of several different forms of cancer, cancer occurring in paired organs such as both kidneys or breasts, several first-degree relatives who have the same disease, evidence of certain birth defects that are associated with cancer, and being susceptible to cancer disorders due to gender, ethnicity, or race. Genetic researchers have identified inherited mutations for most, if not all, cancerous conditions, which means that individuals can identify their risks for the development of cancer with genetic testing. Health care providers are encouraged to strongly recommend **genetic counseling** when the following three criteria are met: the patient has a personal or family history that is consistent with an inherited cancer mutation, the test results will provide definitive information regarding the presence or absence of the disease, and the test results can be used to develop the plan of care.

Tumor Markers

In addition, **tumor markers** have been identified for many malignant conditions that may be helpful in monitoring the tumor burden or identifying a recurrence of the disease; however, in most cases, these markers do not provide definitive details about the primary disease. Some of the more common markers include carcinoembryonic antigen (CEA), cancer antigen 125 (CA125), prostate-specific antigen (PSA), and Estrogen Receptor Assay (ERA). CEA is a blood test that identifies the presence of an antigen that is associated with GI tissue malignancies. It is not specific for identifying a primary site; however, persistent elevations of this marker greater than 10 ng/mL are indicative of significant disease, and levels greater than 20 ng/mL are indicative of metastatic disease. Providers must be aware that cigarette smoking affects the accuracy of this test, and false-positive results are common in smokers. CA125 is also a blood test that is useful for monitoring ovarian cancer, with levels greater than 35 U/mL considered positive. PSA is a blood test that measures an antigen that is present in prostate tumors. Providers understand that false-positives are common in individuals with benign prostatic hypertrophy, and the PSA level can also be falsely elevated if the test sample is drawn immediately after a rectal exam due to possible manipulation of the prostate gland. ERA identifies the presence or absence of estrogen receptors in a malignant tumor. This is an essential pre-treatment assessment because tumors that are estrogen-receptor negative do not respond to hormone therapy, while an estimated 55 percent of estrogen-receptor positive tumors can be effectively treated with hormone therapy.

Basic Patterns of Inheritance

Genetics is the study of heredity, which is the transmission of traits from one generation to the next, and hereditary variation. The chromosomes passed from parent to child contain hereditary information in the form of genes. Each gene has specific sequences of DNA that encode proteins, start pathways, and result in inherited traits. In the human life cycle, one haploid sperm cell joins one haploid egg cell to form a diploid cell. The diploid cell is the zygote, the first cell of the new organism, and from then on mitosis takes over and nine months later, there is a fully developed human that has billions of identical cells.

The monk Gregor Mendel is referred to as the father of genetics. In the 1860s, Mendel came up with one of the first models of inheritance, using peapods with different traits in the garden at his abbey to test his theory and develop his model. His model included three laws to determine which traits are inherited; his theories still apply today, after genetics has been studied more in depth.

1. The **Law of Dominance:** Each characteristic has two versions that can be inherited. The gene that encodes for the characteristic has two variations, or alleles, and one is dominant over the other.

2. The **Law of Segregation:** When two parent cells form daughter cells, the alleles segregate and each daughter cell only inherits one of the alleles from each parent.

3. The **Law of Independent Assortment:** Different traits are inherited independent of one another because in metaphase, the set of chromosomes line up in random fashion – mom's set of chromosomes do not line up all on the left or right, there is a random mix.

Organisms contain a **genotype** and a **phenotype**. The genotype is the DNA present in the cells that code for the genes, and the phenotype is the set of observable traits that are expressed. For example, a brown-eyed girl may have genes for both blue and brown eyes, but the actual physical trait expressed is brown eyes. So, the genotype is blue and brown eyes, but the phenotype is brown eyes.

Dominant and Recessive Traits

Each gene has two **alleles**, one inherited from each parent. **Dominant alleles** are noted in capital letters (A) and **recessive alleles** are noted in lower case letters (a). There are three possible combinations of alleles among dominant and recessive alleles: AA, Aa, and aa. If both alleles are identical, the individual is considered **homozygous**; if the two alleles have different sequences, the individual is considered **heterozygous**. In most genes, one allele is considered more dominant than the other and will mask the appearance of the less dominant, or recessive, allele when there is a heterozygous situation. Dominant alleles, when mixed with recessive alleles, will mask the recessive trait. The recessive trait would only appear as the phenotype when the allele combination is aa because a dominant allele is not present to mask it.

Although most genes follow the standard dominant/recessive rules, there are some genes that defy them. Examples include cases of co-dominance, multiple alleles, incomplete dominance, sex-linked traits, and polygenic inheritance.

In cases of **co-dominance**, both alleles are expressed equally. For example, blood type has three alleles: I^A, I^B, and i. I^A and I^B are both dominant to i, but co-dominant with each other. An I^AI^B has AB blood. With incomplete dominance, the allele combination Aa actually makes a third phenotype. An example: certain flowers can be red (AA), white (aa), or pink (Aa).

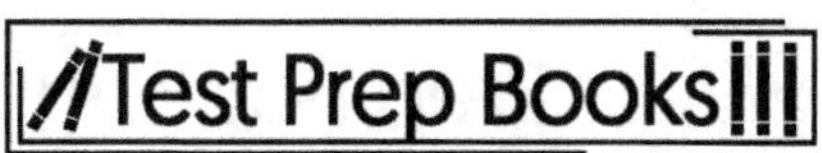

Punnett Square

For simple genetic combinations, a **Punnett square** can be used to assess the phenotypes of subsequent generations. In a 2 x 2 cell square, one parent's alleles are set up in columns and the other parent's alleles are in rows. The resulting allele combinations are shown in the four internal cells.

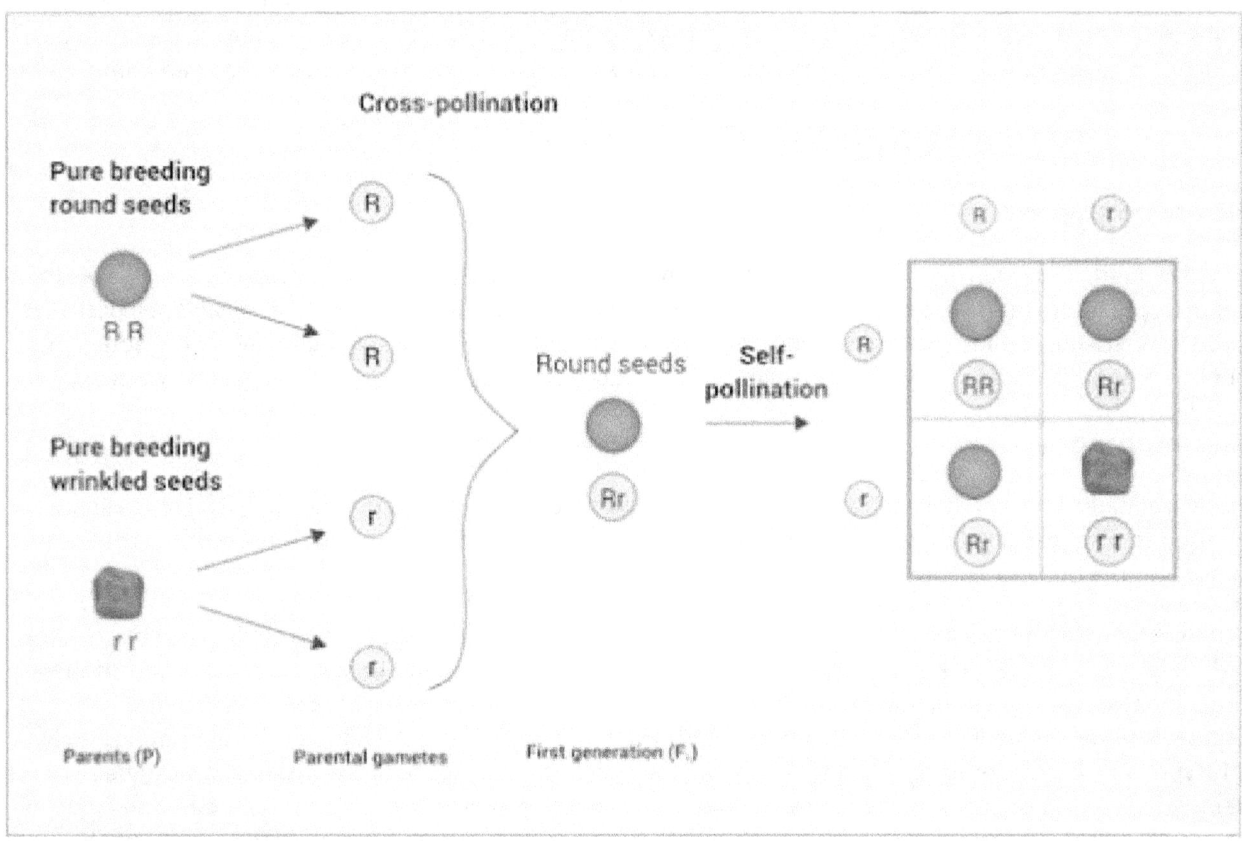

In the example above, two parents with alleles RR and rr, have a 50% chance (2 in 4) of having an offspring with alleles Rr.

Hepatitis Panel

Universal screening for **hepatitis B virus** (HBV) using the surface antigen (HBsAg) is recommended at the first prenatal visit. A triple-panel approach that tests for HBsAg, anti-HBs antibodies, and total anti-HBc antibodies differentiates between active infection and immunity due to vaccination versus previous infection. A positive HBsAg and anti-HBs indicates active acute infection. Conversely, negative HBsAg, positive anti-HBs, and positive anti-HBc represents immunity due to prior infection. Negative HBsAg, positive anti-HBs, and negative anti-HBc denotes immunity achieved through vaccination because the HBV vaccine specifically stimulates production of anti-HBs but not anti-HBc. Importantly, patients found with acute HBV infection as described above should undergo testing for HBV DNA quantification, which measures viral load and allows stratification of the risk of vertical transmission. Crucially, every reputable professional organization and guideline recommends initial hepatitis B immunization at birth for newborns regardless of maternal antenatal HBV testing. This is advised due to the risk of false negative tests and of horizontal transmission from family members or others who are unknowingly infected.

COVID Testing

Nasopharyngeal Swab

The provider will position the patient in a seated position with the head tilted back. After verifying the patency of the nares, the provider will insert the sterile swab 3 to 4 inches into the nasopharynx, rotate the swabs to obtain the sample, remove the swabs, break the tips of the swabs to secure them in the labeled collection sleeve, transport the specimen to the laboratory, and document the collection site and time.

Imaging Studies (common indications)

Ultrasonography

An **ultrasound**, also referred to as a sonograph, is an imaging test that uses high frequency sound waves to create images from inside the body. Ultrasounds can be done on various parts of the body and help visualize blood flow, tissues, tumors, and cysts. One of the most common uses of ultrasound imaging is to detect and monitor pregnancy. Sound waves produce fetal images that can be observed on an ultrasound machine.

Mammography

There are many different diagnostic tests available for innumerable patient conditions. Different mediums are used to diagnose conditions, including blood work, ultrasound technology, x-rays, procedures that put cameras in the body to visualize internal structures, and more.

A comprehensive physical exam is an essential first step in the diagnosis of cancer. Providers use the results of the exam to identify the appropriate diagnostic tests, which are intended to confirm the findings of the screening tests, provide direction for the therapeutic plan, and continue surveillance of recurrent or new disease. A female patient who has discovered a lump in her breasts may be scheduled for a **mammography**. This type of diagnostic procedure is a type of x-ray that visualizes the tissue of the breast. This can help identify lumps that the patient or the practitioner is not able to palpate. The generally agreed-upon guideline for mammography is for it to be performed once every year or two after the age of forty for early breast cancer detection.

Diagnostic studies are often a variation of the screening test. For instance, a **screening mammogram** generally consists of two views—craniocaudal and mediolateral oblique—of each breast, while a **diagnostic mammogram** may use one or more additional views—spot compression and magnification views—to study an identified abnormality.

WHNPs must be prepared to counsel women who receive an abnormal mammogram report. The Breast Imaging-Reporting and Data System (BI-RADS) identifies the results on the following scale: BI-RADS 0, meaning the screening exam is incomplete and more imaging or comparison views are needed; BI-RADS 1, which is normal; BI-RADS 2, when abnormalities are present but are considered benign; BI-RADS 3, when abnormalities are present that are most likely benign, but 6-month follow-up for two years is recommended; BI-RADS 4 and BI-RADS 5, which refer to probable and definite evidence of malignancy respectively and biopsy is recommended; and BI-RADS 6, which refers to findings that have already been previously identified as malignant on a biopsy.

Bone Densitometry

Bone mineral density (**BMD**) is most often measured by **dual-energy X-ray absorptiometry** (**DEXA**) scans. DEXA is an outpatient imaging procedure recommended in all women over age 65, typically biannually. It

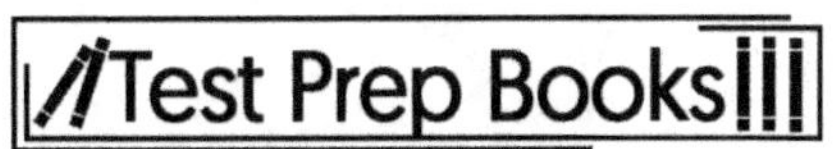

screens for decreased BMD, for which decreased estrogen function after menopause is a major risk factor owing to estrogen's role in promoting osteoblasts and inhibiting osteoclasts. DEXA images are most commonly obtained for the lumbar spine and hip/femoral neck but may also involve the forearm or even the entire skeleton. From these images, a T-score is produced and represents the number of standard deviations from the patient's BMD to that of the appropriate reference population, matched for race and sex. A T-score of −1.0 or greater is normal; a T-score between −1.0 and −2.5 denotes **osteopenia**; and a score of −2.5 or less diagnoses **osteoporosis**. Furthermore, a fragility fracture (that is, a fracture caused by minimal trauma) is also diagnostic for osteoporosis regardless of the T-score. For patients with osteopenia, the **Fracture Risk Assessment Tool** (**FRAX**) score estimates their 10-year risk of fracture by incorporating other risk factors, such as age, sex, BMI, steroid use, and alcohol and smoking histories.

Practice Quiz

1. To diagnose a PE in a patient with renal failure, which type of scan will likely be performed?
   a. Transesophageal echocardiography
   b. CT scan with contrast
   c. MRI of the thoracic cage
   d. V/Q scan

2. What is the significance of a "pertinent negative" documented in the patient's EHR?
   a. The patient was unable to identify symptoms.
   b. The documentation of the physical assessment is incomplete.
   c. The assessment did not identify the symptoms commonly associated with a condition.
   d. The assessed manifestations are inconsistent with the patient's report.

3. Which of the following is NOT identified as one of the five Ps of the sexual history?
   a. Pills—the use of recreational drugs
   b. Prevention of pregnancy
   c. Prevention of sexually transmitted infections (STIs)
   d. Past history of STIs

4. Which of the following cancers is NOT commonly linked to hereditary factors?
   a. Breast cancer
   b. Non-polyposis colon cancer
   c. Cervical cancer
   d. Ovarian cancer

5. Which of the following statements is consistent with disease characteristics that influence the selection and use of a screening test?
   a. The disease is associated with a projected survival rate of greater than five years after diagnosis.
   b. The test can produce positive results before physical symptoms of the disease are present.
   c. The disease must be widely disseminated in the population.
   d. Screening tests for genetically linked diseases are associated with greater specificity.

See answers on the next page

Answer Explanations

1. D: A patient who is in renal failure with a suspected PE will likely undergo V/Q scanning, in which ventilation and perfusion of the lungs are visualized. Transesophageal echocardiography is used for visualizing the back of the heart and is not appropriate in this scenario. CT scanning with contrast is contraindicated, as the patient with renal failure cannot tolerate the dye, which is primarily metabolized by the kidneys. An MRI is not a usual scan for a PE.

2. C: The pertinent negative is a manifestation that is commonly associated with a condition, and the absence of that manifestation is an important consideration in the diagnosis of that condition. The remaining choices are not associated with the concept of the pertinent negative; therefore, Choices *A, B,* and *D* are incorrect.

3. A: Pills is not one of the five Ps of the sexual history. The missing pieces are partners and sexual practices; therefore, the five Ps of the sexual history are partners, sexual practices, prevention of pregnancy, prevention of STIs, and a past history of STIs. Therefore, Choices *B, C,* and *D* are incorrect.

4. C: Cervical cancer is not linked to an inherited gene mutation. Breast and ovarian cancer, Choices *A* and *D*, are linked to inherited mutations in the BRCA1 and BRCA2 genes. Non-polyposis colon cancer, Choice *B*, is caused by inherited mutations in a group of genes affecting DNA repair.

5. B: Screening tests are appropriate for conditions that can be identified and treated before symptoms of the disease are evident, which potentially improves patient outcomes, and in some cases, may prevent the development of cancer. Screening tests are not limited by projected survival rates. Screening tests assume a certain incidence of the disease in the target population; however, widespread incidence is not required for accurate testing. There is no published data to indicate that screening tests are more sensitive to genetic diseases.

Primary Care

Problem Recognition, Management, and Referral (Evaluation, diagnosis, treatment or referral)

The scope of practice for the WHNP in primary care includes caring for patient and families with acute and chronic illnesses. The primary care setting is often the **patient-centered medical home** (PCMH). In the PCMH care delivery model, care is delivered and coordinated by a primary care provider who also provides access to all required specialty referrals. The model also supports care activities that are consistent with the WHNP role, including coaching, information for self-management, personalized care plans, and medication review. The PCMH model does facilitate care for all age groups; however, the most common reason for healthcare visits is the identification and treatment of chronic illnesses.

The WHNP's care of patients with chronic illness is also consistent with the **chronic care model** (CCM), which is reported to be effective in meeting the longitudinal care needs of patients with chronic disease. This model differs from other models in two ways: chronic disease is treated proactively rather than reacting only to periodic crises, and the patient's care is planned and coordinated by an interdisciplinary team rather than a single provider. The implementation of the care model requires six essential resources that collectively contribute to optimal patient outcomes. The resources include:

- Support of the organizational structure
- Availability of sophisticated clinical information software systems that go beyond the electronic health record (EHR)
- Integrated care teams
- Proprietary software systems that provide current clinical guidelines
- Self-management systems for patients that combine education and results tracking for the patient and the provider
- Identification of available community resources

The fully-integrated CCM supports the WHNP's intervention selection and evaluation through the availability of software systems that supply current clinical guidelines, and clinical information systems that can track patient outcomes over time. This advanced data is necessary to maintain the accuracy of the plan for chronic diseases and to assess the effects of the pharmacologic and non-pharmacologic interventions on the patient's clinical outcomes.

The WHNP will provide care for the most commonly occurring chronic diseases, including hypertension, diabetes, asthma, and chronic heart failure. These common diseases often occur together, or one disease may cause another, increasing the complexity of the patient's care. For instance, the patient with diabetes often develops hypertension as a consequence of the chronically elevated blood glucose. The WHNP activities required for the development of the treatment plan include; selection and interpretation of relevant diagnostic tests, identification of appropriate evidence-based pharmacologic and clinical interventions, a patient education exercise that promotes self- management, and appropriate specialty referrals. In the case of diabetes and hypertension, additional diagnostic tests might include coronary angiography to assess the effects of both diabetes and hypertension on the coronary arteries. Pharmacologic interventions might include alterations in insulin management to improve A1C (glycosylated red blood cell) levels. The WHNP can recommend a patient information and tracking system that is either electronic such as

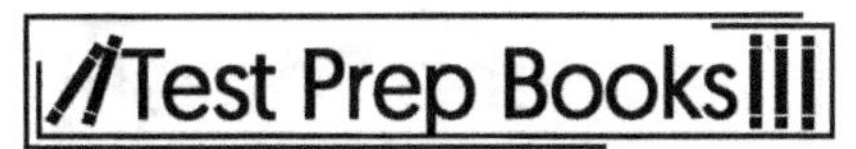

a phone application, or a paper-and-pencil instrument that the patient can review with the WHNP. Specialty referrals for this patient population might be vascular surgeons, ophthalmologists, or cardiologists.

The ongoing systematic evaluation of the plan of care requires the interim assessment of all parameters to track the patient's progress. If the stated goals are not being met, the plan must be modified. One of the essential components of this process is the inclusion of the patient and the patient's family or care providers in goal setting and in the evaluation of the plan. There is evidence that the patient's input into these processes has a direct effect on the patient's adherence and progress in meeting those goals. For instance, if the goal for the patient with diabetes and hypertension is to complete thirty minutes of moderate exercise per day, the patient who has input into setting the goal is more likely to meet the goal. The evaluative process is also used to check the adequacy of care for specific patient populations such as lesbian, gay, bisexual, transgender, and intersex (LGBTQI) patients; homeless patients; and patients for whom English is a second language.

When caring for the patient with chronic disease, the WHNP will use the clinical guidelines to compare the patient's actual and expected manifestations and to modify the clinical and pharmacologic interventions based on the result of that comparison. This longitudinal care plan is reported as the most effective approach to the management of chronic diseases because it assesses not only the current state of the disease, but also provides early recognition of progression or onset of additional manifestations that require intervention. For example, if a patient with hypertension reports the onset of headaches, the WHNP will investigate the reason for the headaches, which could be due to worsening hypertension (HTN) or decreased patient adherence to the drug plan.

The purpose of evaluation is to assess the adequacy of the care plan and to identify any necessary modifications. Assessment of the patients' satisfaction with the care they receive has become a significant issue in primary care and in acute care institutions. The **Centers for Medicare & Medicaid Services (CMS)** commissioned the creation of the Hospital Consumer Assessment of Healthcare Providers and Systems Survey (HCAHPS) for the assessment of patient satisfaction in acute care settings. The survey results are publicized, and exemplary "grades" are tied to monetary awards. Critics of this competitive aspect of the evaluation stress the importance of using the data to improve the relationship between patients and providers and to make substantive changes in the system. Interestingly, the research indicates that three of the five issues that are most important to patients relate to communication and information. WHNPs should understand that patients value comprehensive information related to self-care management and timely communication about their condition above other concerns such as the wait time for the provider.

Skin Conditions

Chronic and Acute Skin Conditions

Vitiligo

Vitiligo is a common hereditary autoimmune disorder that causes a lack of pigmentary cells, leading to demarcated white patches of skin. These patches are commonly round or oval and affect the body symmetrically, exhibiting similar patterns of depigmentation on either side of the body. Vitiligo affects the trunk, hands, neck, and face with periocular and perioral presentations. It is thought to be an autoimmune reaction that attacks melanocytes and reduces the synthesis of melanin. Depigmentation known as the Koebner phenomenon may occur after trauma to the skin and is commonly seen on the knees, elbows, hands, and feet. Depigmentation is often separated into three categories: localized, generalized, and segmental. Vitiligo can develop at any age; however, it is commonly diagnosed in adults between twenty and thirty years old. Diagnosis will usually involve a history of present illness, physical examination, and occasionally a Wood light exam. Treatment involves many modalities, including topical medications (e.g., corticosteroids), laser therapies, phototherapy, and surgery.

Psoriasis

Psoriasis is a chronic condition caused by swelling of the dermal layer of the skin. Patients with psoriasis will present with reddened, circular plaques with white scales. Psoriasis is due to an abnormal growth of the epidermal cells. Cell division in psoriasis occurs within four to five days as opposed to normal regeneration, which occurs within twenty-eight days. Treatment is aimed at reducing the cell turnover rate and decreasing swelling. The condition can be diagnosed by a physical assessment or skin biopsy.

Eczema

Eczema or **atopic dermatitis** is a common skin condition characterized by chronic inflammation as well as itchy, dry, and red skin patches. This rash often results from scratching due to pruritus and is prone to infections. Children are at a higher risk of developing eczema; however, it is seen across all age groups. Genetics and environmental factors play a major role in the development and severity of eczema. Mutations in the filaggrin gene (*FLG*) are linked to an increased risk of eczema due to the lack of filaggrin, which leads to an impaired skin barrier. Environmental factors include stress, chemical product exposure (e.g., soaps or laundry detergents), or exposure to allergens (e.g., pet dander and dust). The rash may be generalized in children and start to localize in adulthood, usually affecting the face, elbows, wrists, and knees. A complete history and physical examination will assist in diagnosis. If necessary, an allergy test may be performed. Treatment involves reducing exposure to any environmental triggers and applying topical anti-inflammatory medications. Keeping the skin hydrated with increased water intake and the application of a fragrance-free ointment is also recommended.

Contact Dermatitis

Contact dermatitis is a skin disease characterized by inflammation caused by irritants or allergens. Irritant contact dermatitis is a skin reaction that develops following direct chemical or friction exposure to the skin. Length, frequency, and type of exposure will determine the extent of irritant contact dermatitis. Allergic contact dermatitis is a type IV hypersensitivity reaction, which occurs when the skin is exposed to allergens such as poison ivy, nickel, and formaldehyde. Both irritant and allergic contact dermatitis present with erythematous vesicles or pustules that are pruritic, inflamed, and painful. A complete history of medication usage, chemical exposure, and environmental exposure is necessary for diagnosis, along with a physical exam. Patch testing is often used to diagnose the cause of allergic contact dermatitis. Treatment involves avoiding the irritant or allergen identified along with applying topical corticosteroids. Antihistamines may be prescribed for pruritus, and occasionally systemic steroids may be necessary, depending on the severity of the reaction.

Tinea

Dermatophyte infections are fungal infections that subsist from keratin and therefore involve skin, nails, and hair. Transmission of dermatophytes can occur from direct contact via person to person, animals, or soil or indirectly through carrier objects (e.g., hats and hair brushes). There are many different types of dermatophyte or "tinea" infections, such as tinea capitis, tinea corporis, tinea barbae, tinea faciei, tinea manuum, tinea cruris, tinea pedis, and tinea unguium.

Tinea capitis is an infection of the hair shaft and follicle which causes alopecia to occur. This is commonly seen in pediatrics and is typically passed indirectly through fomites. KOH microscopy, Wood's lamp exams, and fungal culture are all utilized to confirm diagnosis. Treatment requires oral antifungal agents, such as Griseofulvin.

Tinea corporis, also known as **ringworm**, is characterized by a circular rash with raised erythematous borders. This condition is commonly seen on the extremities, face, or trunk. A complete history and physical exam are necessary for diagnosis along with a KOH microscopy. Treatment includes topical antifungals and protocols to keep skin dry.

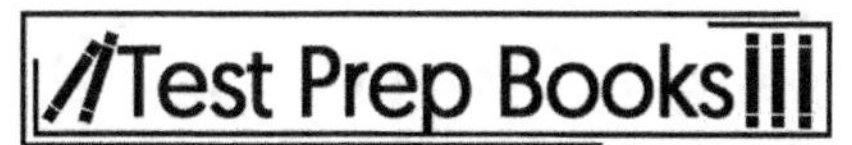

Tinea barbae is commonly seen in adult males and affects the skin and hair follicle of the beard or mustache. Pustules, erythema, and scaling are all symptoms of tinea barbae. Diagnosis includes complete history and physical exam, followed by a course of oral antifungals.

Tinea faciei involves red patches on the face, which may be pruritic in nature. Diagnosis follows a clinical exam and KOH microscopy. Topical antibiotics are usually used in treatment, along with keeping the area dry.

Tinea manuum involves one or both hands and is common in patients who suffer from tinea pedis. Dry, scaly palms with hyperkeratosis are commonly seen with this condition. Topical antifungals are used along with lactic acid creams.

Tinea cruris, also known as jock itch, is characterized by a pruritic rash that affects the groin, inner thighs, abdomen, and buttocks. The condition is commonly seen in conjunction with tinea pedis. Treatment includes low-dose corticosteroids, possible oral antifungals, and keeping the area dry.

Tinea pedis, commonly known as athlete's foot, is a pruritic scaly rash typically seen between the fourth and fifth toes but may also affect the soles or sides of feet. Topical antifungals should be applied to all affected areas.

Tinea unguium is a nail infection that is more common in patients with tinea pedis, advanced age, or diabetes. A fungus such as yeast or mold may be the cause of tinea unguium. Diagnosis involves a clinical exam as well as periodic acid-Schiff staining of the infected toenail clipping. Treatment takes three to four months for fingernails and four to six months for toenails using systemic doses of itraconazole or terbinafine.

Lesions

Paying close attention to any alterations in the skin is of particular importance, as these changes may be telltale signs of potentially life-threatening conditions such as skin cancer. Abnormal growths, such as bumps, patches, or discolored moles, can be indicative signs of **skin cancer**. Receiving an early diagnosis and effective treatment are crucial to the individual's overall health and well-being. Some forms of skin cancer include basal cell carcinoma (BCC), Actinic Keratoses (AK), squamous cell carcinoma (SCC), and melanoma.

Actinic Keratoses

Actinic keratoses (AKs) are skin lesions that result from sun exposure. They are themselves benign but are considered premalignant due to the roughly 8 percent chance of transformation into SCC. They typically manifest as irregular, scaly plaques or papules in areas of sun exposure, such as the face, scalp, arms, and hands. Risk factors include male sex, older age, immunosuppression, occupations such as farming or construction, or outdoor sports such as golf, tennis, or baseball. Depending on the lesion, treatment options include surveillance, medications such as 5-fluorouracil and imiquimod, cryotherapy, curettage, or surgical excision. Counsel patients on sunscreen use and the need for regular full-body skin examinations, especially if treatment is deferred.

Basal Cell Carcinoma

Basal cell carcinoma (BCC) is the most common skin cancer in America, though metastasis and death due to BCC is rare. Cumulative UV light exposure is the most significant risk factor; however, up to 20 percent of BCCs arise in areas without UV exposure. Presentation typically occurs about 20 years after UV damage, and sun exposure during childhood and adolescence poses a particularly high risk. Nodular BCC is the most common variant, but superficial, pigmented, and morphea-like BCC may also occur. Classic findings include a shiny papule or nodule with rolled borders, telangiectasias, and a pink or flesh-colored central hue. Biopsy via shave, punch, or excision is required for definitive diagnosis, and referral to dermatology is appropriate in most cases. Treatment typically involves surgical excision. Fortunately, the 5-year cure rate is over 95 percent. Patients must be educated on sunscreen use and absolute avoidance of tanning beds.

Squamous Cell Carcinoma

Squamous cell carcinoma (SCC) is the second most common skin malignancy behind basal cell carcinoma and shares many of the same risk factors. SCCs may arise from actinic keratoses or may occur at a site with no previous lesion. This cancer classically presents as a hyperpigmented papule or plaque with overlying scale and possible associated erythema or pruritus. Providers should refer these patients to dermatology for biopsy and excision; sentinel lymph node biopsy and/or computed tomography (CT) imaging may also be indicated for evaluation of lymph node metastasis. Surgical excision remains the first-line treatment for SCC, such as with Mohs micrographic surgery. As with any other cutaneous malignancy, sunscreen use, avoidance of tanning beds, and regular dermatology follow-up are crucial.

Melanoma

Melanoma represents the most dangerous form of skin cancer, with high risk of metastasis and subsequent mortality. Risk factors include UV damage from either sun exposure or tanning bed use, fair complexion, and family history. Any observed skin lesions should be assessed using the ABCDE mnemonic for asymmetry, border irregularity, color variation, diameter over 6 mm, and evolving. Concerning lesions warrant prompt dermatology evaluation as well as evaluation for metastases with CT, positron emission tomography (PET), and/or ultrasound. Primary tumors require surgical excision along with possible chemotherapy and radiation, depending on metastasis. Prognosis worsens with increased tumor depth and spread, with stage IV melanoma carrying a 5-year survival rate as low as 30 percent. Providers in all clinical specialties must educate patients on sunscreen use, absolute avoidance of tanning beds, and regular skin checks by both the patient and his or her provider.

HEENT Conditions

Many diagnoses can apply to the head, ears, eyes, nose, and throat (HEENT) system. These organs all work together to provide various sensory functions and are among the first organs to indicate illness.

Conjunctivitis

Conjunctivitis, more commonly known as pink eye, is a broad term used to describe inflammation or swelling of the corneal surface and inner eyelids. Conjunctivitis causes the eye to appear bright red or pink and irritated. Thick discharge is also associated with conjunctivitis, especially upon waking. If caused by bacteria or viruses, conjunctivitis is highly contagious and spreads quickly through direct contact. Allergies or reactions to contact lenses or other eye products can also cause conjunctivitis; these cases are not contagious. Most will clear up on their own, but cases resulting from bacteria often require topical antibiotics.

Rhinitis

Allergic rhinitis is a condition in which the mucous membranes inside the nose become irritated and swollen due to an airborne allergen. Common airborne allergens are pollen and pet dander. Patients will have symptoms such as nasal itching, sneezing, coughing, and headache. If not treated, allergic rhinitis can progress to a sinus infection, or sinusitis. Treatment is aimed at suppressing the allergic response with antihistamine medications.

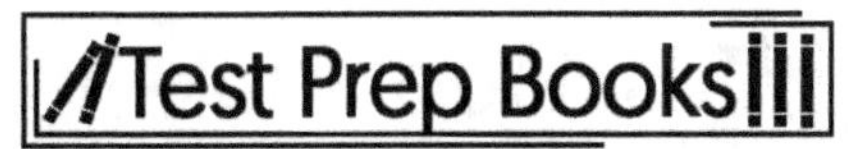

Pharyngitis

The throat is known as the oropharynx and includes the tonsils, which are part of the lymphatic system. One of the most common complaints in primary care is sore throat, or **pharyngitis**. Infections are usually the cause for inflammation of the oropharynx mucosa. The most common cause of bacterial pharyngitis is B-hemolytic streptococcus, or **group A streptococcus** (**GAS**). Prompt treatment of GAS is necessary to avoid complications, such as an abscess, rheumatic fever, or glomerulonephritis. Fever is a key symptom in patients with GAS. Practitioners should inspect the oral cavity for any exudate, lesions, or enlarged papillae. The tonsils, if present, should be observed and graded accordingly. A grade of 4 on the tonsillar scale requires rapid attention because they can obstruct the airway. Yellow tonsillar exudate may be present in GAS. If GAS is suspected, a throat swab should be obtained and sent for analysis of streptococcal antigens. A throat culture will provide the gold standard for diagnosis. Exudate and crusting should be removed from lesions prior to swabbing.

Sinusitis

Sinusitis refers to infections of the membrane lining of the air passages around the nasal cavity. This is a fairly common condition that often presents after another respiratory illness, such as a cold, which causes the sinuses to become filled with mucus and fluid. If these fluids remain stagnant, they are susceptible to breeding bacteria in the space. Sinusitis events can last anywhere from one to two weeks and may require the use of antibiotics if the event is determined to be bacterial in origin. Untreated, however, bacteria and viruses in the sinus cavities can travel to the brain and cause serious repercussions.

Otitis

Otitis Externa

Ear wax, or cerumen, protects the ear canal from foreign bodies. Prolonged water exposure can decrease cerumen and cause irritation. This may lead to a condition known as swimmer's ear, or **otitis externa**. The practitioner should inspect the external ears for pain, lesions, or swelling in the opening of the ear canal. These may be indicative of a bacterial infection. Practitioners should also palpate the ears and pre-auricular lymph nodes. Tenderness may be felt when otitis is present.

Otitis Media

Otitis media is an infection of the middle ear that is most commonly seen in infants and toddlers but may occur at any age. The cause of infection may be bacterial, viral, or both. The most common bacterial causes are *Streptococcus pneumoniae*, *Haemophilus influenzae*, and *Moraxella catarrhalis*. Common viral pathogens include respiratory syncytial virus, coronavirus, influenza, and adenovirus. Risk factors for the development of otitis media include immunodeficiencies, anatomic abnormalities of the palate or inner ear, cochlear implants, vitamin A deficiency, allergies, GERD, and second-hand tobacco smoke exposure. Ear pain is often the first sign of otitis media, and the patient may also experience ear pressure, tinnitus, headache, and fever.

Antibiotics are often prescribed to treat the infection, especially in patients less than two years old. The first-line antibiotic treatment for patients who do not have a penicillin allergy is amoxicillin. For patients who are allergic to penicillin, azithromycin, clarithromycin, or cefdinir may be considered. In cases of chronic or recurring infections, a tympanocentesis may be used to collect middle ear fluid for culture and sensitivity testing. Patients who have experienced four or more ear infections within twelve months can be considered candidates for tympanostomy tubes according to the American Academy of Pediatrics guidelines.

Respiratory Conditions

The respiratory system consists of the airway, lungs, and respiratory muscles. The airway is composed of the pharynx, larynx, trachea, bronchi, and bronchioles. The lungs contain air-filled sacs called alveoli, and they are covered by a visceral layer of double-layered pleural membrane. The intercostal muscles are located between the ribs, and the diaphragm separates the thoracic cavity from the abdominal cavity.

On inspiration, the airway transports the outside air to the lungs, while the expired air carries the carbon dioxide that is removed by the lungs. The alveoli are the site of the exchange of carbon dioxide from the systemic circulation with the oxygen contained in the inspired air. The muscles help the thoracic cavity to expand and contract to allow for air exchange.

The respiratory rate in the infant gradually decreases from a normal of thirty to forty breaths per minute, until adolescence when it equals the normal adult rate of twelve to twenty breaths per minute. Pulmonary function declines after the age of sixty because the alveoli become larger and less efficient, and the respiratory muscles weaken.

Asthma

Pulmonary ventilation is the movement of air in and out of the lungs. The upper airways help facilitate air into the lower airways. Air travels through a series of bronchial tubes and ends in clusters known as alveoli. Gas exchange occurs within these clusters. If the bronchial tubes become narrow or obstructed, oxygen cannot fill the lungs. **Asthma** is a condition that causes inflammation of the airways due to an inhaled trigger. Environmental triggers activate the immune response, which in turn causes the inflammation of the airways. There are many risk factors that can lead to asthma. Family history of asthma increases the likelihood of developing the condition.

According to the American Lung Association, a person is three to six times more likely to develop asthma if one of their parents has the condition. The immune response is stimulated when a virus enters the body. Viruses that attack the lungs cause inflammation of the airways and produce more mucus in an attempt to trap foreign bodies. The accumulation of this mucus narrows the airways, making pulmonary ventilation difficult. Practitioners should ask patients about their smoking habits. Smokers have a higher probability of developing asthma. Cigarette smoke irritates the airways. Irritation leads to the activation of the immune response, and the airways become swollen. Other lung irritants include air pollution, dust, mold, chemical fumes, and pollen. Questions regarding the patient's living conditions, occupational hazards, and exposure to environmental factors should be addressed during a health history.

Patients with asthma will have exacerbations that cause them to have trouble breathing, wheezing, a cough, and tightness in the chest. Pulsus paradoxus, or a greater than ten-point fall in systolic BP while breathing in, is a sign of an asthmatic attack, along with tachycardia, tachypnea, and use of accessory muscles to breath. A diagnosis of asthma will be made based on the patient's clinical presentation, their history of symptoms, and pulmonary function tests. They will be treated with inhaled beta-2 agonists and inhaled corticosteroids, as well as monitoring and controlling their exposure to their asthmatic triggers or the substances in their environment that cause exacerbations.

Status Asthmaticus

Acute severe asthma attacks, also known as **status asthmaticus**, are repeated, back-to-back asthma attacks that are not responding to the usual treatment of bronchodilators. Status asthmaticus is an emergency that requires special medical treatment to resolve.

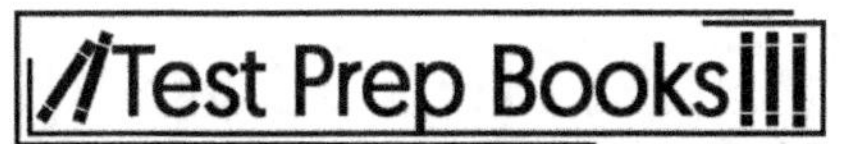

A patient experiencing a severe asthma attack that is unresponsive to bronchodilators may have chest tightness, severe shortness of breath, a dry cough, and wheezing. Their airway is undergoing bronchospasm, inflammation, and mucus plugging, all of which contribute to difficulty breathing. The patient's lungs may be retaining carbon dioxide, resulting in hypoxemia and respiratory failure.

Often a respiratory illness is the triggering factor in status asthmaticus, occurring a few days before the attack. This weakens the body's immune defenses, leading to exacerbation of asthma. Other triggers may include exposure to allergens or irritants in the environment with an especially potent effect.

In the emergency treatment of a patient with status asthmaticus, subcutaneous epinephrine may be used. Alternatively, terbutaline may be used, as it has fewer cardiac effects such as tachycardia. Albuterol that has been nebulized may be administered alongside nebulized ipratropium. Corticosteroids such as prednisone should be given to decrease the systemic inflammatory response. If a bacterial infection seems to be part of the patient's presentation, antibiotics may be used. Supplemental oxygen will be part of the patient's therapy as well.

If the patient is unresponsive to all the above treatments and respiratory function continues to decline, noninvasive positive pressure ventilation or mechanical ventilation will be considered to stabilize the patient, restore ventilation and oxygenation, and prevent further complications such as cardiac arrest.

Bronchitis

Bronchitis is inflammation of the bronchial tubes (bronchi), which extend from the trachea to the lungs. It is one of the top five reasons for visits to healthcare providers and can take between ten days and three weeks to resolve. Common causes of bronchitis include respiratory viruses (such as influenza A and B), RSV, parainfluenza, adenovirus, rhinovirus, and coronavirus. Bacterial causes include *Mycoplasma species, Streptococcus pneumoniae, Chlamydia pneumoniae, Haemophilus influenzae,* and *Moraxella catarrhalis.* Other causes of bronchitis are irritants such as chemicals, pollution, and tobacco smoke.

Signs and symptoms of bronchitis can include:

- Cough (most common symptom) with or without sputum
- Fever
- Sore throat
- Headache
- Nasal congestion
- Rhinorrhea
- Dyspnea
- Fatigue
- Myalgia
- Chest pain
- Wheezing

Bronchitis is typically diagnosed by exclusion, which means tests are used to exclude more serious conditions such as pneumonia, epiglottitis, or COPD. Useful diagnostic tests include a CBC with differential, a chest x-ray, respiratory and blood cultures, PFTs, bronchoscopy, laryngoscopy, and a procalcitonin (PCT) test to determine if the infection is bacterial.

Treatment of bronchitis is primarily supportive and can include:

- Bedrest
- Cough suppressants, such as codeine or dextromethorphan

- Beta-2 agonists, such as albuterol for wheezing
- Nonsteroidal anti-inflammatory drugs (NSAIDs) for pain
- Expectorants, such as guaifenesin

Although bronchitis should not be routinely treated with antibiotics, there are exceptions to this rule. It's reasonable to use an antibiotic when an existing medical condition poses a risk of serious complications. Antibiotic use is also reasonable for treating bronchitis in elderly patients who have been hospitalized in the past year, have been diagnosed with congestive heart failure (CHF) or diabetes, or are currently being treated with a steroid.

Upper Respiratory Infection (URI)

The treatment of **URIs** is a common occurrence in primary practice. The initial step involves the identification of the cause of the condition, which is most often viral, but may also be due to bacterial invasion or the result of an allergic reaction. URIs include the following conditions:

- Nasopharyngitis
- Pharyngitis
- Rhinosinusitis
- Epiglottitis
- Laryngotracheitis (croup)

Each of these conditions is caused by specific viruses, bacteria, and environmental agents; however, these conditions are most often caused by a limited number of viruses, which include the following:

- Rhinoviruses
- Coronaviruses
- Adenoviruses
- Coxsackieviruses

The infecting agents gain entrance to the body by direct contact or droplet infection. After the initial inoculation, there are physical, mechanical, and immune system barriers to the development of the conditions. For instance, the hairs lining the nose, the mucous covering all structures, the immune cells of the tonsils and adenoids, and the normal flora of the upper respiratory tract all function in different ways to decrease the progression of the disease. Pathogens that manage to overcome these defenses trigger the inflammatory response that is responsible for the manifestations associated with the individual conditions. When body tissues are injured, histamine, bradykinin, and prostaglandins are released, causing the capillaries to leak fluid into the wound. These chemicals also attract phagocytes that neutralize the infecting agents. The inflammatory response follows a precise sequence that first includes the identification of the harmful agents by the cell surface pattern receptors of the immune cells. The next step of the sequence is the activation of the inflammatory pathways, which is followed by the release of inflammatory markers and the stimulation of the release of the inflammatory cells.

Risk factors for the development of URIs include the following:

- Close contact with children in a group setting or within a family
- Inflammation from an additional source such as asthma
- Travel, due to the exposure to large groups of people
- Smoking and exposure to second-hand smoke, which damages the protective effects of mucous
- Immunocompromise from corticosteroid treatment, or due to stem cell or organ transplant
- Anatomic changes or trauma that alters the upper airways
- Carrier state—carriers of group A Streptococcus have frequent viral URIs

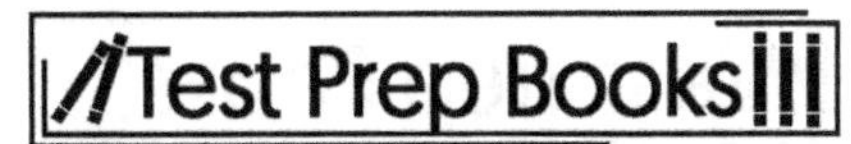

In most cases, URIs are mild and self-limiting; however, in susceptible populations such as infants and the elderly, additional complications can include epiglottitis and pneumonia, which are both life-threatening. The manifestations result from the inflammatory changes in the nasal mucosa and the remainder of the nasopharynx. The differential diagnosis is among the common cold, an allergic reaction, and influenza. The presence or absence of fever is one of the defining characteristics because it is rare with the common cold and the allergic response, but it is common with the influenza virus. General manifestations include rhinorrhea, dry cough, nasal congestion, watery eyes, possible headache and myalgias, and sore throat. The WHNP will assess the presenting manifestations, establish the diagnosis, and institute the appropriate therapy.

Cardiovascular Conditions

The cardiovascular system includes the heart, the blood vessels, and the blood. The heart is a muscle that has four "chambers," or sections. The three types of blood vessels are: the arteries, which have a smooth muscle layer and are controlled by the nervous system; the veins, which are thinner than arteries and have valves to facilitate the return of the blood to the heart; and the capillaries, which are often only one-cell thick. Blood is red in color because the red blood cells (RBCs) contain hemoglobin, which is a red pigment as well a protein that transports oxygen.

The deoxygenated blood from the body enters the heart and is transported to the lungs to allow the exchange of waste products for oxygen. The oxygenated blood then returns to the heart, which pumps the blood to the rest of the body. The arteries carry oxygenated blood from the heart to the body; the veins return the deoxygenated blood to the heart, while the actual exchange of oxygen and waste products takes place in the capillaries.

The fetal cardiac system must undergo dramatic changes at birth as the infant's lungs function for the first time. Cardiovascular function remains stable until middle age, when genetic influences and lifestyle choices may affect the cardiovascular system. Most elderly people have at least some indication of decreasing efficiency of the system.

Hypertension

Hypertension (**HTN**) is an abnormally high BP (140/90 mmHg or higher). The diagnosis is based on two or more accurate readings that are elevated. Essential, or primary, HTN, which is the most common form of the disease, is defined as elevated blood pressure that has no other identifiable cause such as renal disease. Secondary HTN that is due to other conditions is less common but is more difficult to treat successfully. Multiple factors—including genetic history; patients' sodium intake, which increases water reabsorption and increases cardiac output; and adrenergic balance—may be responsible for the development of essential HTN. Although the mechanism associated with any possible genetic link has not yet been identified, an estimated 30 to 50 percent of all cases of HTN are due to inherited variants. The role of the renin-angiotensin-aldosterone system in the pathogenesis of HTN has been widely studied, and medications have been developed to counter the effects of this process; however, these treatments have not prevented nor controlled HTN in every patient. There is also a cohort of patients that experience progressive disease even with treatment that includes all available therapies.

Other researchers believe that there is an immune component involved as well. In this model, oxidation of lipids, sympathetic nervous system activation, and noradrenergic stimuli are thought to activate the T-cells, which then infiltrate target organs such as the kidney and the vasculature, resulting in severe HTN. Additional research is aimed at identifying the role of epigenomic regulation, which includes a series of cellular mechanisms that alter the activity of genes without causing alterations in the DNA sequence. There is growing evidence that two of these processes—DNA methylation and histone modification—can contribute to the development of HTN due to changes in the walls of the vasculature. The purpose of this research is to develop novel therapies to treat the large majority of patients with HTN that progress to target organ disease. The result of all of these influences is changes in the arteries that prompt systemic vasoconstrictive stimulation in addition to changes in the function of the endothelium that are responsible for the vascular resistance and the thickening of the vascular wall that increases the systolic blood pressure.

In addition to persistent elevations in diastolic and systolic blood pressure, the manifestations associated with this slowly progressive process can include alterations in kidney function, retinopathy, left ventricular hypertrophy leading to stroke and heart failure, peripheral arterial vascular disease, and aneurysms. Unfortunately, the disease is called the "silent killer" for good reason because the earliest manifestations of the disease are not evident to the patient even though the target organs are being damaged. This means that the opportunity for early intervention may be lost. If the patient is already experiencing visual alterations or headaches prior to being evaluated for the presence of HTN, the patient has already sustained organ damage, which also can affect the effectiveness of the treatment plan. WHNPs should understand that prevention is the key to treating HTN.

Variables

Blood pressure (BP) is the product of cardiac output (CO) multiplied by systemic vascular resistance (SVR); *BP = CO × SVR*. CO is the volume of blood being pumped by the heart in one minute. It is the product of HR multiplied by SV; *HR × SV = CO*. SV is the amount of blood pumped out of the ventricles per beat.

SVR is related to the diameter of blood vessels and the viscosity of blood. The narrower the vessels or the thicker the blood, the higher the SVR. Conversely, larger-diameter vessels and thinner blood decrease SVR.

Mechanism

For HTN to develop, there must be a change in one or more factors affecting SVR or CO and a problem with the control system responsible for regulating BP. The body normally maintains and adjusts BP by either increasing the HR or the strength of myocardial contraction or by dilating or constricting the veins and arterioles.

When veins are dilated, less blood returns to the heart, and subsequently, less blood is pumped out of the heart. The result is a decrease in CO. Conversely, when veins are constricted, more blood is returned to the heart, and CO is increased. The arterioles also dilate or constrict. An expanded arteriole reduces resistance, and a constricted arteriole increases resistance. The veins and arterioles impact both CO and SVR. The kidneys contribute to the maintenance and adjustment of BP by controlling Na^+, chloride, and water excretion and through the RAAS. Management of HTN will focus on one or more of the factors that regulate BP. Those regulatory factors are SVR, fluid volume, and the strength and rate of myocardial contraction.

Classification

HTN is classified as primary or secondary depending on the etiology. In primary HTN, the cause is unknown, but the key factors include problems related to the natriuretic hormones, RAAS, or electrolyte disturbances. Primary HTN is also known as essential or idiopathic HTN.

In secondary HTN, there is an identifiable cause. Associated disease states include kidney disease, adrenal gland tumors, thyroid disease, congenital blood vessel disorders, alcohol abuse, and obstructive sleep apnea. Products associated with secondary HTN are nonsteroidal anti-inflammatory drugs (NSAIDs), birth control pills, decongestants, cocaine, amphetamines, and corticosteroids.

HTN normally increases with age, and it is more prominent among African Americans.

BP is classified according to treatment guidelines as normal, elevated blood pressure (prehypertension), Stage 1 HTN, and Stage 2 HTN. Normal blood pressure is a systolic reading of <120 mmHg AND diastolic reading of <80 mmHg. Elevated blood pressure (referred to as prehypertension) is defined as a systolic reading ranging from 120 to 129 mmHg AND a diastolic reading maintaining <80 mmHg. Stage 1 HTN includes either a systolic reading ranging from 130 to 139 mmHg OR a diastolic reading ranging from 80 to 89 mmHg. In the more severe Stage 2 HTN, the systolic reading is 140 mmHg or higher OR the diastolic reading is 90 mmHg or higher.

Sequelae

Systolic pressure is the amount of pressure exerted on arterial walls immediately after ventricular contraction and emptying. This represents the highest level of pressure during the cardiac cycle. Diastolic pressure is the amount of pressure exerted on arterial walls when the heart is filling. This represents the lowest pressure during the cardiac cycle. In general, hypertension increases the risk of cardiovascular disease; however, diastolic hypertension specifically poses the greatest risk.

Prolonged HTN damages the delicate endothelial layer of vessels. The damaged endothelium initiates the inflammatory response and clotting cascade. As mentioned, the diameter of veins, arterioles, and arteries changes SVR. When SVR is increased, the heart must work harder to pump against the increased pressure. In other words, the pressure in the LV must be higher than the pressure being exerted on the opposite side of the aortic valve by systemic vascular pressure. The ventricular pressure must overcome the aortic pressure for contraction and ventricular emptying to occur. When the myocardium works against an elevated systemic pressure for a prolonged period of time, the LV will enlarge, and HF may ensue.

Risk Factors

There are both modifiable and nonmodifiable risk factors associated with the development of HTN. Modifiable risk factors include obesity, a sedentary lifestyle, tobacco use, a diet high in sodium, dyslipidemia, excessive alcohol consumption, stress, sleep apnea, and diabetes. Age, race, and family history are nonmodifiable risk factors.

Treatment

First-line treatments include lifestyle changes and pharmacologic therapy.

Initial therapy includes diuretics, CCBs, ACE inhibitors, and ARBs. Diuretics decrease fluid volume, while CCBs decrease myocardial contractility. Both ACE inhibitors and ARBs interfere with the RAAS by preventing the normal mechanism that retains fluids and narrows blood vessels. The result is decreased volume and SVR.

Summary

The astute WHNP will conduct an in-depth patient interview to identify prescribed and illicit drug use, alcohol and tobacco use, family history, sleep patterns, and dietary habits. Patient education should include information about the Dietary Approach to Stop Hypertension (DASH) diet and alcohol in moderation with a limit of one to two drinks per day. Aerobic exercise and resistance training three to four times weekly for an average of 40 minutes is recommended. Information about prescribed hypertensive medications should also be reviewed with the patient.

Hypertensive Crisis

A **hypertensive crisis** is defined as a BP higher than 180/120 mmHg. BP must be lowered quickly to prevent end organ damage. Pregnancy, an acute MI, a dissecting aortic aneurysm, and an intracranial hemorrhage are associated with a hypertensive crisis. The therapeutic goal is to reduce the BP by 25 percent within the first hour of treatment, with a continual reduction over the following 2 to 6 hours and an ongoing reduction to the target goal over a period of days. Short-acting antihypertensive medications administered intravenously is the primary treatment.

Thromboembolic Disease

In the simplest terms, a **thrombus** is a blood clot that forms in a vein. Clots can be caused by either a fat globule, gas bubble, amniotic fluid, or any foreign material that gets into the bloodstream. A DVT usually forms in the leg. A thrombus becomes an embolus when a fragment dislodges and travels through the circulatory system. The embolus will remain in the circulatory system until it reaches a vessel too narrow for its passage. An embolism occurs when the embolus lodges and prevents blood flow. In the cardiac cycle, veins begin at the capillary bed and get progressively larger as they return deoxygenated blood to the right side of the heart. From the right side of the heart, blood flows to the lungs.

A pulmonary embolism (PE) occurs when the embolus, or a fragment of the embolus, becomes lodged in the pulmonary circulation. A DVT frequently results in a PE. A fat embolism may form when fat globules pass into the small vessels and damage the endothelial lining. As the fat breaks down to free fatty acids, it causes toxic damage. When the damage occurs in the lungs, acute respiratory failure ensues.

Mechanism

A strong clinical link exists between clot formation and atherosclerosis, PAD, diabetes, and other factors contributing to heart disease. Anything that damages a vein's endothelial lining may cause a DVT to form. Damage to vessel lining can occur from smoking, cancer, chemotherapy, injury, or surgery. In addition to a damaged endothelial layer, increased age, dehydration, and viscous or slow-flowing blood increase the risk of DVT formation. Factors that slow blood flow are prolonged bed rest, sitting for extended periods, smoking, obesity, and HF. In the presence of atrial fibrillation, the atria do not empty adequately. Blood pools in the upper chambers, increasing the risk for clots to form.

Closed long-bone fractures carry a high risk for a fat embolism to develop because when the bone marrow is exposed as a result of a fracture, its particles can enter the bloodstream. Orthopedic procedures, a bone marrow biopsy, massive soft tissue injury, and severe burns are also associated with the development of an embolus. In addition, there are nontraumatic conditions associated with a fat embolism, such as prolonged corticosteroid therapy, pancreatitis, liposuction, fatty liver, and osteomyelitis.

Women who are pregnant or taking oral contraceptives are at risk for the development of an embolus. Estrogen increases plasma fibrinogen, some coagulation factors, and platelet formation, which lead to the hypercoagulability of the blood. During pregnancy, the expanding uterus can slow blood flow in the veins. The combined effects of hypercoagulability and slowed blood flow exacerbate the risk. During delivery, an embolus can form from the amniotic fluid and travel through maternal circulation. Therefore, during pregnancy and the subsequent postpartum period, women are at increased risk for DVT formation.

Symptoms

Swelling of the leg below the knee is a common symptom of a DVT. There may also be redness, tenderness, or pain over the area around the clot, but a DVT may be asymptomatic. When a DVT becomes a PE, the patient may experience difficulty breathing and a rapid HR. Reported symptoms may include chest pain, coughing up blood, fainting, and low BP. There is a 24- to 72-hour latent period from injury to onset in the development of a fat embolism.

Diagnosis and Treatment

The clinician will consider presenting signs and symptoms, the patient's and family's medical history, and an ultrasound to evaluate blood flow to identify a DVT. The differential diagnoses are pneumonia and a thrombus. A vena cava filter may be placed in the inferior vena cava to capture a clot or fragments. In life-

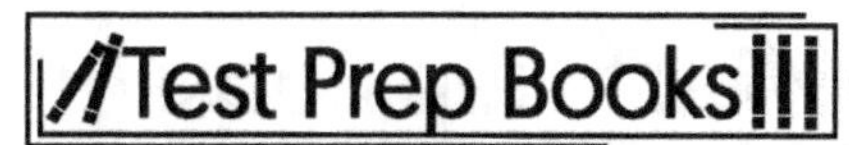

threatening situations such as a PE, an IV thrombolytic may be used to break up the clot. Indications for thrombolytic therapy are chest pain lasting longer than 20 minutes, ST elevation in two leads, and less than 6 hours from the pain's onset. However, thrombolytic medications are absolutely contraindicated in a patient with active bleeding. Prior to the administration of a thrombolytic, the international normalized ration (INR) must be calculated to determine clotting time. In healthy people, an INR of 1.1 or below is considered normal. An INR range of 2.0 to 3.0 is an effective acceptable therapeutic range for people taking warfarin.

For long-term management, patient education should include anticoagulant medication therapy, the use of compression stockings, and avoidance of tight clothing. Patients should be instructed to regularly elevate their feet, avoid prolonged periods of sitting, and increase their exercise to counteract slowed blood flow.

Hyperlipidemia

Lipid-lowering medications are used for the treatment of high blood lipids (**hyperlipidemia**), including high cholesterol (hypercholesterolemia) and high triglycerides (hypertriglyceridemia). Although a patient with hypercholesterolemia typically will not experience symptoms, the condition leads to the accumulation of fatty deposits in the blood vessels and liver, called atherosclerotic plaques. As time progresses, the deposits slow, impede, or block the flow of blood through the vessels. When blood flow is compromised to the heart muscle, ischemic heart disease can result. If the blood flow to the brain decreases, there is a possibility of ischemic stroke. Compromised blood supply in peripheral tissues and limbs can cause the development of peripheral vascular diseases (PVD). Lifestyle changes, such as a healthy diet and regular exercise, can significantly reduce the risk of hypercholesterolemia, even in the presence of predisposing genetic risk factors. Total cholesterol is determined from two components: high-density lipoproteins (HDL) cholesterol, considered the "good" cholesterol, and low-density lipoproteins (LDL) cholesterol, considered the "bad" cholesterol. Although it is helpful to keep a lower total cholesterol level for health and reduced disease risk, it is more critical to keep the ratio of HDL to LDL elevated.

Examples of lipid-lowering agents include the following:

- Statins: pravastatin, simvastatin, atorvastatin, rosuvastatin
- Cholesterol absorptions inhibitors: ezetimibe, cholestyramine, colestipol
- Fibrates: Gemfibrozil, fenofibrate

Gastrointestinal Conditions

The gastrointestinal system includes the mouth, pharynx, esophagus, stomach, small intestine, large intestine, and sigmoid colon. The entire system forms a twenty-four-foot tube through which ingested food passes. Digestion begins in the mouth, where digestive enzymes are secreted in response to food intake. Food then passes through the esophagus to the stomach, which is a pouch-shaped organ that collects and holds food for a period of time. The small intestine begins at the distal end of the stomach. The lining of the small intestine contains many villi, which are small, hair-like projections that increase the absorption of nutrients from the ingested food. The large intestine originates at the distal end of the small intestine and terminates in the rectum. The large intestine is four feet long and has three segments, including the ascending colon along the right side, the transverse colon from right to left across the body, and the descending colon down the left side of the body, where the sigmoid colon begins.

The enzymes of the mouth, stomach, and the proximal end of the small intestine break down the ingested food into nutrients that can be absorbed and used by the body. The nutrients are absorbed by the small intestine. The large intestine removes the water from the waste products, which forms the stool. The muscle layer of the large intestine is responsible for peristalsis, which is the force that moves the waste products through the intestine.

The function of the digestive system declines more slowly than other body systems, and the changes that most often occur are the result of lifestyle issues or medication use.

Upper GI Disorders

Gastroesophageal Reflux Disorder (GERD)

In **gastrointestinal reflux disorder** (**GERD**), the lower esophageal sphincter does not close properly, which causes the contents of the stomach to back up into the esophagus. This leads to irritation, which is why the common symptoms of GERD include heartburn, coughing, nausea, difficulty swallowing, and a strained voice. There are many factors that can cause or exacerbate GERD including obesity, pregnancy, eating a large meal, acidic foods, a hiatal hernia, and smoking. Lifestyle modifications such as avoiding trigger foods, losing weight (if obesity is a component), decreasing meal size, and trying not to lie down immediately after eating, can reduce symptoms. Gastric acid neutralizers/suppressants either neutralize stomach acid or decrease acid production, and therefore, can also be used to provide relief of symptoms associated with hyperacidity.

Peptic Ulcer Disease

Ulcers of the GI tract are categorized as to the anatomical site of injury. **Gastric ulcers** are located in the body of the stomach, and **peptic ulcers** are located in the duodenum. The presenting symptom is abdominal pain 2 to 4 hours after eating for duodenal ulcers, in addition to hematemesis and melena. The defect is due to erosion of the mucosal lining by infectious agents, most commonly *H. pylori;* extreme systemic stress such as burns or head trauma; ETOH abuse; chronic kidney and respiratory disease; and psychological stress. If left untreated, the mucosal erosion can progress to perforation, hemorrhage, and peritonitis.

Laboratory studies include examination of endoscopic tissue samples for the presence of the *H. pylori* organism, urea breath test, CBC, stool samples, and metabolic panel. Endoscopy, which is used to obtain tissue samples and achieve hemostasis, and double barium imaging studies made be obtained. The treatment depends on the extent of the erosion and will be focused on healing the ulcerated tissue and preventing additional damage. The treatment protocol for *H. pylori* infection includes the use of a PPI, amoxicillin, and clarithromycin for a minimum of 7 to 14 days. Subsequent testing will be necessary to ensure that the organism has been eradicated. Patients infected with *H. pylori* also must discontinue the use of NSAIDs or continue the long-term use of PPIs. Surgery may be indicated for significant areas of hemorrhage that were not successfully treated by ultrasound, and the procedure will be specific to the anatomical area of ulceration.

Cholecystitis

Cholecystitis is defined as an inflammation of the gallbladder. It is most often due to blockage of the cystic duct by gallstones. The condition may be complicated by the presence of perforation or gangrene of the gallbladder. Common risk factors include increasing age, female gender, obesity or rapid weight loss, and pregnancy. Symptoms include colicky epigastric pain that radiates to the right upper quadrant that may become constant, a palpable gallbladder, jaundice, nausea, vomiting, and fever. Providers understand that the elderly and chronically ill children may present with atypical manifestations of cholecystitis. Presenting symptoms in elderly patients may be limited to vague complaints of localized tenderness; however, the condition can rapidly progress to a more complicated form of cholecystitis due to infection, leading to gangrene or perforation of the gallbladder. This risk is increased in elderly patients with diabetes. Children with sickle cell disease, congenital biliary defects, or chronic illness requiring total parenteral nutrition (TPN) therapy may present with generalized abdominal pain and jaundice.

Diagnostic studies include routine lab tests, liver function tests, and abdominal ultrasounds. Additional imaging studies may be required; however, ultrasound is very sensitive for cholecystitis, does not expose the patient to radiation, and is readily available in hospitals. Treatment options depend on the severity of symptoms. Acalculous cholecystitis may progress quickly to perforation and gangrene of the gallbladder

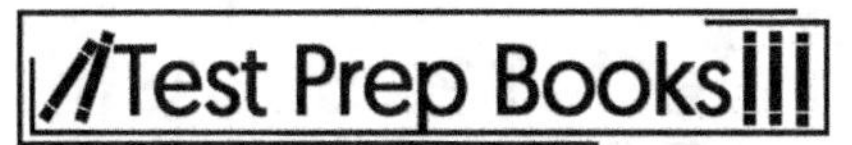

requiring emergency intervention, while uncomplicated cases of acute cholecystitis can be treated with bowel rest, intravenous (IV) fluids, and short-term antibiotic therapy. Providers understand that elective laparoscopic cholecystectomy is the procedure of choice, with the rate of conversion to open cholecystectomy at 5 percent; however, emergency laparoscopic cholecystectomy is associated with a 30 percent conversion rate.

Early recognition and intervention are required due to the rapid progression of acute acalculous cholecystitis to gangrene and perforation.

Upper GI Bleeding

Gastrointestinal (GI) bleeding is defined according to the area of the defect. **Upper GI bleeding** occurs superiorly to the junction of the duodenum and jejunum. **Lower GI bleeding** occurs in the large and small intestine. Conditions associated with an upper GI bleed include esophageal varices, gastric and duodenal ulcers, cancer, and Mallory-Weiss tears. Risk factors include age, history of gastroesophageal reflux disorder (GERD), use of nonsteroidal anti-inflammatory drugs (NSAIDs) and steroids, and alcoholism. Acute presenting manifestations include hematemesis, melena, hematochezia, and lightheadedness or fainting. The diagnosis is made by the patient's history and physical examination, routine lab studies including complete blood count (CBC) and coagulation tests, endoscopy, and chest films. Treatment is specific to the cause; for example, peptic ulcer disease will be treated with the appropriate antibiotic and a proton-pump inhibitor (PPI).

Lower GI Disorders

Constipation

When stool does not get properly eliminated or is hard to pass, patients will present with **constipation**. Constipation is a common symptom that can have many etiologies. The provider should establish the patient's bowel habits, asking about frequency and characteristics of stool. Constipation is defined as passing fewer than three stools per week or having difficulty passing stool. Patients should be asked about changes from baseline and their definition of constipation. Questions about diet preferences can be a factor in diagnosing constipation. Acute constipation is a sudden change from the patient's normal bowel habits. Persistent constipation can last weeks and increases in frequency. Chronic constipation is a long-term dysfunction in bowel elimination.

Providers should assess for presence of bowel sounds and passing of gas; inspect the abdomen for symmetry, distention, bulges, or visible peristalsis; and inquire about abdominal fullness or bloating, accompanying nausea or vomiting, use of laxatives, and current diet. Interventions focus on optimization of laxatives and stool softeners, as well as counseling to increase dietary fiber, oral fluids, and activity.

Hemorrhoids

Hemorrhoids are swollen veins in the rectum or anus, often caused by increased pressure from straining during bowel movements, prolonged sitting, pregnancy, or obesity. Common signs and symptoms include pain, swelling, itching, and bleeding during bowel movements. Diagnosis typically involves a physical examination, and healthcare providers may use procedures such as anoscopy for a more detailed assessment. A complete blood count to assess for anemia may be necessary in patients who also complaint of lethargy as blood loss from hemorrhoids can be significant over time. Treatment ranges from conservative measures to surgical options. Initial management often includes lifestyle changes such as increasing fiber intake, drinking more water, and avoiding straining during bowel movements. Over-the-counter topical treatments and warm baths can be used to alleviate symptoms. In more severe cases, procedures like rubber band ligation, sclerotherapy, and hemorrhoidectomy may be recommended.

Irritable Bowel Syndrome (IBS)

Irritable Bowel Syndrome (IBS) is a common gastrointestinal disorder characterized by abdominal pain and altered bowel habits. Etiology of the condition is often unknown, but contributing factors include disconnection in the gut-brain axis, altered gastrointestinal motility, and increased sensitivity to gastrointestinal stimuli. Signs and symptoms vary but commonly include abdominal pain, bloating, gas, and diarrhea or constipation (sometimes alternating between the two). The condition may be triggered by stress or by certain foods. Commonly reported foods that may elicit or worsen symptoms are gluten-containing foods, dairy, citrus fruits, cabbage, legumes, and carbonated beverages. Patients should be educated to keep a food diary to try to identify contributing dietary causes. Diagnosis of IBS typically involves a thorough medical history, physical examination, and ruling out other conditions through tests like blood work or colonoscopy. The gold standard for diagnosis is to evaluate clinical symptoms using the Rome IV diagnostic criteria.

Treatment focuses on symptom management through dietary changes (e.g., low-FODMAP diet), medications (e.g., antispasmodics, laxatives, or antidiarrheal agents), and lifestyle modifications (e.g., stress management, regular exercise). In some cases, therapies such as cognitive behavioral therapy (CBT) may be beneficial.

Lower GI Bleeding

Gastrointestinal (GI) bleeding is defined according to the area of the defect. Lower GI bleeding occurs in the large and small intestine. Causative factors for a lower GI bleed include anatomical defects such as diverticulosis, ischemic events of the vasculature related to radiation therapy or other embolic events, cancer, and infectious or noninfectious inflammatory conditions. Manifestations that are specific to the cause and location of the hemorrhage include melena, maroon stools or bright red blood, fever, dehydration, possible abdominal pain or distention, and hematochezia. Common diagnostic studies include routine lab studies, endoscopy, radionucleotide studies, and angiography. Treatment is focused on the identification and resolution of the source of the bleeding and correction of any hematologic deficits that resulted from the hemorrhage.

Genitourinary Conditions

The urinary system includes the kidneys, ureters, bladder, and urethra. The kidneys are a pair of bean-shaped organs that lie in the peritoneal cavity just below and toward the rear of the liver. The nephron is the functional unit of the kidney, and there are about 1 million nephrons in each of the two kidneys. The ureters are hollow tubes that allow the urine formed in the kidneys to pass into the bladder. The urinary bladder is a hollow mucous lined pouch with the ureters entering the upper portion, and the urethra exiting from the bottom portion. The urethra is a tubular structure lined with mucous membrane that connects the bladder with the outside of the body.

In addition to the formation and excretion of the waste product urine, the nephron of the kidney also regulates fluid and electrolyte balance and contributes to the control of blood pressure. The ureters allow the urine to pass from the kidneys to the bladder. The bladder stores the urine and regulates the process of urination. The urethra delivers the urine from the bladder to the outside of the body.

The lifespan changes in the urinary system are more often the result of the effects of chronic disease on the system, rather than normal decline.

Urinary Tract Infection (UTI)

Urinary tract infections or **UTIs** can be divided into two categories: lower and upper. Upper UTIs affect the kidneys and can be called pyelonephritis. Lower UTIs affect the bladder, urethra, or prostate and can be

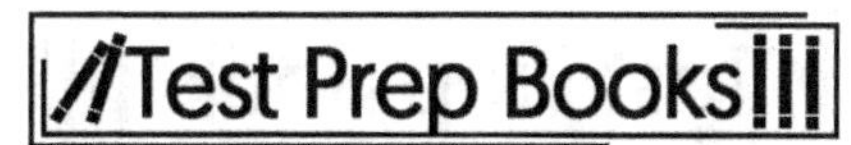

called cystitis, urethritis, or prostatitis. Differentiating between the specific types of UTIs in clinical practice can be difficult to do and thus the broad term of UTI usually refers to an infection of the kidneys or bladder.

There are many causative organisms involved in UTIs, but the most commonly seen UTIs are caused by a bacterial infection. Fungal infections, usually arising from the candida species, are also a possibility, as well as parasites and viruses.

An infection that affects the urethra specifically, called urethritis, is likely a result of a sexually transmitted disease (STD).

A urinary tract infection that was caught as a result of a urinary catheter insertion is called a **catheter-associated urinary tract infection** (**CAUTI**). The provider must take special care to use proper aseptic technique when inserting a catheter, remove catheters as soon as they are no longer needed, and follow facility procedure when deciding if a patient actually needs a catheter in the first place. Many patients have catheters that may not need them, setting them up for a hospital-acquired infection.

Patients who have contracted a UTI may be asymptomatic for some time before the UTI is detected. When they are symptomatic, they may present with a fever, altered mental status, hypotension, dysuria, and lower abdominal pain.

Urine will be cultured and, in the case of patients with indwelling catheters, the catheter tip will be cultured as well to obtain diagnosis of UTI. Antibiotic therapy is common in the treatment of UTI, depending on the cause.

Cystitis

Cystitis is inflammation of the bladder that is often caused by a bacterial infection. Cystitis can also refer to irritation of the bladder from other causes, such as radiation therapy, hygiene products, or long-term catheter use. It presents with symptoms of a urinary tract infection, including a painful or burning sensation with urination, frequent urge to urinate, foul-smelling and cloudy urine, pelvic discomfort, fever, and hematuria. Women, especially post-menopausal women, tend to be more commonly impacted. Other risk factors include being sexually active, use of a diaphragm, pregnancy, being immunocompromised, long-term catheter use, and urinary outlet dysfunction. Cystitis caused by a bacterial infection should be treated with antibiotics. Non-infectious causes should be treated with supportive measures, including encouraging fluid intake, urinating often and as soon as possible after sex, wiping front to back, favoring showers over baths, and avoiding irritating products such as deodorant in the genital area.

Urethritis

Fungal infections, usually arising from the candida species, parasites, and viruses can also cause UTIs. An infection that affects the urethra specifically, called **urethritis**, is likely a result of a sexually transmitted disease (STD).

Pyelonephritis

Urinary tract infections (UTIs) are the result of bacteria that are introduced into the urethra and infect the bladder. UTIs that are not treated promptly may ascend through the urinary tract. Infection that reaches the kidneys is termed **pyelonephritis**. Patients with pyelonephritis may exhibit fever and blood in the urine. Women are more at risk for UTIs due to the short length of the internal urethra. In the older adult population, an atypical sign may be confusion. Providers should assess for costovertebral angle tenderness by indirectly percussing the lower back. Pain or tenderness when the area is struck may be a sign of a kidney infection. Non-pharmacological management includes increasing fluid intake, while pharmacological treatment includes antibiotics. Diagnostic studies include a urinalysis to check for the presence of WBCs and nitrites. A culture and sensitivity test should be performed to determine the type of bacteria for proper antibiotic selection.

Renal Stones

Nephrolithiasis is defined as the process of stone or calculi formation in the pelvis of the kidney. The pain associated with this condition is referred to as renal colic and most often reflects the stretching and distention of the ureter when the stone leaves the kidney. The most common cause is insufficient fluid intake that concentrates stone-forming substances in the kidney. In order of occurrence, calculi are composed of calcium (75 percent) due to increased absorption of calcium by the GI tract, struvite (15 percent) as a result of repeated UTIs, uric acid (6 percent) due to increased purine intact, and cysteine (1 percent) due to an intrinsic metabolic defect in susceptible individuals. In addition, AIDS medications, some antacids, and sulfa drugs are also associated with stone formation. Renal calculi are more common in men than women, are associated with obesity and insulin resistance, and have a familial tendency.

Diagnosis is based on the patient's history and physical examination. Common lab studies include CBC, coagulation studies, kidney function tests, and C-reactive protein. Imaging studies may include ultrasonography, KUB films, and CT scans. Treatment options are based on the likelihood that the stone will be expelled spontaneously from the urinary system, given the size and location of the stone. Common interventions include aggressive fluid management, antimicrobial therapy, and pain management. If necessary, to prevent mechanical damage to the organs or the progression of the condition to urosepsis, the stone may be surgically removed, or the patient may undergo extracorporeal shock wave lithotripsy. Care is focused on preventing damage to the urinary tract, restoring fluid volume, managing pain, and preventing progression of the illness to systemic urosepsis. Patient education regarding the essential follow-up care is critical to the prevention of recurrent calculi formation.

Urinary Incontinence

The inability of the body to control voluntary sphincters is known as incontinence. One form of incontinence is the inability to control urine excretion, or **urinary incontinence**. An acute form of incontinence is known as transient incontinence, which lasts 6 months or less. Intra-abdominal pressure causes another form of urinary incontinence known as stress incontinence. Overflow incontinence occurs when the bladder is filled and can no longer hold urine. Functional incontinence is the lack of proper toileting. Reflex incontinence occurs when the body cannot feel the release of urine. Total incontinence happens when the urine loss is continuous and the patient does not have the ability to stop its flow.

Mixed incontinence occurs when a patient experiences one or more types of incontinence. Many factors can contribute to urinary incontinence. Some are medically induced, others are due to illness or an acute change in health status, and some are psychologically driven. Patients who are dehydrated may require intravenous fluids that increase fluid volume in the body. Diuretic medications that treat HTN are used to excrete excess fluid from the systemic circulation. This increases urine volume in the bladder. Activities that produce pressure in the intra-abdominal cavity, such as sneezing or coughing, can lead to stress incontinence. Obesity and pregnancy increase the weight that is pressed onto the bladder and can also lead to stress incontinence. The bladder empties when the stretch receptors along the bladder wall are activated by urine. The stretch receptors are controlled by the nervous system.

Patients who have spinal cord injuries or nerve damage do not have an intact nervous system, leading to overflow, or reflex incontinence. Patients who have conditions affecting orientation can have functional incontinence. Dementia, Alzheimer's, acute psychotic episodes, or confusion may lead to decreased toileting. Patients may not utilize the restroom appropriately and suffer incontinence in inappropriate places. Patients who suffer trauma or develop cancers in the pelvic area may have a urostomy. Artificial openings do not have sphincters. A urostomy does not provide control over urine excretion and is a form of total incontinence.

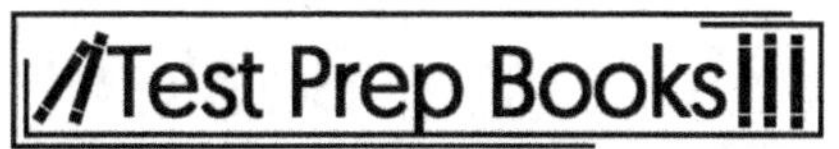

Musculoskeletal Conditions

The musculoskeletal system consists of the bones, muscles, tendons, ligaments, and connective tissues that function together, providing support and motion of the body. The layers of bone include the hard exterior compact bone, the spongy bone that contains nerves and blood vessels, and the central bone marrow. The outer compact layer is covered by the strong periosteum membrane, which provides additional strength and protection for the bone. Skeletal muscles are voluntary muscles that are capable of contracting in response to nervous stimulation. Muscles are connected to bones by tendons, which are composed of tough connective tissue. Additional connective tissues called ligaments connect one bone to another at various joints.

In addition to providing support and protection, the bones are important for calcium storage and the production of blood cells. Skeletal muscles allow movement by pulling on the bones, while joints make different body movements possible.

The two most significant periods of bone growth are during fetal life and at puberty. However, until old age, bone is continually being remodeled. Specialized cells called osteoclasts break down the old bone, and osteoblasts generate new bone. In the elderly, bone remodeling is less effective, resulting in the loss of bone mass, and the incidence of osteoporosis increases. These changes can result in bone fractures, often from falling, that do not heal effectively. Muscle development follows a similar pattern with a progressive increase in muscle mass from infancy to adulthood, as well as a decline in muscle mass and physical strength in the elderly.

Back Pain

Ankylosing Spondylitis

Ankylosing spondylitis is a type of inflammatory arthritis that directly affects the vertebral column of the spine by causing discs to fuse. This compromises the structural integrity of the spine and results in kyphosis, a spinal curve that causes the patient to stoop over. Ankylosing spondylitis is characterized by slow onset lower back and hip pain and blurry vision. Severe cases can affect the ability of the ribcage to expand in order to allow full lung capacity, which can impair efficient and adequate respiration in patients. Inflammation of major cardiac arteries is also associated with ankylosing spondylitis. This condition is most commonly treated with immunosuppressant medications, tailored physical therapy, and non-steroidal anti-inflammatory drugs.

Herniated Disc Disease

Herniated disc disease, also called a slipped or ruptured disc, occurs when the nucleus pulposus (gel in the center of the disc) leaks through a weak area or tear in the annulus fibrosus (outer layer of the disc). This leads to the compression of neighboring nerves, causing numbness, weakness, and pain. Herniated discs are most commonly seen in the lumbar and cervical spine. Causative factors include degeneration of the discs through age, trauma, forceful injury, repetitive stress, or overuse. The patient's chief complaint is most often shooting pain that follows the distribution of the affected nerve (e.g., a patient with a lumbar herniated disc would experience sciatica). Other symptoms include numbness, weakness, a positive straight leg raise, and symptoms that worsen with sitting or bending and improve with laying down or walking.

Physical examination for diagnosis should include a thorough neurological exam, assessing for any motor weakness, sensory deficits, or abnormal reflexes (e.g., L5 radiculopathy with a weak foot dorsiflexion or decreased sensation to foot). The preferred imaging option for diagnosis is an MRI, as it is able to highlight the size, location, and severity of the herniation. Electromyography and nerve conduction studies may be helpful to assess the severity of nerve damage or for patients with persistent symptoms despite treatment.

For most patients, medical management will be conservative with rest and activity modification or reduction. NSAIDs can help to reduce pain and inflammation. Physical therapy may also be beneficial to strengthen the surrounding supportive muscles. Corticosteroids can be injected into the epidural space to reduce severe inflammation and/or pain. Muscle relaxers are beneficial to help reduce muscle spasms associated with herniated discs. Approximately ninety percent of patients see improvement within six to twelve weeks with conservative treatment measures. However, when these interventions are unsuccessful and symptoms persist, surgical intervention via a discectomy, laminectomy, or spinal fusion may be necessary.

Scoliosis

Scoliosis is a condition characterized by an abnormal lateral curvature of the spine of more than ten degrees. It is most often diagnosed in children or teens; however, the condition can present in adulthood, especially in cases where neuromuscular or degenerative disorders are present. Multiple causes of scoliosis exist, including idiopathic (which is the most common). Neuromuscular scoliosis is caused by weakened muscles due to neurological disorders like cerebral palsy and polio. Degenerative (adult-onset) scoliosis is caused by the degenerative spinal changes associated with age, leading to decreased structural integrity of the spine. Congenital scoliosis occurs during fetal development, during which vertebral anomalies like hemivertebrae occur. Other causes of scoliosis include infections (e.g., Pott's disease), tumors, and trauma (e.g., fractures).

Patients with scoliosis will present with an abnormal posture, including uneven shoulders, unilateral rib hump, and uneven hips; these deformities are most noticeable when the patient bends over (referred to as the Adam's test). Patients may also complain of back pain, numbness, tingling, and weakness in more severe cases. X-rays are the imaging option of choice to diagnose scoliosis, where the Cobb angle is used to determine the degree of the curvature (greater than ten degrees is abnormal, indicating scoliosis). An MRI may be used to assess for the presence of neurological damage and to rule out any spinal tumors or infections.

Medical management is conservative for mild cases and may only require observation. For teenagers with moderate scoliosis (Cobb angle of twenty-five to forty-five degrees), a brace, such as a Boston brace or thoracolumbosacral orthosis, may be used to prevent the spinal curvature from progressing. Physical therapy, including Schroth therapy, is also used to improve posture and muscle strength. NSAIDs are recommended for mild to moderate pain, while muscle relaxers are recommended for severe pain. For severe cases of scoliosis (Cobb angle of forty-five to fifty degrees), surgical intervention in the form of spinal fusion, vertebral osteotomy, or growing rods may be necessary. Routine follow up visits to monitor disease progression are recommended.

Spinal Stenosis

Spinal stenosis refers to the narrowing of the spinal canal, which most commonly occurs in the lumbar and cervical spine as a result of structural changes and places pressure on the spinal cord and/or nerves. There are three categories of change that contribute to spinal stenosis: degenerative, congenital, and acquired. Examples of degenerative changes include intervertebral disc degeneration, face joint arthritis, and/or ligamentum flavum hypertrophy. Congenital factors may not present with symptoms until later in life, when degenerative changes associated with age exacerbate the already restricted spinal area. Acquired factors include trauma (e.g., spinal fractures), spinal tumors, infection, and inflammation. The most common symptoms include pain in the affected region of spine, neurogenic claudication, and cervical myelopathy.

Physical assessment to confirm diagnosis should look for postural abnormalities, spinal tenderness, muscle atrophy, nerve root compression, positive straight leg raise test, and gait or balance troubles. MRI is the diagnostic imaging of choice to visualize the spinal cord, ligaments, and nerve roots as well as the degree of compression. An X-ray may also be used to assess any degenerative changes. Conservative medical management is initially used and includes NSAIDs for pain and inflammation reduction, muscle relaxants for

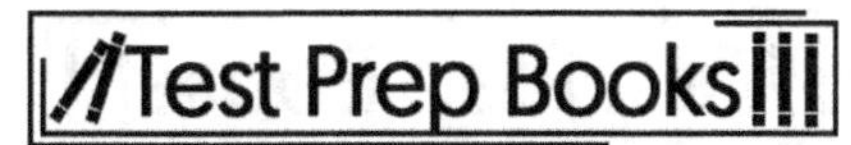

spasms contributing to pain, gabapentin or pregabalin for neuropathic pain, and epidural steroid injections to reduce inflammation around the nerves. Physical therapy is also recommended to strengthen back and abdominal muscles to support posture. A spinal brace or lumbar corset may also be used to provide stability and support. Activity modification and weight loss can reduce symptom exacerbations. If conservative interventions fail or neurological deficits are present, surgical intervention (e.g., decompressive laminectomy, spinal fusion, or microdiscectomy) may be necessary.

Osteoarthritis

Loss of cartilage and hypertrophy of bones leads to a condition known as **osteoarthritis**. There are two types of osteoarthritis. Idiopathic osteoarthritis is associated with an increase in age, wear and tear of the joints, and joints that are not aligned properly. Traumatic osteoarthritis results from mechanical stress, professional athletic activities, running, joint instability, inflammation in the joints, certain medications, and metabolic disorders. Patients who experience osteoarthritis may have pain at the joints that presents as a deep ache. Joint movement may increase the pain and can cause numbness to extremities. Joints may also be stiff, and patients may exhibit decreased range of motion to the affected joints.

In addition, joints may be visibly enlarged due to overgrowth of bone. Osteoarthritis is a non-inflammatory disease process. The bones become exposed due to loss of cartilage. Osteoarthritis is progressive and may begin at the age of forty. It is one of the leading disabilities and pain-inducing conditions in the elderly population. Risk factors include obesity, sedentary lifestyle, chronic gout, and coexisting rheumatoid arthritis. Providers will note stiffness to the joints, limited range of motion, pain, asymmetry in the joints, impaired gait, and visible deformities. X-rays, CT scans, MRIs, and bone density scans can all help diagnose osteoarthritis. Treatment is aimed at restoring function via physical therapy and resting the joints when not in use. Medications include pain relievers and nutritional supplements.

Sprains and Strains

A **sprain** occurs when a ligament is overstretched during events such as twisting or falling. Sprains are graded on a scale from I–III (mild to severe). A Grade I (mild) sprain is when the ligament fibers are stretched or minimally torn, with the ligament remaining intact and absence of joint instability. A Grade II (moderate) sprain is when there is a partial tear in the ligament, resulting in moderate symptoms and some loss of function. A Grade III (severe) sprain is when there is a complete ligament rupture with severe symptoms and total loss of function.

A **strain** occurs when a muscle and/or tendon is overstretched due to overuse or repetitive movements. Strains are also graded on a scale from I–III (mild to severe). With a Grade I (mild) strain, the muscle fibers are overstretched with minimal or no tearing, resulting in symptoms that are mild and strength that is almost normal. A Grade II (moderate) strain occurs when the muscle fibers are partially torn, causing some challenges in using the affected muscle. A Grade III (severe) strain is a completely ruptured muscle and/or tendon, leading to severe pain and swelling with a total loss of function.

Both sprains and strains present with localized pain and swelling, decreased mobility, and weakness. Tenderness will be present in the affected area. Ligament-specific tests, such as the anterior drawer test for the ACL or the Lachman test for the knee, may be used. Strains should be assessed for a rupture. An MRI is the diagnostic imaging option of choice to assess soft tissue injuries and identify the presence of any tearing or swelling. Acute medical management entails the RICE protocol: rest, ice, compression, and elevation. Pain can be managed with NSAIDs, muscle relaxers, and topical analgesics. Physical therapy is also recommended to improve strength and range of motion. For Grade III sprains that have not healed successfully with conservative interventions, surgical intervention (e.g., arthroscopic tendon repair) may be necessary. Patient education on sprain and strain prevention should also be provided, including insights on warming up effectively before exercise, benefits of muscle strengthening, and appropriate footwear to reduce the risk of injury.

Neurologic/Psychiatric Conditions

The two parts of the neurologic system are the central nervous system, which contains the brain and spinal cord, and the peripheral nervous system, which includes the ganglia and nerves. The cerebrospinal fluid and the bones of the cranium and the spine protect the brain and spinal cord. The nerves transmit impulses from one another to accomplish voluntary and involuntary processes. The nerves are surrounded by a specialized myelin sheath that insulates the nerves and facilitates the transmission of impulses.

The nervous system receives information from the body, interprets that information, and directs all motor activity for the body. This means the nervous system coordinates all the activities of the body.

The fetal brain and spinal cord are clearly visible within six weeks after conception. After the child is born, the nervous system continues to mature as the child gains motor control and learns about the environment. In the well-elderly, brain function remains stable until the age of eighty, when the processing of information and short-term memory may slow.

Headaches

Cluster Headaches

Cluster headaches are characterized by recurrent, unilateral headaches that usually affect one eye or one temple. They occur in "clusters" over a period of days, weeks, or months with a coinciding period of remission. There is no exact cause; however, hypothalamic dysfunction, trigeminal nerve activation, endorphin dysregulation, and genetic predisposition are all attributed to cluster headaches. Cluster headaches typically affect individuals between twenty and forty years of age, with smoking and alcohol consumption increasing risk.

Diagnosis for cluster headaches includes the following criteria: severe, unilateral temporal pain lasting fifteen minutes to three hours; headaches at least once every other day (up to eight per day); autonomic symptoms (e.g., lacrimation or rhinorrhea); restlessness or agitation during headaches; and cluster periods of attacks with a remission of at least one month. Acute medical management includes oxygen therapy, sumatriptan, and local anesthetic administration. Long-term and preventive management includes the use of verapamil and corticosteroids. Occipital nerve or sphenopalatine ganglion blocks may be used to provide pain relief. Patients should be educated on avoiding triggers and implementing proper sleep hygiene habits to help prevent attacks.

Migraines

Migraine headaches are often preceded by an aura, which may be visual or sensory. The pulsatile pain associated with migraine headaches is described as throbbing and constant and most often localizes to one side of the head. Other manifestations include photophobia, sound sensitivity, nausea and vomiting, and anorexia. The pain increases over a period of one to two hours and then may last from 4 to 72 hours. The exact cause of the migraine headache syndrome is not well understood; however, there is strong evidence of a genetic link and some support for the role of alterations in neurovascular function and neurotransmitter regulation. Risk factors include elevated C-reactive protein and homocysteine levels, increased levels of TNF-alpha and adhesion molecules (systemic inflammation markers), increased body weight, hypertension, impaired insulin sensitivity, and coronary artery disease. The diagnosis is determined by the patient's history, laboratory testing for inflammatory markers, and imaging studies and lumbar puncture, as indicated by the severity of the patient's condition.

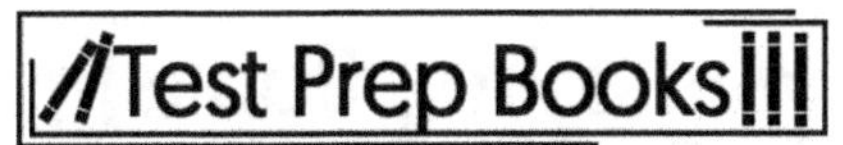

The treatment for migraine headaches may be preventive, therapeutic, and/or symptomatic. Medications used to prevent migraine headaches are used for those patients with chronic disease who have fourteen or more headaches per month. Antiemetics are used to lessen nausea and vomiting, while opioids may be prescribed even though their use in migraine management is not recommended. The care of the patient with a migraine headache is focused on establishing the differential diagnosis and correcting fluid volume alterations that may result from vomiting. Although most patients who seek care are diagnosed with migraine headaches, the importance of early intervention for temporal arteritis, stroke, or brain tumor requires a prompt diagnosis.

Tension Headaches

Tension headaches are the most common type of headache, characterized by bilateral, non-pulsating head pain and causing a tight band or pressure experience in the head. There is no exact cause; however, muscle tension, central sensitization, neuromuscular dysfunction, psychological stress, and genetic predisposition are linked to tension headaches. The most common triggers are stress and anxiety. Sleep disturbances, poor posture, prolonged repetitive neck muscle strain, and environmental factors (e.g., bright lights or loud noises) can also trigger a tension headache. Criteria for diagnosis includes mild to moderate bilateral, tightening/pressing, and non-pulsating pain lasting between thirty minutes and seven days; additional criteria include absence of symptom aggravation with physical activity and lack of associated nausea, vomiting, or aura. Tension headaches can either be episodic (occurring less than fifteen days per month) or chronic (occurring more than fifteen days per month for at least three months).

Medical management includes the use of acetaminophen and NSAIDs for pain relief, with tramadol or low-dose opioids for cases of severe pain. Muscle relaxers can help with muscle tension. Preventive treatment options include tricyclic antidepressants, selective serotonin reuptake inhibitors (SSRIs), anticonvulsants, or Botox. Biofeedback, cognitive behavioral therapy, physical therapy, and acupuncture can also be used to relieve pain and reduce the severity or frequency of headaches. Patients should be educated on the benefits of stress management, a regular sleep schedule, exercise, and proper posture.

Temporal Arteritis

Temporal arteritis, also known as giant cell arteritis, is an inflammatory disorder of unknown origin that manifests as inflammatory changes in the intima, media, and adventitia layers of the artery as well as scattered accumulations of lymphocytes and macrophages that result in ischemic changes distal to the damaged areas. The condition is more common in women over fifty years of age, and current research indicates that infection and genetics also may be related to the development of the disease. The onset may be acute or insidious, and common signs and symptoms include head pain, neck pain, jaw claudication (jaw pain caused by ischemia of the maxillary artery), visual disturbances, shoulder and pelvic girdle pain, and general malaise and fever. The condition is diagnosed by a patient history of the onset of the headaches or the change in the characteristics of the headache in patients with chronic headaches, elevated ESR, and temporal artery biopsy that confirms the diagnosis. The condition is immediately treated with steroids if possible, or alternatively with cyclosporine, azathioprine, or methotrexate.

The onset of ophthalmic alterations requires emergency care because any loss of vision before treatment is initiated will be irreversible. In addition, if treatment is delayed beyond two weeks after the onset of the initial vision loss, vision in the unaffected eye will be lost as well. Additional complications are related to steroid therapy and include stroke, myocardial infarction, small-bowel infarction, vertebral body fractures, and steroid psychoses. Even with successful treatment that prevents irreversible vision alterations, the patient with temporal arteritis has a lifelong risk of inflammatory disease of the large vessels.

Psychosocial/Mental Health Disorders

Screening Tools

There are a number of **mental health screening tools** that can assist a provider in developing a plan of care or referring patients to other specialties. The Generalized Anxiety Disorder 7-item (GAD-7) scale is a 7-question tool that aids in recognizing the severity of behaviors and thought processes. Similarly, the Patient Health Questionnaire-9 (PHQ-9) is a 9-question tool that explores behaviors and treatment response for depressive disorders. The Columbia-Suicide Severity Rating Scale (C-SSRS) is a questionnaire that is available in multiple languages to conduct a suicide assessment. Substance use is screened using tools such as the Alcohol Use Disorders Identification Test (AUDIT) and the Car, Relax, Alone, Forget, Friends, Trouble (CRAFFT) tool for adolescents, which focuses on areas related to their perception of drug usage.

Anxiety Disorders

Anxiety and panic attacks are characterized by extreme, sudden, and often unpredictable feelings of paralyzing fear, nervousness, and discomfort. These situations are often debilitating for the individual experiencing them, with some reporting symptoms such as chest pain, the inability to breathe, and feeling a sense of impending death. Other common symptoms include overwhelming dizziness, nausea, sweating, trembling, accelerated heart rate, and feelings of "checking out" from reality. For a true medical diagnosis, four or more of these symptoms must be present. Typically, these episodes can last anywhere from 10 minutes to over an hour. Individuals who experience an anxiety or panic attack for the first time may be unfamiliar with the event, and it can warrant a trip to the healthcare facility. Consequently, it is important for providers to know how to address these situations to help the patient to receive proper, adequate, and cost-efficient treatment in the future. It is important to show support and compassion toward the patient's feelings, even if the patient's fears seem irrational.

For recurrent anxiety and panic attacks, medication and/or psychotherapy is often needed to support the patient's quality of life. Selective serotonin reuptake inhibitors (SSRIs) are often prescribed to help manage anxiety symptoms. Common SSRIs used for anxiety include names include fluoxetine, sertraline, paroxetine, and escitalopram.

Bipolar Disorder

Bipolar disorder is characterized by extremes in mood, energy, and functioning. The individual tends to experience manic periods, marked by highly energetic, almost frenzied behaviors and excitable moods, as well as depressive periods, marked by lethargy, sadness, and isolation. Clinically, manic periods must last at least a week and depressive periods at least two weeks for an individual to be diagnosed with bipolar disorder. Bipolar is a brain disorder that may be caused by physiological distinctions in the brain or genetics. It is often treated with mood-stabilizing medications in conjunction with psychotherapy. Common medications to manage symptoms of bipolar disorder include lithium and valproate.

Due to the nature of the disorder, the extremes experienced by an individual with bipolar disorder can result in a trip to the emergency department or other acute care facility. Individuals experiencing a manic period are at risk of engaging in impulsive behaviors, such as drug abuse, violence, unsafe sexual encounters, and following through with suicidal thoughts. Individuals experiencing a depressive period are also at risk of having suicidal thoughts or tendencies due to a marked increase in feelings of hopelessness. Individuals with bipolar disorder can also experience periods of psychosis and have delusions or hallucinations. WHNPs should be prepared to show sympathy and compassion while still being firm and direct with the patient. Patient behavior will likely be unpredictable, especially if he or she is in a manic phase.

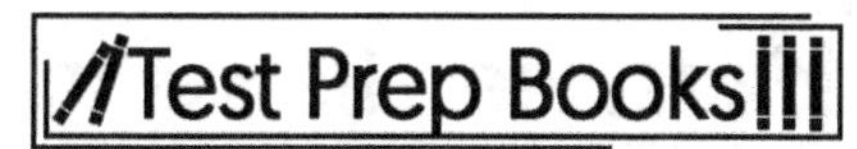

Depression

Depression is characterized by feelings of lethargy; hopelessness; an inability to derive pleasure from once pleasurable activities; problems with sleep, eating, and substances; and/or sexual dysfunction that lasts longer than two weeks. It can be caused by genetics, an imbalance of neurochemicals, or situational contexts. Depression often presents differently in men, women, children, and older adults. Men tend to exhibit increased anger and irritability, while women tend to feel sad, worthless, and guilty. Women tend to internalize symptoms and experience depression at a higher rate and frequency than men due to unique societal issues, hormonal changes, and other factors. Children present symptoms of depression through isolation, anxiety, or acting out. Older adults are more prone to hide symptoms of depression, attribute the feelings to another health problem, or be taken less seriously than other age demographics. It should be noted that these are generalizations and not hard rules, as depression can have a different clinical presentation depending on the specific patient.

Depression is usually managed through psychotherapy and sometimes medication. Common medications to treat depression include SSRIs, like those used to treat anxiety. Depression can also be treated with serotonin and norepinephrine reuptake inhibitors, such as duloxetine and venlafaxine. When these options don't work, tricyclic antidepressants may be prescribed. Because they tend to have more intense side effects, tricyclic antidepressants are not usually prescribed unless other options have been exhausted. Even with medication, some periods of depression can become so intense and unmanageable that the patient enters a major depressive episode or has suicidal ideation. In this context, emergency services are usually needed. It is important to show the depressed patient reassurance, comfort, and support, including directly asking the patient what would help comfort and support him or her during this time. Noting verbal and nonverbal communication will help determine if the patient is at risk for suicide and how severe that risk might be. A critical factor of assessing a potentially suicidal patient is inquiring if there is a suicide plan in place.

The WHNP should assess patients for suicidal ideation using nonjudgmental, therapeutic methods that support the patient in being honest with the healthcare staff. This should include clear, direct questions related to plan, intent, and history of attempts. Euphemisms should not be used. If the patient is determined to be high risk, this should be communicated with the healthcare team and the patient should not be left alone until further assessment by a social worker or psychiatry specialist can take place. Patient safety attendants are often utilized in hospitals for this purpose.

High-risk patients must be continually monitored, and their environment should be adapted for safety. In the hospital, this can mean removing cords, tubing, sharp items, and anything that could be used to cause harm. A patient's belongings should be checked for weapons and hoarded medications, which need to be removed if found. The WHNP should work with the patient to create a safety plan and explain the precautions to the patient and the family. When administering medications, the nurse should ensure the medicine is taken promptly by the patient and not being stored for a future attempt. Social work should be involved, and discharge planning should include family and caregivers.

Homicidal and Suicidal Ideation

Homicidal ideation is characterized by recurrent thoughts of homicide and is an immediate cause for concern or emergency intervention. Homicidal ideation can consist of fleeting, ambiguous thoughts of homicide or long-term, detailed plans that are made with the intention of following through to completion. It often stems from another psychological disorder in which delusions or hallucinations may be present, such as bipolar disorder or schizophrenia. Other risk factors include a tendency toward violence or hostile behavior, victimization, and head injury; however, it is important to note that individuals who experience homicidal ideation can often be normal, otherwise healthy people who may be triggered by distress (e.g., betrayal). Consequently, it can be hard to detect and manage unless the individual makes direct comments about his or her homicidal thoughts or documents it in some other way (e.g., comments on social media, drawings, or journaling).

Suicidal ideation refers to having thought of suicide. It is often a component of another mental health diagnosis in an individual, such as depression. It can range from a spectrum of fleeting suicidal thoughts without a plan of action (also referred to as passive suicidal ideation) to suicidal thoughts with a plan of action (also referred to as active suicidal ideation). Suicidal ideation, like homicidal ideation, is an immediate cause for concern and emergency intervention. Risk factors for suicidal ideation include family history, above-average number of negative life experiences, chronically high levels of stress, inability to cope with or manage stressors, mental illness, guns in the home, domestic violence, and imprisonment. Men are more likely to experience suicidal ideation than women. Medical personnel should note patient symptoms associated with depression, comments made about death or dying, history of or visible marks from past suicide attempts, marks from self-harm, mood swings, extreme anxiety, and intense negative emotions. Suicide attempts that are not fatal can result in severe consequences, such as brain damage or falling into a long-term coma.

Obsessive-Compulsive Disorder

Obsessive-compulsive disorder (OCD) is a chronic mental health disorder that presents with recurring intrusive thoughts and repetitive behaviors that significantly impair daily functioning. Contributing factors include serotonin dysregulation, family history of OCD, stress, trauma, and abnormalities in the orbitofrontal cortex, cingulate gyrus, and basal ganglia. The hallmark characteristics of OCD include obsessions or intrusive thoughts (e.g., fear of harm or intense need for symmetry/order) and compulsions or repetitive behaviors (e.g., handwashing or mental rituals). Diagnosis criteria from the DSM-5 include the presence of both obsessions and compulsions that are time-consuming, and the individual's attempt to suppress or counteract these urges with a different thought or action. Screening tools, such as the Yale-Brown Obsessive-Compulsive Scale, may also be used. Cognitive behavioral therapy directed toward exposure and response prevention is the hallmark treatment for OCD. SSRIs may also be used for symptom management.

Post-Traumatic Stress Disorder (PTSD)

PTSD is a disorder that develops in some people who have experienced a shocking, scary, or dangerous event. People who have PTSD may feel stressed or frightened even when they are not in danger. Fear triggers many split-second changes in the body to help defend against danger or to avoid it. This fight-or-flight response is a typical reaction meant to protect a person from harm. Most people recover from initial symptoms naturally but those who continue to be diagnosed with PTSD.

Symptoms usually begin within 3 months of the traumatic incident, but may occur later. Symptoms must last more than a month and be severe enough to interfere with relationships or work to be considered PTSD. The course of the illness varies, and it may become chronic. Some people recover within 6 months, while others have symptoms that last much longer. Re-experiencing symptoms may cause problems in a person's everyday routine. The symptoms can start from the person's own thoughts and feelings. Words, objects, or situations that are reminders of the event can also trigger re-experiencing symptoms.

To be diagnosed with PTSD, an adult must have all of the following for at least 1 month:

- At least one re-experiencing symptom
- At least one avoidance symptom
- At least two arousal and reactivity symptoms

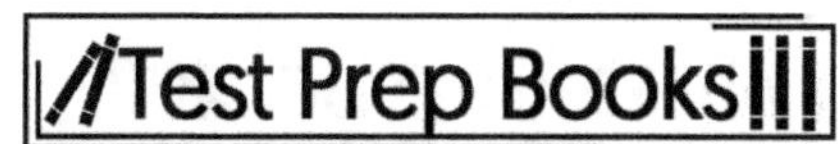

- At least two cognition and mood symptoms
- Re-experiencing symptoms include:
  - Flashbacks—reliving the trauma over and over, including physical symptoms like a racing heart or sweating
  - Bad dreams
  - Frightening thoughts

Avoidance symptoms include staying away from places, events, or objects that are reminders of the traumatic experience and avoiding thoughts or feelings related to the traumatic event. Things that remind a person of the traumatic event can trigger avoidance symptoms. These symptoms may cause a person to change their personal routine. For example, after a bad car accident, a person who usually drives may avoid driving or riding in a car.

Arousal and reactivity symptoms include: being easily startled, feeling tense, having difficulty sleeping, and having angry outbursts. Arousal symptoms are usually constant, instead of being triggered by things that remind one of the traumatic events. These symptoms can make the person feel stressed and angry. They may make it hard to do daily tasks, such as sleeping, eating, or concentrating.

Cognition and mood symptoms include: trouble remembering key features of the traumatic event, negative thoughts about self or the world, distorted feelings like guilt or blame, and loss of interest in enjoyable activities. Cognition and mood symptoms can begin or worsen after the traumatic event, but are not due to injury or substance use. These symptoms can make the person feel alienated or detached from friends or family members.

Anyone can develop PTSD at any age. This includes war veterans, children, and people who have been through a physical or sexual assault, abuse, accident, disaster, or many other serious events. According to the National Center for PTSD, about 7 or 8 out of every 100 people will experience PTSD at some point in their lives. Women are more likely to develop PTSD than men, and genes may make some people more likely to develop PTSD than others.

The main treatments for people with PTSD are medications, psychotherapy, or both. Everyone is different, and PTSD affects people differently so a treatment that works for one person may not work for another. It is important for anyone with PTSD to be treated by a mental health provider who is experienced with PTSD. Some people with PTSD need to try different treatments to find what works for their symptoms. As genetic research and brain imaging technologies continue to improve, scientists are more likely to be able to pinpoint when and where in the brain PTSD begins. This understanding may then lead to better targeted treatments to suit each person's own needs or even prevent the disorder before it causes harm.

A 2012 study of 395 military veterans with PTSD found a link between risk-taking behavior and the disorder. In addition to the above forms of riskiness, vets with PTSD have a propensity for firearms play, potentially endangering their lives. People with PTSD have already survived dangerous situations and risk-taking behavior may give such individuals the feeling that they have more control over their present circumstances than those that led to them developing PTSD. Recognizing this propensity in their personality may help patients with risk-taking behavior, thus being the first step in remediating the problem. Behavioral and cognitive therapy, as well as psychological drugs such as antidepressants, may also aid in the treatment of this behavior.

Psychosis

Psychosis is a broad term encompassing any mental condition in which the individual experiences thoughts or exhibits behaviors that indicate a detachment from reality. Psychosis can be its own diagnosis or a part of another mental health issue. It is often associated with schizophrenia, a cognitive disorder characterized by episodic hallucinations and delusions. Acute or short-term episodes of psychosis may be seen in patients diagnosed with bipolar disorder; episodes can also stem from drug abuse, especially in patients who have used methamphetamines, cocaine, or LSD.

Psychosis can be characterized by abnormal or awkward social behavior, indecipherable verbal communication or writing, catatonia, visual or auditory hallucinations, and/or extreme paranoia. Individuals experiencing psychotic episodes are often brought to the emergency department by concerned friends, family, or legal professionals, as they may pose a threat to themselves or others while detached from reality. It is important to rule out any concerns or influences of a physiological nature (such as head trauma or a brain tumor) before diagnosing the patient as having a psychotic episode. The patient should be approached gently and asked about the delusions in a neutral manner (without openly denying or accepting the patient's storyline), and all effort should be made to not excessively stimulate or frighten the patient.

Schizophrenia

Schizophrenia is a mental disorder that results in psychosis, paranoia, delusions, hallucinations, and other dissociations with reality. It is a disorder that often significantly impairs the patient's ability to function in normal, daily routines and typically requires complex medical interventions. Patients often need long-term support and may not be able to live independently at any point during their lifetime. However, early intervention may reduce the disease's progression and severity. Typical onset varies by sex, but most patients are diagnosed in their 20s. Risk factors for schizophrenia include family history, a difficult prenatal environment (e.g., experiences that negatively impact brain and nervous system development), and drug use during the adolescent years. Deeply stressful, traumatic events can also trigger the onset of symptoms.

Without intervention or support, many patients with schizophrenia experience intense suicidal ideation and mood disorders. Psychosocial obstacles—such as loss of work and relationships, homelessness, and financial hardship—are also common. Patients are often unable to take care of their basic living needs (such as hygiene) or are disinterested in doing so. Treatment includes psychiatric therapy and anti-psychotic medications. Family therapy is also recommended, as the diagnosis can place strain on caretakers and other close relatives. In severe cases, the patient may need a long-term residential program that offers varying degrees of intervention.

Endocrine Conditions

The glands of the endocrine system include the pituitary, thyroid, parathyroid, adrenal, and reproductive glands, as well as the hypothalamus, the pancreas, and the pineal body. The function of the system is to synthesize and secrete hormones that control body growth, sexual function, and metabolism, which is the production and use of energy by the body. The thyroid gland, located on either side of the trachea, regulates energy production, or the rate at which the body uses ingested food to support body functions. The parathyroid, located on the upper margin of the thyroid gland, regulates calcium levels by the activation of Vitamin D, which increases intestinal absorption of calcium, and by regulating the amount of calcium that is stored in the bones or excreted by the kidneys.

The adrenal glands, located on the upper margin of the kidneys, consist of the adrenal cortex and the adrenal medulla. The hormones secreted by the adrenal cortex are necessary for life and include: cortisol, or hydrocortisone, which regulates the breakdown of proteins, carbohydrates, and fats for energy production and the body's response to stress; corticosterone, which works with cortisol to regulate the immune system; and aldosterone, which contributes to blood-pressure control. The adrenal medulla secretions, including adrenaline, regulate the body's reaction to stress known as the fight-or-flight response. The ovaries secrete estrogen and the testes secrete testosterone, which regulate sexual maturation and function. The pancreas, located in the right upper quadrant of the abdomen, secretes the insulin that regulates blood sugar, in

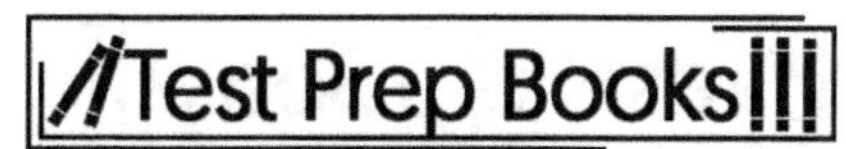

addition to other hormones that regulate water absorption and secretion in the intestines. The pineal gland, located in the center of the brain, secretes melatonin, which regulates the circadian rhythm or sleep cycle.

The nervous system connects each of these glands to the hypothalamus and the pituitary gland. The hypothalamus senses alterations in hormone secretions in all of these organs and conveys those messages to the pituitary gland, which then stimulates each specific organ to either increase or decrease secretion of the relevant hormone. This feedback system is necessary for homeostasis.

Diabetes Mellitus

Type 1 Diabetes

Type 1 diabetes is a genetically-linked autoimmune disease that is characterized by damage to the beta cells of the pancreas due to the autoimmune response that results in the hyposecretion of insulin. There is evidence that environmental factors such as viruses or β cell stress due to obesity, puberty, trauma, infections, and glucose overload can also contribute to the onset of type 1 diabetes. The combination of these two elements triggers the formation of autoantigens on the surface of normal β cells, which stimulates the production of autoantibodies that eventually destroy the β cells.

The destruction of the β cells and the cessation of insulin secretion can be evident at any age, but the most common age at onset in the United States is 14 years old. Many adults that present with manifestations of diabetes are told that they have type 2 diabetes because there is a misconception that the onset of type 1 diabetes always occurs at an earlier age. Providers are encouraged to assess the serum C-peptide level, which is a by-product of insulin production that contains a short chain of amino acids. It is released from the β cells at the same time that insulin is secreted, and the levels of C-peptide and insulin are equal, which means that the C-peptide level is a way to assess the adequacy of insulin secretion.

The early manifestations associated with type 1 diabetes include the following:

- The 3 P's—polydipsia, polyphagia, and polyuria
- New onset of bed wetting in children
- Unintended weight loss
- Mood changes
- Fatigue
- Blurred vision

These manifestations are general and might be missed; however, the classic three P's together are specific for type 1 diabetes and will prompt further investigation. The progressive manifestations are the result of persistent elevations of the serum glucose levels on the vasculature of the eye, the kidney, and the cardiovascular system. The patient may experience some or all of the following: retinopathy with visual defects, kidney failure, poor wound healing, stroke, and peripheral vascular disease of the lower extremities. In addition, damage to the peripheral nerves results in neuropathy, which causes pain and puts the patient at an increased risk for falls. Patients with type 1 diabetes receive daily insulin injections or have a pump that can be programmed to release insulin continuously and/or as needed based on the patient's specific needs and blood glucose levels.

Type 2 Diabetes

Type 2 diabetes is due to inadequate secretion of insulin and cellular insulin resistance. The β cells do produce insulin, but the amount is not sufficient to meet the patient's metabolic needs and/or the body is not effective at using the insulin that is produced. **Insulin resistance** is defined as cellular resistance to the uptake of insulin. The early manifestations of type 2 diabetes are similar to those of type 1 diabetes, and if untreated the complications associated with type 2 diabetes will be similar to those of type 1 diabetes. Many patients with type 2 diabetes are treated successfully with a modified diet, weight loss, and increased exercise, whereas others require oral hypoglycemic agents. This form of diabetes is reversible, whereas type 1 diabetes is not reversible.

Hypoglycemia

In the body, a normal amount of blood glucose is necessary as an energy source for metabolic processes. The brain relies on glucose as an energy source to perform its functions. The term "blood sugar" refers to the amount of glucose circulating in one's blood at any given time. A normal blood sugar before a person eats falls into the 70 mg/dl to 99 mg/dl range. After one eats, blood sugar rises, but should be no more than 140 mg/dl a few hours after a meal. When the blood glucose level falls below 50 mg/dl, this is considered **hypoglycemia**, or low blood sugar.

Hypoglycemia may occur with or without symptoms. The body has a number of regulatory activities that are performed to correct low blood sugar. As a compensatory mechanism, the levels of glucagon and epinephrine may rise, and growth hormone and cortisol levels may increase. These regulatory mechanisms may occur and correct the hypoglycemia before any noticeable symptoms arise.

Symptoms of hypoglycemia are reflective of the autonomic activity occurring within the body. The patient may be sweating, feel warm, or experience nausea, anxiety, and palpitations. The patient may be trembling, complain of headache, experience blurry or double vision, become confused, slur their speech, or even begin to have a seizure or enter a comatose state. Many of these symptoms are caused by the lack of blood glucose to the brain, causing neurological symptoms.

The cause of an acute hypoglycemic state is almost always drug-induced, especially if the patient is receiving insulin therapy. Overtreatment with insulin without proper balance with the patient's mealtime schedule will result in hypoglycemia. Patients in the hospital setting often fall victim to hypoglycemia due to an ever-changing schedule of tests, procedures, and periods of time where they are required to fast.

Treatment of hypoglycemia usually includes administration of dextrose or some other form of sugar. Oral glucagon is an option in the alert patient who can swallow. Symptoms should be corrected upon normalization of blood sugar.

Hyperglycemia

Hyperglycemia, or a random blood sugar reading not affected by a recent meal that is greater than 200 mg/dL, is often a symptom of insulin resistance or insulin deficiency. Insulin resistance and deficiency are the key factors producing diabetes types I and II, hence hyperglycemia is a trademark of these two diseases.

When insulin does not properly regulate the level of blood glucose circulating, blood sugar rises to unhealthy levels. This produces a sequela of complications, as well as some unpleasant symptoms in the patient experiencing hyperglycemia.

The most commonly-associated symptoms of hyperglycemia are polydipsia and polyuria, in which a person is drinking and then urinating copious amounts of fluids. A patient might also experience nausea, warmth, and blurred vision. The high level of circulating blood sugar puts the patient at risk for bacterial and fungal infections, as these organisms feed on and thrive in environments where there are high levels of glucose.

Prolonged polyuria will result in dehydration, as evidenced by tachycardia, hypotension, fatigue, and weakness in the patient. These are serious complications that will be treated with fluid resuscitation and electrolyte correction if imbalances exist. High blood glucose will be treated with insulin therapy, including oral antihyperglycemics, and injectable glucagon.

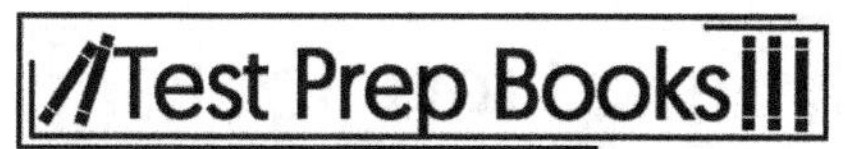

Diabetic Ketoacidosis (DKA)

A patient diagnosed with diabetes mellitus may be prone to a complication of this condition called **diabetic ketoacidosis** (**DKA**), which is a medical emergency. While DKA can develop in both type 1 and type 2 diabetes mellitus, it is more common for the type 1 diabetic. The process of developing DKA is a complex metabolic pathway in which the body seeks alternative energy sources to glucose, resulting in an acidotic state.

At the beginning of DKA, the body is in a state of insulin deficiency. This at times happens because of diabetes mellitus, and the body must compensate in attempts to restore homeostasis. The body begins to metabolize triglycerides and amino acids to create energy. In a normal state, the body breaks down glucose as an energy source. However, when insulin is deficient and blood glucose supply is constantly in flux, as is the case with diabetes mellitus, the body searches for an alternative, more stable energy source.

The breakdown of triglycerides and amino acids then causes an increase in serum levels of glycerol and free fatty acids as a byproduct of lipolysis, or fat breakdown. Serum alanine also rises, as a byproduct of muscle breakdown, to provide another energy source when the body cannot find enough glucose. This rise in alanine and glycerol stimulates the liver to produce its own glucose as an energy source. Glucagon, which is produced in the pancreas and used as an emergency source of energy when outside glucose sources drop, rises to excessive levels and stimulates free fatty acids to be converted to ketones. This process is called ketogenesis and is normally blocked by sufficient levels of insulin. Ketogenesis results in ketoacids, such as acetone, which create the acidic environment of DKA. Acetone is released from the body by way of respiration, which is why a patient with DKA has a "fruity" smell to their breath.

When the blood sugar rises during DKA, it causes substantial amounts of fluids to be excreted through the urine, called osmotic diuresis. This leads to fluid and electrolyte imbalances. Potassium levels must be carefully monitored during DKA. They may not initially fall in serum tests because, despite great loss of potassium through the urine, there is also a great release of potassium from the cells into the bloodstream. Potassium will be ushered back into the cells when insulin levels return to normal.

Presenting symptoms of DKA include polyuria, polydipsia, nausea, abdominal pain, fruity breath odor, confusion, and hyperglycemia. Diagnosis will be made based on symptoms and measurements of arterial blood gases. Presence of ketones in the bloodstream (ketonemia) or urine (ketonuria), hyperglycemia, and an anion gap of >20 mEq/L are considered positive diagnostic signs of DKA. Metabolic acidosis, as evidenced by hypocapnia and arterial pH <7.3, can also be diagnostic signs for DKA.

During diabetic ketoacidosis management, the care team works to reduce unpleasant symptoms while closely monitoring blood glucose levels, intake and output, diabetic diet, vital signs, and level of orientation. Emergency treatment of DKA will include insulin administration, correction of fluid and electrolyte imbalances (especially potassium), and possibly bicarbonate to correct severe cases of acidosis. Most facilities have policies in place for DKA, with the key components including isotonic saline, potassium to replace deficit, and IV insulin at low doses once potassium is within normal range. Frequent blood sugars and ABGs will be drawn per institution protocol. Monitoring serum sodium, potassium, and chloride are also crucial in the medical management of the DKA patient.

Hyperosmolar Hyperglycemic State (HHS)

A patient with type 2 diabetes has an impaired response to insulin, as the cells have developed a resistance to insulin. When blood sugar rises to unhealthy levels, it stimulates the kidneys to excrete large amounts of urine, a condition called polyuria. The blood volume is thus depleted, causing a state of dehydration and abnormal serum concentration. Concentration of the blood creates a hyperosmolar state in the bloodstream. When the blood is concentrated yet not acidotic as a result of fat cells breaking down, it is called **hyperosmolar hyperglycemic state** (**HHS**).

HHS can result from a patient not taking their prescribed diabetic medications appropriately, causing a hyperglycemic state. At other times, an infection or illness unrelated to diabetes mellitus may cause a hyperglycemic state. Corticosteroids are known to cause a rise in blood sugar; thus, their use must be administered with caution in high-risk individuals. If the patient also suffers from high blood sugar and has been prescribed diuretics, a hyperosmolar state may result. Unlike DKA that typically develops quickly, HHS can gradually progress over days. While hyperglycemia is commonplace for both DKA and HHS, the patient with HHS will have severe hyperglycemia—potentially exceeding 1000 mg/dL.

The concentrated blood of HHS will primarily cause neurological deficits such as confusion, disorientation, drowsiness, and even coma. Certain patients will experience seizures or stroke-like syndromes. Death may occur if HHS is left untreated. HHS will be diagnosed based on symptoms of confusion and blood tests to look for hyperosmolarity of the blood, as well as decreased blood volume signaling dehydration. Treatment will occur via intravenous (IV) therapy to correct fluid and electrolyte imbalances. Treatment of HHS is very similar to treatment of DKA.

Thyroid Disorders

Hyperthyroidism

Hyperthyroidism, often seen in the autoimmune condition of Grave's disease, leads to symptoms of nervousness, weight loss, increased appetite, tachycardia, heat intolerance, hand tremor, protruding eyes, and warm, moist skin. In the severe case of thyroid storm or thyrotoxic crisis, the WHNP should pay close attention to the presence of palpitations, fever, and delirium. Care measures involve ensuring balanced nutrition with a high-caloric diet during this hyperbolic state and monitoring vital signs as well as cardiac output. Laboratory testing may reveal decreased thyroid-stimulating hormone (TSH) and elevated or normal levels of triiodothyronine (T3) and thyroxine (T4). Medication management involves propranolol, propylthiouracil, methimazole, and iodine. If exophthalmos is present, the WHNP should ensure that conjunctivas remain moist and recommend eye drops if necessary. Interventional therapies could include radioiodine ablation and thyroidectomy. In the event of a total thyroidectomy, the patient will then have hypothyroidism, requiring lifelong treatment with thyroid hormone replacement.

Hypothyroidism

Hypothyroidism, often seen in the autoimmune condition of Hashimoto's thyroiditis, leads to symptoms of fatigue, weight gain, loss of appetite, bradycardia, cold intolerance, puffy face, and dry skin. In the severe case of myxedema coma, the WHNP should assess for hypotension, hypothermia, hypoglycemia, enlarged tongue, and slow, slurred speech. Laboratory testing may reveal elevated thyroid-stimulating hormone (TSH), along with either reduced or normal levels of triiodothyronine (T3) and thyroxine (T4). Thyroxine hormone replacement is typically delivered via natural or synthetic preparations. Close monitoring for signs and symptoms of hyperthyroidism during treatment should be maintained.

Thyroiditis

Thyroiditis refers to an inflammatory condition of the thyroid gland, which occurs most often as a result of autoimmune disease such as Hashimoto's disease. Additional causative factors include those related to infection (e.g., subacute or infectious thyroiditis), specific drugs (e.g., amiodarone, lithium), radiation, and postpartum status. Women and those between thirty and fifty years of age are most commonly affected. Symptoms of the condition typically follow a pattern: thyrotoxicosis (overactive thyroid), hypothyroid (underactive thyroid), and euthyroid (return to normal). During thyrotoxicosis, symptoms can consist of tachycardia, anxiety, tremors, weight loss, sweating and insomnia. On the other hand, the hypothyroid phase will result in fatigue, depression, weight gain, dry skin, and constipation.

Diagnostic workup should include laboratory testing, including thyroid-stimulating hormone (TSH), T3, and T4 to evaluate thyroid function as well as C-reactive protein (CRP) and Erythrocyte sedimentation rate (ESR)

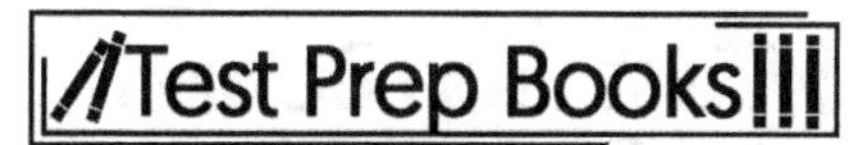

levels to evaluate inflammation. Additional diagnostic testing measures consist of thyroid ultrasound, antibody testing, and radioactive iodine uptake testing. Treatment will be guided by the type and phase of thyroiditis; hyperthyroid states can be treated with beta blockers, while hypothyroid states can be treated with levothyroxine. Infectious causes of thyroiditis require treatment with antibiotics along with NSAIDS for relief of pain associated with the condition. Postpartum thyroiditis will often resolve on its own or require supplementation with levothyroxine for a period of time. For drug-induced cases, the patient's medication will either be switched to a different drug, or the same medication will be continued alongside levothyroxine treatment.

Thyroid Nodules

Thyroid nodules, which refer to a lump found within the thyroid gland, are a common yet important patient complaint that requires investigation. While the vast majority of thyroid nodules are benign, around five percent will be associated with thyroid cancer. The condition is typically asymptomatic; however, in some cases patients may complain of possible pressure in the anterior neck region. Risk factors include older age, female gender, and history of iron-deficiency anemia, uterine fibroids, or radiation to the thyroid. Physical assessment should include palpation of the thyroid gland to determine the presence, characteristics, and size of the nodule. Thyroid nodules may consist of either a single or multiple masses, as well as be either solid or filled with fluid. Those at greatest risk of being identified as malignant will consist of a single, firm, and fixed nodule that is greater than four centimeters in size. Diagnostic workup should include laboratory testing, beginning with a thyroid stimulating hormone (TSH) to evaluate thyroid function. Additional diagnostic testing measures consist of thyroid ultrasound and fine-needle aspiration for further evaluation of the nodule and to guide treatment. For benign cases, the nodule will continue to be monitored on a regular basis with no initial treatment required. In cases where the nodule causes dysfunction of the thyroid gland, radioactive iodine may be used to reduce their size. In malignant or severe cases which interfere with breathing or swallowing, surgical removal will be advised.

Goiter

A **goiter** refers to any enlargement in the thyroid gland. Goiters can occur in healthy thyroids or in thyroids producing abnormal levels of hormones. Their presence can indicate a lack of iodine, an autoimmune disease, an injury, or cancer.

Thyroid Cancer

Thyroid cancer is rare but can result in goiters and thyroid dysfunction. Thyroid cancer is more common in people who have nodes or goiters already present on the thyroid, which later turn malignant. The disease is also more prevalent in people who have been exposed to radiation. Thyroid cancer is usually treated through surgery, and thyroid hormone replacement therapy is a part of follow-up treatment.

Hematologic Conditions

The hematopoietic system, a division of the lymphatic system, is responsible for blood-cell production. The cells are produced in the bone marrow, which is soft connective tissue in the center of large bones that have a rich blood supply. The two types of bone marrow are red bone marrow and yellow bone marrow.

The red bone marrow contains the stem cells, which can transform into specific blood cells as needed by the body. The yellow bone marrow is less active and is composed of fat cells; however, if needed, the yellow marrow can function as the red marrow to produce the blood cells.

The red bone marrow predominates from birth until adolescence. From that point on, the amount of red marrow decreases, and the amount of yellow marrow increases. This means that the elderly are at risk for conditions related to decreased blood-cell replenishment.

Common Anemias

Approximately eight percent of the body's total weight is blood volume. Blood is a connective tissue that carries important nutrients throughout the body. Oxygen is transported via the blood and helps perfuse the extremities and vital organs. Red blood cells (RBCs) are typically in the shape of a disc and are concave to allow the maximum amount of oxygen to be transported. Vitamins and minerals, specifically folic acid and vitamin B12, aid in the maturity of RBCs. A lack of vitamins and minerals will decrease the life span of RBCs and can alter their size and shape. A reduction in the number of RBCs will reduce the amount of oxygen that is transported throughout the body. Inadequate oxygenation of the tissues due to decreased RBCs or hemoglobin is termed **anemia**.

Diagnosing anemia is typically done through a serum CBC by looking closely at the hemoglobin and hematocrit. For non-pregnant adult females, anemia is generally diagnosed when the hemoglobin is <11.9 g/dL and/or the hematocrit is <35%. For males, anemia is generally diagnosed when the hemoglobin is <13.6 g/dL and/or the hematocrit is <40%.

Often anemia is not a disease in and of itself but rather a symptom of an underlying disorder. The medical provider will investigate possible underlying causes of the anemia in order to determine and treat the etiological factors.

There are three broad categories of anemias, not including blood loss: microcytosis, normocytosis, and macrocytosis. In microcytosis, including iron-transport deficiency, lead toxicity, sickle cell disease, and thalassemia, the heme and globin synthesis is defective or deficient; this results in RBCs that are smaller in size than usual. In normocytosis, the RBC is normal in size but deficient in quantity. Examples of normocytic anemias include anemia of chronic disease and aplastic anemia acquired from primary bone marrow disorders. Macrocytosis, caused by abnormal DNA synthesis, leads to large RBCs that do not have sufficient oxygen-carrying ability. Mean corpuscular volume (MCV) is a vital serum measurement that can give insight to the average size of the patient's RBCs.

The symptoms commonly experienced by patients with anemia include fatigue, weakness, difficulty breathing during exercise, and a pale skin tone. Pallor, or paleness, can be assessed in a dark-skinned patient by looking at the bottoms of their feet, palms, lips, buccal mucosa, and conjunctiva of the eye. Dark-skinned patients will usually have a warm tone, but when anemic or cyanotic, they will have a more gray or ashen hue.

The treatment of anemia will depend on the underlying cause and the severity of the patient's condition. If the patient is anemic because of massive blood loss, blood transfusions will be required. If the anemia is caused by deficient erythropoiesis, the process by which blood is formed, drugs like erythropoietin will be used to stimulate blood production.

Common types of blood products include whole blood, packed red blood cells (PRBC), fresh frozen plasma (FFP), platelets, and albumin. Complications of a blood transfusion include mild-moderate allergic reaction, anaphylactic reaction, acute hemolytic reaction, febrile non-hemolytic reaction (FNHTR), septic reaction, transfusion-associated circulatory overload (TACO), and transfusion-related acute lung injury (TRALI). If signs of a serious reaction are noted, the nurse should stop the transfusion, keep intravenous access while running the normal saline (through different tubing), and call the provider. Epinephrine should be available for administration if the patient shows signs of anaphylaxis.

Although blood transfusions may be the recommended lifesaving treatment for patients who are low on one, many, or all components of blood, not all patients will accept blood products for a variety of reasons. One of the most common reasons for refusal of blood products is religious beliefs, such as those of Jehovah's Witnesses. Others may refuse blood products due to risks of infection or previous adverse reactions to blood

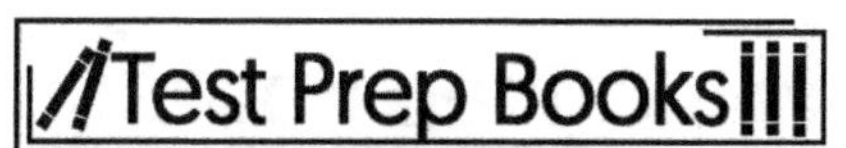

products. Regardless of the reason for refusal, it is important that the patient is fully educated on why the physician is recommending blood product transfusion and the risks of not accepting the transfusion. Ultimately, the patient's decision should be respected, and blood products should not be given to any patient who refuses them. The care team may look into alternative solutions, such as autotransfusion, pharmacologic erythropoiesis, iron supplementation, or other treatments for the cause of anemia. The WHNP should advocate for the patient's autonomy and ensure that they are provided with the education needed to make an informed decision.

Iron Deficiency Anemia

Iron-deficiency anemia results from an insufficient amount of iron intake. Dietary habits are important to assess to determine whether a patient is ingesting a sufficient amount of nutrients. Vegetarians are at risk for iron-deficiency anemia. Iron is not as well absorbed from vegetables and grains as it is from meats. Patients who suffer from alcoholism or GI disorders such as Crohn's or celiac disease do not absorb enough nutrients from the small intestine. Symptoms of iron-deficiency anemia include fatigue, shortness of breath, dizziness, and increased heart rate.

Practitioners will observe pale mucous membranes and brittle hair and nails in patients with iron-deficiency anemia. Blood work will aid in the diagnosis. A complete blood count will reveal a low RBC count and decreased levels of hemoglobin and hematocrit. Iron studies will show a ferritin level below 12 mcg/L and decreased serum iron and transferrin levels. Treatment is aimed at increasing iron-rich foods and prescribing iron supplements.

Folate Deficiency Anemia

Folic acid deficiency anemia is due to a decrease in folic acid levels that interferes with the DNA synthesis and maturation of RBCs. Pharmacological treatment is aimed at increasing folic acid levels. Oral folate is recommended. Serum folic acid levels should increase within a period of 3 to 4 months.

Thalassemia

Thalassemia is an inherited condition in which the body does not produce enough hemoglobin. Severity depends on the hemoglobin chain and the number of genes impacted. Alpha-thalassemia occurs when the four genes involved in the making of the alpha hemoglobin chain are mutated. If one is impacted, the patient will have no symptoms but will be a carrier. Severity increases with each impacted gene; however, when all four are mutated, the result is typically stillbirth. Beta-thalassemia results when there are mutations to the two genes that make up the beta hemoglobin chain. With one mutated gene, symptoms are mild, whereas two mutated genes result in moderate to severe anemia.

Symptoms of thalassemia are typical of anemia, including fatigue, shortness of breath, and paleness, along with jaundice, abdominal pain and swelling, and slow growth in infants and children. People with a family history of thalassemia and those of Mediterranean, Asian, African, and Middle Eastern descent are at higher risk. Diagnosis is completed through family history, iron studies, hemoglobin electrophoresis, CBC, and DNA analysis to confirm mutations. Treatment is typically dependent on severity of symptoms, with blood transfusions and iron chelation therapy being the most prevalent treatments. In severe cases, a bone marrow transplant may be indicated if an appropriate match can be found

Rheumatologic Conditions

Anemia of Chronic Disease

Anemia of chronic disease (ACD) results from a host of different chronic diseases, including infection, autoimmunity, malignancy, and organ dysfunction. Overall, chronic kidney disease (CKD) causes ACD most often. Signs and symptoms resemble other forms of anemia: fatigue, weakness, dyspnea, chest pain, dizziness, and even syncope. Review of labs may reveal microcytosis, but ACD characteristically often features a normal MCV. Chronic diseases frequently increase hepatic production of hepcidin, which diminishes intestinal iron absorption. Chronic inflammation may also promote erythrocyte destruction. Crucially, tissue hypoxia due to anemia stimulates renal production of erythropoietin; however, in CKD, the kidneys' response to this stimulus is blunted, making anemia highly prevalent in patients with CKD and end-stage renal disease (ESRD). As a result, patients with ESRD on hemodialysis frequently receive erythropoietin replacement.

Common Autoimmune Disorders

Fibromyalgia

Fibromyalgia is a chronic pain disorder which affects both the central nervous system and musculoskeletal system. It is most commonly seen in women between thirty and sixty years old and in combination with comorbidities like irritable bowel syndrome, depression, postural orthostatic tachycardia syndrome, and chronic fatigue syndrome. Because fibromyalgia causes abnormal processing of the nociceptive signals in the brain and spinal cord, patients experience pain at a lower threshold level than usually experienced. Abnormalities are also present in the neurotransmitters responsible for pain and mood regulation, such as serotonin, dopamine, and norepinephrine. Dysregulation of these neurotransmitters can also contribute to pain, depression, and anxiety. Another primary symptom of fibromyalgia is nonrestorative sleep, including slow-wave and REM sleep disruptions, leading to significant fatigue and further contributing to chronic pain. However, the hallmark symptom is widespread pain; this is experienced bilaterally, above the waist, and in the neck and back for at least three months.

Diagnosis is made via exclusion, as there are no specific tests that can confirm diagnosis. Differentials to consider include rheumatoid arthritis, systemic lupus erythematosus, hypothyroidism, and multiple sclerosis. Lab tests, such as a CBC or CRP, may be used to rule out other inflammatory diseases. Thyroid function tests can be used to rule out thyroid issues, while rheumatoid factor with anti-cyclic citrullinated peptide (anti-CCP) antibodies can be used to rule out autoimmune diseases.

Medical management includes acetaminophen or NSAIDs for pain; however, these are usually not highly effective for the widespread pain seen in fibromyalgia. Opioids also show limited benefit for fibromyalgia pain and are usually not recommended for pain management due to the risk of dependence. Some antidepressants, such as amitriptyline, can be used in low doses to help with sleep disturbances and possibly pain. Selective serotonin-norepinephrine reuptake inhibitors (SSRIs), like duloxetine, may be used to help with depression as well as pain. Anticonvulsants, such as pregabalin and gabapentin, can also be used to treat fibromyalgia pain since they modulate pain pathways and are beneficial for nerve and generalized pain. Nonpharmacological interventions such as cognitive behavioral therapy, physical therapy, exercise, and good sleep hygiene may also prove beneficial in managing symptoms.

Chronic Fatigue Syndrome

Chronic fatigue syndrome (CFS) is a complex multisystem disease of multifactorial origin, though its full pathophysiology remains poorly understood. It is characterized by severe post-exertional fatigue and malaise, possibly accompanied by headaches and muscle or joint pain. Some patients also experience dysregulated sleep habits, including daytime drowsiness and nighttime sleeplessness. Theorized causes include increased oxidative stress, autoimmunity and abnormal immunoglobulin function, central nervous system inflammation leading to altered glial cell function, and hypocortisolism. CFS is a diagnosis of exclusion for which the following three symptoms should be present for at least 6 months, with at least half the time featuring moderate or severe symptoms: fatigue, post-exertional malaise, and unrefreshing sleep. Furthermore, one of two other symptoms must be present for confirmation: cognitive impairment and/or worsening of symptoms with upright posture (that is, orthostatic intolerance). Treatment may involve nonpharmacologic measures such as cognitive behavioral therapy or medications such as tricyclic

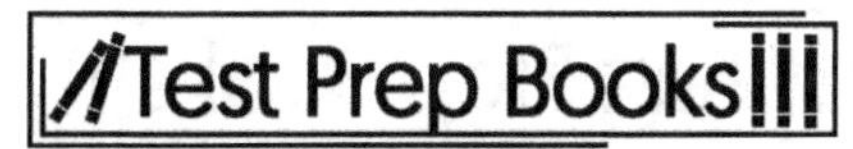

antidepressants, selective serotonin reuptake inhibitors (SSRI)/serotonin–norepinephrine reuptake inhibitors (SNRIs), corticosteroids, and/or NSAIDs for pain. Special efforts should be given to attentiveness and emotional support for patients affected by CFS.

Rheumatoid Arthritis (RA)

Rheumatoid arthritis is an autoimmune disorder that causes cartilage between joints to become inflamed. This is often most noticeable and painful in the hands and fingers but can also affect joints throughout the body. Rheumatoid arthritis is different than traditional arthritis (osteoarthritis), which results from the wear and breakdown of cartilage between joints over time or with overuse. Since it can affect all areas served by the immune response, patients may also experience vision, heart, and skin problems. Due to the extreme swelling of the joints, limbs can become permanently deformed, and patients may be unable to perform basic functions like holding items. Rheumatoid arthritis is primarily treated with immunosuppressive drugs, but lifestyle changes, such as eliminating processed grains and sugars, can help alleviate symptoms as well.

Systemic Lupus Erythematosus (SLE)

Systemic lupus erythematosus (SLE) is an autoimmune disease in which the immune system attacks tissues throughout the body, causing damage and widespread inflammation. This can affect any of the organs in the body, including the skin, heart, lungs, liver, kidneys, nervous system, and digestive system. Because of this, symptoms can be varied and systemic. For example, should the disease attack the nervous system, the patient may present with fatigue, headaches, seizures, and memory problems. Should it attack the heart, the patient may present with palpitations, murmurs, and arrythmias.

Diagnosis of SLE can be a lengthy process, as the patient may present with many seemingly unrelated symptoms. Depending on presentation, the patient may have basic laboratory work, imaging of various organs, ECG, EEG, or biopsies completed. SLE is more definitively diagnosed with a positive antinuclear antibody test along with clinical findings.

Treatment for SLE is much like that of other autoimmune disorders, in that it involves suppression of the overactive immune system along with treatment of the damage it has caused to the body. Patients with SLE may be given NSAIDs for pain management and to decrease inflammation. They may also be placed on steroids for inflammation and immunosuppressants to decrease immune response. Those at risk of blood clots may also be placed on anticoagulants. Treatment beyond this varies significantly depending on the organs affected. For example, if the disease is affecting the heart, the patient may require antihypertensives, antiarrhythmics, or even procedures like valve replacements. Those who have had kidney damage due to lupus may end up requiring hemodialysis or kidney transplantation.

Management of the SLE patient is also multifaceted. The patient may be admitted to the hospital for disruption of any number of their organ systems. This will require thorough head-to-toe assessment and continuous monitoring. Additionally, WHNPs should be aware that those on immunosuppressants are at greater risk of infection, and thus, providers should be especially careful about infection prevention with SLE patients. Finally, WHNPs should provide thorough education to the SLE patient, informing them about infection prevention, the need to wear protective garments, when to seek emergency care, and how to decrease adverse outcomes by maintaining a healthy diet, exercising (when possible), and avoiding drugs, alcohol, and smoking.

Health Screening, Education, and Counseling (Risk Assessment, Disease Prevention, Counseling and National Screening Guidelines)

One of the main goals of primary care is to prevent illness and disease. Limiting hospitalizations, readmissions, and reducing healthcare costs is the responsibility of healthcare practitioners. Preventive care can decrease the presence of chronic illness. Annual wellness visits are useful to discuss concerns, perform screening, and obtain laboratory data that can help generate an educational plan. Early treatment or lifestyle modifications can prevent complications of disease processes. There are three levels of disease prevention. Primary prevention is geared toward education and preventing the development of disease and includes minimizing environmental or external factors. Secondary prevention includes screening for illness when patients present with an early manifestation or detection of an asymptomatic disease. Tertiary prevention includes managing a current disease process in order to prevent future complications.

Obtaining a health history is crucial during a wellness visit. Many of the modifiable risk factors can be determined from exploring dietary habits, activity levels, environment, smoking, and drug usage. During an annual wellness visit, vital signs are an important screening tool. Blood pressure monitoring is essential in the early diagnosis of HTN and cardiovascular diseases. Cholesterol levels can alert a practitioner about the patient's risk of a cardiac event. Early detection of dyslipidemia can be corrected by lifestyle modifications, such as a healthy diet and regular exercise.

Immunization schedules should be shared with patients and vaccinations encouraged if they meet the criteria. Wellness visits for patients with female anatomy should include a pelvic exam and Pap smear at least every two to three years if no abnormalities exist. Education on monthly breast self-exams should be provided. **Mammograms** are a screening tool that can detect breast cancer. Mammograms are encouraged every one or two years beginning at age fifty. In male patients, screening for prostate cancer with a PSA test can begin at age fifty-five. Education on monthly testicular self-exams should be provided to male patients. Screening for bone health can be done by ordering a bone mineral density scan. Women are more prone to osteoporosis and are encouraged to get screened beginning at age fifty, while men are encouraged to begin screening at age seventy.

Age-Appropriate Primary, Secondary, and Tertiary Prevention

Primary Prevention

Primary prevention focuses on health interventions and lifestyle practices that prevent the initial occurrence of an illness. Immunization is an example of primary prevention that is applicable to all age groups. Children are immunized against communicable diseases; adults are immunized against the flu virus; and elderly adults are immunized against the flu virus, pneumonia, and herpes zoster. Additional primary prevention measures for children include assessments of all developmental milestones. These assessments aim at early intervention in the case of any abnormal findings. These assessments also include identification of effective parenting behaviors to support both physical and cognitive development of the child. Beginning as early as the six-month well-child visit, it is important to discuss literacy and the importance of reading to children at an early age. Primary prevention in all populations includes healthy lifestyle practices such as exercise, weight management, and blood pressure control. Because of the onset of chronic diseases, these behaviors become even more important as people age.

Primary prevention measures may also include complementary alternative medicine (CAM) therapies such as acupuncture, tai chi, and massage. The term "alternative" medicine is now more commonly identified as "integrative" medicine as these therapies have become more widely accepted. All these primary prevention

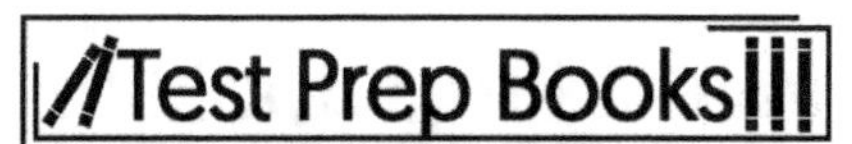

measures require reinforcement to be effective, and now patients have access to wellness coaches who make frequent personal contact with patients to encourage adherence to activities such as exercise and weight management. Insurance coverage for primary prevention measures has also increased because prevention measures are less expensive than the treatment of hypertension, the effects of obesity, and cardiovascular disease. Additional sources of information and support for the success of primary prevention include the government-supported Bright Futures initiative, which addresses primary preventive measures for infants, children, and adolescents.

Secondary Prevention

Secondary prevention focuses on early detection and prompt intervention for patients who have a disease, illness, or injury to prevent it from progressing. For example, breast self-exams may identify early lumps and catch an early stage of breast cancer so that treatment can be started before the disease has time to progress. Blood pressure screening can identify early changes that can be treated successfully, which limits systemic changes associated with hypertension and the possible progression to cardiovascular disease. The WHNP in the medical home will promote secondary prevention for pre- and post-menopausal women and assessment of cardiac risk in all adults. Medicare offers patient reimbursement for completion of the annual wellness visit, which provides the WHNP the opportunity to reinforce the need to employ all three forms of prevention.

The assessment measures can also be used to address a specific health hazard that has the potential to affect large populations. For instance, if the city water supply is contaminated by heavy metals, health officials will conduct testing to assess the effects on the group. The criteria for secondary prevention assessment measures include broad application, adequate sensitivity and specificity, and reasonable cost. An example of this cost-benefit analysis is the comparison of the routine guaiac exam for fecal occult blood (FOBT) versus the fecal immunological test for occult blood (FIT). Recent research has found no statistically significant difference between the results for these assessment measures; however, the FIT test costs approximately twenty times more than the FOBT. That means that the FIT measure is not appropriate as a secondary prevention measure in the general population.

Common secondary preventive measures for infants include anticipatory guidance for safety, feeding and nutrition counseling, and assessment for altered parenting. Bright Futures provides a timeline for secondary prevention measures for all children and adolescents, which provides parent and child educational resources for conditions that may include obesity, dental disease, and behavioral issues.

Tertiary Prevention

Tertiary prevention focuses on reducing the negative impact that a disease or illness has on a patient who is currently experiencing the issue. Tertiary preventive measures may involve treatment or rehabilitation actions that decrease the impact of deficits associated with acute or chronic disease and maximizing the patient's recovery potential. Effective tertiary prevention limits the negative effects of disease, improves quality of life indicators, and limits disease progression. This last requires minimizing potential risk factors and developing a relapse plan for disease progression. Tertiary prevention in infants often addresses genetic alterations such as hip dysplasia, which is treated initially with the application of the Pavlik harness. Children and adolescents also benefit from assessment and treatment of the adverse effects of diseases such as asthma or traumatic injuries. Adolescents and teens who engage in unsafe behaviors such as smoking, recreational drugs, or unprotected sex, require tertiary prevention measures including education and treatment of possible sexually-transmitted diseases (STDs).

Participation in cardiac rehabilitation, quit smoking programs, and medically managed weight loss programs are examples of tertiary prevention for adults that focus on minimizing the effects of an existing disease or eliminating unsafe behavior. Tertiary prevention can improve surgical outcomes; for example, it can consist of preoperative physical therapy for common orthopedic surgeries such as arthroplasty of the knee or hip or correction of scoliosis. Minimizing the effects of existing diseases becomes more complex and potentially less successful in the elderly, who may have multiple chronic conditions. Tertiary prevention programs may be focused on a population group. For instance, the incidence of Lyme disease is higher in New England than in other regions of the United States. Population-specific treatment plans are in place to minimize the long-term effects of the disease, which can include facial nerve palsy and arthritis.

Cancer

Screening Tests

Screening tests provide early detection of treatable diseases, which provides the opportunity for more timely interventions, such as lifestyle changes and medical treatments, that are often more effective in the early stages of the disease. The screening tests are most effective if individuals begin testing at the recommended age and continue with follow-up exams as necessary. Colonoscopy is recommended beginning at age 50, with repeat testing every 10 years if the results are normal. There is debate about the age at which women should have the first screening mammogram; however, many authorities agree that women should have an initial exam at 40 and repeat the exam yearly. The timing for a Pap smear is also debated by some authorities. According to the current American College of Obstetricians and Gynecologists (ACOG) recommendations, women between 21 and 29 years of age should receive a Pap smear every three years, while women between 30 and 35 years of age have three options. These options include a Pap smear every three years, HPV co-testing every five years, or a Pap smear and HPV co-testing every five years. Annual full-body dermatology exams are also recommended as an important safeguard against skin cancer, which is the most common form of cancer in humans.

Early detection can also prevent the onset of the disease. For example, polyps of the large intestine can be identified and removed during a colonoscopy, which eliminates the progression of the polyps to colon cancer. There are rigorous criteria for screening tests that include measurements of sensitivity, specificity, positive predictive value, negative predictive value, and acceptability. Sensitivity is defined as the ability of the test to identify cancer in individuals who have the disease. Specificity refers to the validity of negative test results, which means that individuals who do not have cancer will have negative results. Positive predictive value is a measure of the probability that an individual who tests positive actually has cancer. In contrast, the negative predictive value measures the probability that an individual who tests negative does not have the disease. WHNPs understand that the interpretation of these two predictive values is dependent on the prevalence of the disease in the population. Acceptability refers to the willingness of people to agree to be tested. Additional criteria for screening tests include consideration of costs, availability of the necessary technology and trained personnel, and sufficient follow-up resources for patients with the disease.

Staging and Histological Grading

Stage 0	Stage I	Stage II	Stage III	Stage IV
Early stage	Localized	Early Locally Advanced	Late Locally Advanced	Metastasized
Cancer cells are in their original place of formation	*Tumor has grown but has not spread to another location*	*Tumor has grown and spread to nearby tissue and possibly close lymph nodes*	*Tumor has grown more and spread further within the region*	*Cancer has spread past the region to distant areas of the body*

Malignancies are staged according to the tumor size and the presence or absence of lymph node involvement and metastasis. The **TNM system** is used to standardize the reporting of the patient's disease. The "T"

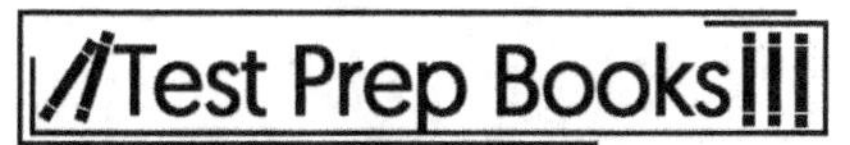

classifies the size of the tumor from no tumor detectable to tumor in situ, or T1–T4. The "N" classifies lymph node involvement from N1 or N2—not able to identify or no nodes identified—to N3, which signifies the number of involved nodes. The "M" classifies the presence or absence of distant metastasis from not able to detect metastasis to no metastasis identified to M1, which indicates the presence of distant metastasis.

Tumor cells are also graded in terms of the degree to which the cellular structure deviates from the originating cell structure. **Well-differentiated** cells that more closely resemble the cell of origin are associated with a more favorable prognosis because the cells tend to grow and metastasize more slowly. The source of the original cell structure cannot be identified in **poorly differentiated** tumor cells which means that their behavior will be unpredictable and most likely harmful to the patient. These standardized details are used to develop an individualized plan of care based on treatment results from similar cancers and to predict the prognosis and possibility of recurrence or recovery. The scores of this general **grading system** range from GX (grade cannot be determined) to G4 (undifferentiated), which correlates with a high-grade tumor. This grading system is essential to the treatment of certain cancers including breast cancer, prostate cancer, primary brain tumors, and soft tissue sarcomas.

In addition, there are several condition-specific grading systems that compare the patient's tumor with different categories of normal cells. The **Nottingham Scale** is used in the diagnosis of breast cancer to compare tubule structure, size and shape of the nucleus, and the number of proliferating cells. The **Gleason scale** is used to grade cellular structure of a prostate tumor and is reported according to the similarities between the normal cells and the tumor cells. The **Byrne scale** is used to classify oral squamous cell carcinoma.

Prevention Strategies

Common cancer prevention strategies include dietary and lifestyle changes, detection and treatment of precancerous conditions with preventative medications, and surgical procedures. Although the strength of the supporting evidence may vary for these preventive measures, there is irrefutable evidence that smoking, including contact with second-hand smoke, and exposure to occupational and environmental carcinogens are associated with an increased risk for the development of cancer.

The other universally recommended lifestyle behaviors aimed at prevention include UV protection for the skin, weight management, and regular exercise. Although there is conflicting evidence of the benefits of specific foods for the prevention of specific cancers, there is general agreement that a calorie-controlled diet that includes generous amounts of fresh fruits and vegetables and avoids excess salt, red meats, processed meats, and alcohol provides the best possible level of prevention. Exercise guidelines are aimed at weight management and the reduction of the accumulation of abdominal fat, which is identified as a risk factor for several cancers, including endometrial, pancreatic, and colorectal cancers. Chemopreventive medicines, such as tamoxifen, raloxifene, and aspirin, may be used to reduce the risk of cancer in individuals with high-risk genetic profiles. Furthermore, surgical procedures, such as a bilateral mastectomy and ovarian ablation, may be considered to eliminate the risk of breast cancer in susceptible women.

Diabetes

Screening Tests

A **Hemoglobin A1C** test measures the percentage of hemoglobin molecules that are coated or glycated with glucose. Hemoglobin molecules are located in the red blood cell, which has a lifespan of 110 to 120 days; therefore, the hemoglobin A1c test measures the average blood sugar for a three-month period. The normal A1c level is less than 5.7 percent; levels between 5.7 percent and 6.4 percent indicate prediabetes and levels greater than 6.5 percent indicate diabetes. Elevated HGB A1c levels must be confirmed with additional testing before treatment is initiated. The provider will inform the patient that fasting is not required, process the sample, and document results.

Prevention Strategies

Advanced practice nurses provide various types of counseling to patients. Counseling arises from the need to educate patients on certain risks and conditions that can affect their health decisions. For example, as part of the non-drug therapy for Type 2 diabetes, counseling is necessary to help patients understand the important diet and lifestyle modifications. Patients with Type 2 diabetes should try to decrease their consumption of processed foods, simple carbohydrates and refined sugars, and overall caloric intake, while increasing physical activity. These interventions help to decrease the requirement of antidiabetic medications and prevent long-term diabetes-related complications.

Cardiovascular Disease

Screening Tests

The most effective screening for **cardiovascular disease** (**CVD**) in the general population involves screening for the established CVD risk factors, including hypertension, hyperlipidemia, obesity, and diabetes. BP should be monitored at least every 3 to 5 years from ages 18 to 39 and at least annually thereafter. Screening for hyperlipidemia should occur at least every 5 years in adults. For diabetes, screen for hyperglycemia at age 35 and at least every 3 years thereafter. Monitor weight at each annual visit. The frequency of the above screenings should increase if patients already have or develop risk factors for CVD and in those with a family history of CVD regardless of current individual risk factors. Additionally, counseling on physical activity, diet, and complete avoidance or cessation of tobacco use is a cornerstone of CVD prevention.

Prevention Strategies

Both modifiable and non-modifiable risk factors can affect cardiovascular function. Diet and physical activity are among the most prominent modifiable risk factors to address with patients at risk for cardiovascular disease development. Practitioners should ask patients about their dietary habits. Diets that are high in saturated and trans fatty acids can lead to high levels of cholesterol. High levels of cholesterol increase blood lipid levels, leading to the development of atherosclerosis. Atherosclerosis is fatty plaque formation inside the vessel walls that causes narrowing and decreased blood flow.

Physical activity helps control high blood pressure, lower cholesterol, and decrease body weight. All of these benefits help maintain an intact cardiovascular system. The American Heart Association recommends adults get at least 2½ hours of aerobic activity each week. Smoking also increases the risk of cardiovascular disease. Cigarette smoke damages the tissue within the lungs, and the subsequent inflammation narrows the airways. Nicotine also increases the heart rate and blood pressure, which can affect perfusion throughout the body. Non-modifiable risk factors, such as family history and age, also contribute to the development of cardiovascular disease. As people age, the flexibility and elasticity of the blood vessels decreases. Blood travels slower through hardened vessels. Patients should be asked about family history and heart disease. Patients have a higher risk of developing cardiovascular disease if their immediate family members suffer the same diagnosis.

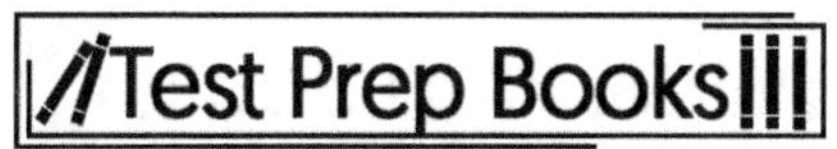

Cardiovascular Risk Reduction in Children

The risk for the development of cardiovascular disease in children should be discussed by the practitioner with young patients and their parents. Many of the modifiable cardiovascular risk factors for adults also apply to the pediatric population. Education on healthy diets is an intervention that may help decrease the prevalence of heart disease in children. Recognizing the food groups that increase heart health, such as fruits, vegetables, and whole grains, can help minimize the popularity of saturated fat ingestion. Physical activity is another factor that contributes to cardiovascular health. The American Heart Association recommends that children between the ages of 6 and 17 perform moderate to vigorous physical activity for at least 60 minutes a day. Patients in these developmental groups are of school age. The practitioner can encourage extracurricular activities, such as sports, that will allow for an increase in physical activity. Careful attention should be given when asking teenagers about their drug and alcohol use. Adolescents may be hesitant to answer questions if a parent is present. Providing education on the cardiovascular effects of smoking will help encourage a truthful answer to these questions.

Hyperlipidemia

Screening Tests

While some guidelines differ mildly regarding lipid screening, the consensus holds that screening for hyperlipidemia via lipid panel should occur between ages 9 and 11, between ages 17 and 21, and at least every 5 years thereafter. In patients with known hyperlipidemia, family history of the condition, or other risk factors for CVD, providers should check lipid panels more frequently. Goal lab values include maintaining low-density lipoprotein (LDL or "bad cholesterol") below 100 mg/dL, high-density lipoprotein (HDL or "good cholesterol") above 60 mg/dL, total cholesterol below 200 mg/dL, and triglycerides below 150 mg/dL.

Prevention Strategies

Few realities in medicine are as well-established as that of hyperlipidemia directly increasing the risk of CVD. Thus, preventing hyperlipidemia is desirable because this directly reduces a patient's CVD risk. The two cornerstones of prevention are diet and exercise. Specifically, a diet high in whole grains, fruits, vegetables, and lean meat while being low in sodium, processed and sugary foods, and red meat is highly recommended for prevention of hyperlipidemia and thus CVD. Additionally, it is recommended that patients complete at least 30 minutes of moderate- to high-intensity exercise at least 5 times per week. These measures, along with absolute avoidance of smoking, effective management of stress, and control of other risk factors, will help mitigate the risk of hyperlipidemia and its numerous related complications.

Obesity/Weight Management

Obesity

Obesity is a complex condition characterized by excessive body fat, often resulting from a combination of genetic, environmental, and behavioral factors. It is typically diagnosed using the Body Mass Index (BMI), a measurement calculated from a person's weight and height. A BMI of thirty or higher indicates obesity. Individuals with obesity will have an increase in body weight, a high waist circumference, and associated health issues such as fatigue, joint pain, and sleep apnea. Obesity significantly raises the risk for numerous health conditions, including type 2 diabetes, cardiovascular disease, certain cancers, and mental health disorders. The patient's medications should be evaluated for those that may be contributing to weight gain, such as gabapentin, antidepressants, or mood stabilizers.

A multidisciplinary approach is required for obesity treatment, often including a primary care provider and dietician as well as physical therapy and mental health counselling. Lifestyle modifications such as a balanced, calorie-controlled diet and regular physical activity are essential first steps, and behavioral therapy may help patients develop healthier habits as well as improve their mental well-being. Prescription medications or weight-loss surgery may be recommended for individuals with severe obesity or for those who have not succeeded using lifestyle changes alone. Regular follow up and support are crucial for long-term success in managing obesity and its associated health risks.

Bariatric Complications

Bariatric surgery is increasingly being performed in the medically complicated obese population as convincing data continue to mount, documenting the success of surgery not only in achieving meaningful weight loss but also in correcting obesity-related illnesses. The 4 most common bariatric surgical procedures are: laparoscopic adjustable gastric banding, vertical sleeve gastrectomy, Roux-en-Y gastric bypass, and biliopancreatic diversion with duodenal switch.

Bariatric surgery is increasingly being accepted as a viable treatment for managing the growing obesity epidemic. Surgery can provide a sustainable, long-term option for weight loss. The prevalence of obesity (body mass index [BMI] ≥30 kg/m2) has stabilized at 35% in the United States since 2003. However, it is estimated that only 1% of eligible patients are undergoing surgical intervention. One barrier to accepting surgery may be the false notion of unacceptable risks and high rate of complications associated with surgery.

Obesity is associated with multiple medical comorbidities, including type 2 diabetes mellitus, cardiovascular disease, dyslipidemia, hypertension, cholelithiasis, gastroesophageal reflux disease, obstructive sleep apnea, degenerative joint disease, lower back pain, and cancer. In addition, obesity is associated with an increase in early mortality. The estimated number of annual deaths attributed to obesity in US adults is 280,000.

In 1991, the National Institutes of Health consensus panel developed a set of recommendations regarding which patients should be considered for bariatric surgery. These recommendations included the criteria that patients have a calculated BMI of at least 40 kg/m2 or a BMI of at least 35 kg/m2 with significant obesity-related comorbidities. Along with the increased volume of surgical procedures, a dramatic decrease in mortality and complications related to surgical intervention has been achieved, as demonstrated in a recent meta-analysis showing a mortality rate of 0.08% within 30 days and 0.31% after 30 days. Complication rates from bariatric operations have progressively fallen from 10.5% of cases in 1993 to 7.6% of cases in 2006, with the majority of complications now being minor.

Osteoporosis

Osteoporosis is a metabolic bone disorder that presents with decreased bone mineral density, leading to the deterioration of the bone tissue, subsequent fragility, and increased fracture risk. Most often, this disease progresses unknowingly and is only identified after a fracture occurs. This disease is most commonly seen in older adults, more specifically postmenopausal women, because of the hormonal impacts on the bones. In postmenopause, women experience a decrease in estrogen, which causes an increase in bone resorption. For older men, testosterone decrease causes a decrease in bone formation. Low calcium intake also contributes to a decrease in bone resorption (less calcium available for bone mineralization). Other risk factors include a family history of osteoporosis, hormonal changes (e.g., menopause, low testosterone, and/or hyperparathyroidism), low body weight (usually indicating low bone mass), certain medications (e.g., glucocorticoids, anticonvulsants, and proton pump inhibitors), certain chronic conditions (e.g., rheumatoid arthritis, hyperthyroidism, and diabetes), smoking, high alcohol intake, and previous history of fractures.

Because osteoporosis is usually asymptomatic, a diagnosis may be made at the time of a fracture (most commonly the back, hips, and wrists). Vertebral fractures may present with back pain, decreased height, and kyphosis. Bone mineral density testing via a DEXA scan is the hallmark diagnostic method. The T-score is a

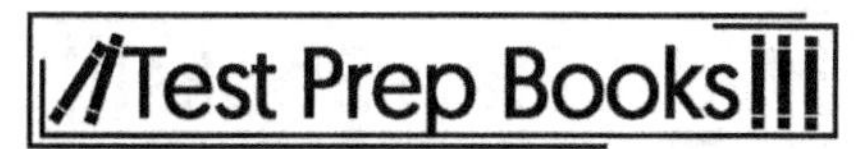

bone density score rated against the bone mass of a healthy thirty-year-old. With osteoporosis, the T-score is -2.5 or less.

Medical management includes the use of bisphosphonates (e.g., alendronate) to inhibit bone resorption by osteoclast inhibition and selective estrogen receptor modulators (e.g., raloxifene) to mimic estrogen's bone-protective effects without the side effects of hormone therapy. Other medications that may be used include calcitonin, denosumab, teriparatide, and abaloparatide. Hormone replacement therapy may be necessary for younger postmenopausal women; however, this may increase their risk of breast cancer. Nonpharmacological interventions include calcium supplementation (1,200 milligrams daily with 800–1,000 IU daily of vitamin D), weight-bearing exercises like walking, and maintaining a safe environment to reduce the risk of falls and subsequent fractures. Routine DEXA and bone mineral density scans should be completed to monitor for any changes.

Healthy Lifestyles

Health promotion refers to the process of encouraging patient attitudes and behaviors that contribute to disease prevention and health maintenance. The World Health Organization (WHO) broadens that focus to include environmental and social conditions that can affect at-risk populations. Practice guidelines that are consistent with the **Health Promotion Nursing Theory** have provided a framework for nursing practice. This theory is based on four general assumptions: individuals continually attempt to influence their own behavior; individuals interact with and exert effects on the environment; health professionals are part of the patients' environment and therefore have the ability to bring about changes in patient behavior; and changed behavior occurs when individuals initiate changes in their patterns of interaction with the environment. According to this model, health professionals are uniquely qualified to provide patients with evidenced-based recommendations for beneficial healthcare practices, which may include regular exercise, weight management and nutritional plans, and smoking cessation. This teaching/learning process may occur in a "health fair" in the community, group sessions in the outpatient clinic, or one-to-one provider-patient encounters in a variety of care settings. WHNPs also participate in health promotion activities that address the needs of the larger community by active involvement in the legislative process.

Diet and Exercise

Advanced practice nurses have various roles in preventing illness and disease. One of the main goals is to promote primary care and screening to a community population. One way the advanced practice nurse promotes health is by providing lifestyle recommendations. Obesity is one of the most significant health issues in the nation. Subsequently, it can lead to complications, such as diabetes, hypertension (HTN), mobility problems, psychosocial ailments, and respiratory and cardiovascular disorders. Assisting patients with formulating healthy eating plans includes recommendations such as limiting high-fat, sugar-rich foods; decreasing alcohol consumption; and incorporating complex carbohydrates to reduce energy intake.

In conjunction with portion control, exercise and activity are promoted. Recommendations are given based on the patient's ability to tolerate physical exercise.

Nutrition

Basic Nutritional Elements

Carbohydrates

Carbohydrates are organic (containing carbon) compounds that are converted into energy for the body. They may be simple, such as refined table sugar, or complex, such as pasta, rice, and fiber.

Fats

Fats are lipid-containing compounds that are necessary for cell wall integrity, energy storage, and protection of all body organs against injury. **Cholesterol** is a body fat that exists in two forms: **low-density lipoprotein** (**LDL**) and **high-density lipoprotein** (**HDL**). LDLs are associated with the formation and progression of **atherosclerosis**, which is a build-up of lipid cells in the vasculature that results in hypertension and cardiovascular disease. Fats are also classified by the configuration of the hydrogen bonds and are classified as **saturated fats**, which are solid at room temperature, or **unsaturated fats**, which are liquid at room temperature. Research indicates that replacing saturated fats with unsaturated fats in the diet facilitates the removal of excess cholesterol from the body. Fats are contained in dairy and animal products, nuts, and vegetable oils. Current recommendations include a consuming a balanced diet that provides unsaturated fats and limited animal fats.

Proteins

Proteins are also organic compounds that contain carbon, hydrogen, and oxygen and form amino acids, the building blocks of the protein molecule. There are nine essential amino acids that must be consumed because the body cannot synthesize them. A **complete protein** consists of all nine essential amino acids, while an **incomplete protein** is deficient in one or more of the essential amino acids. Proteins are essential for all intracellular processes and as enzymes that facilitate all chemical reactions in the body. Nutritional sources of protein include animal products, dairy products, beans, and tofu.

Minerals/Electrolytes

Mineral/electrolytes are metals and nonmetals, including sodium, potassium, chloride, phosphorus, magnesium, calcium, and sulfur. They are necessary for fluid balance, transmission of nervous impulses, bone maintenance, blood clotting, healthy teeth, and protein synthesis and cardiac-impulse conduction. Minerals and electrolytes are generally consumed in adequate amounts from a balanced diet.

Vitamins

Vitamins are organic compounds that are necessary for blood clotting, immune function, maintenance of teeth, and the action of enzymes. There are two classes of vitamins. **Fat-soluble vitamins**, including A, D, E, and K, can be stored in excess in the body in the event of excessive intake. **Water-soluble** vitamins, including B-complex and C, are not stored in the body and ingested amounts greater than body requirements will be excreted in the urine. Vitamins are present in fruits, vegetables, fish, organ meats, and dairy.

Fiber

Dietary fiber is composed of complex carbohydrates and other plant substances that are not broken down by the digestive enzymes. Fiber can be water soluble or insoluble, and both forms contribute to the normal function of the gastrointestinal system. **Soluble fiber** that is present in oatmeal, blueberries, nuts, and beans facilitates the excretion of cholesterol, controls abrupt increases in blood glucose levels, and contributes to normal bowel function. The **insoluble fiber** that is present in whole grains, the skin and seeds of many fruits, and brown rice improves bowel function and also contributes to a feeling of fullness following food intake, which can lead to modest weight loss.

Water

Making up about 75 percent of the body, water is a vital necessity to human life. Water feeds cells and organs, creates a lubricant around the joints, and regulates body temperature. It is also important to digestion, as water moves food through the intestines.

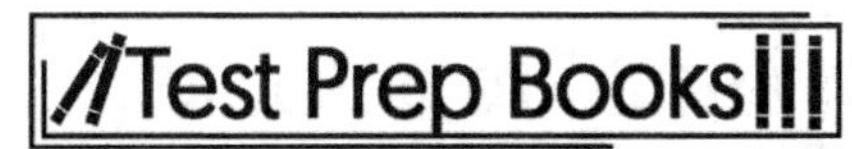

Function of Dietary Supplements and Herbs

Dietary supplements and herbs contain various nutrients that are intended to compensate for inadequate dietary intake of those elements. These products should be used with care by anyone who also takes prescription medications because adverse interactions between the two are common.

Special Dietary Needs

Weight Control

Weight control requires a balanced diet that is calorie controlled and combined with adequate aerobic exercise. Current research indicates that the consumption of sugar and white flour, rather than dietary fats, is the greatest dietary threat to successful weight management.

Diabetes

Diabetes requires a balanced diet that is carbohydrate controlled. Diabetes may be due to a lack of insulin production by the pancreas or cellular insensitivity to the insulin that is present in the bloodstream. The controlled intake of carbohydrates limits the amount of insulin that is necessary to protect the body against the side effects of chronically elevated blood glucose levels.

Cardiovascular Disease/Hypertension

Cardiovascular disease most often is accompanied by excess fluid volume that is manifested by hypertension and edema. The condition requires a balanced diet that is sodium controlled, with adequate fluid intake.

Hypertension is associated with fluid volume excess, which means that excess dietary sodium and fluid should be avoided.

Cancer

Cancer may affect multiple body systems, which means that the diet should be balanced with additional calories to meet energy needs.

Food Sensitivity/Intolerance

Lactose sensitivity/intolerance results from the deficiency of the enzyme lactase, which is necessary for the breakdown or digestion of lactose, a sugar found in dairy products. This deficiency can result in stomach bloating, nausea, vomiting, and diarrhea following the ingestion of dairy products.

Gluten-free diets must be free of wheat, barley, and rye in any form. This means that, in addition to bread, all processed foods must be avoided. **Gluten intolerance** may be a symptom of celiac disease, which affects the absorption of food in the small intestine, or an allergic response to wheat gluten; however, it is most commonly due to the lack of a necessary digestive enzyme. Possible manifestations include stomach bloating, diarrhea, fatigue, and weight loss.

Food allergies can be related to one or several foods for a given patient. The allergic responses can range from mild to life threatening. The diet must be balanced and free of the allergens.

Eating Disorders

Eating disorders are psychologically induced alterations in nutrition. The most common disorders include anorexia nervosa, bulimia, and binge-eating disorder. **Anorexia nervosa** is seen most commonly in young women and is manifested by a fear of gaining weight and refusal to eat. The effects of this self-imposed starvation can vary from mild nutritional deficits to cardiac failure and death. **Bulimia** is also related to the fear of gaining weight and is manifested by the intake of large amounts of food followed by self-induced vomiting or purging, fasting, and depression. Bulimic patients can sustain significant damage to the mouth and teeth as a result of the effects of gastric acids associated with the vomiting. Binge eating occurs in men and women and is manifested by the regular episodes of the consumption of large amounts of food that are followed by feelings of depression. These individuals are often obese and relate these episodes to being out of control. In general, these diseases are difficult to resolve, and relapses are common.

Stress Management

Stress management is a crucial piece of overall patient well-being. Poorly managed stress has the potential to cause significant health decline. When conducting an assessment, the provider must carefully approach the topic of stress management. Since many of life's stressors cannot be completely changed, the provider will be best served to listen actively, remarking about how certain activities or situations can worsen health conditions. Odd work hours, late night shifts, or working multiple jobs can negatively impact sleep patterns. Without restorative sleep, the patient will have difficulties focusing on treatment-plan adherence. As the lack of sleep continues, the patient can begin to lose focus on a previous goal of maintaining healthy lifestyle choices and return to easier high-risk behaviors.

Once the topic of known sources of stress has been initiated, the provider can go one step further to inquire what steps have been taken to ameliorate those stressors. Next, the patient can be encouraged to state how they have worked to manage the stressors and what has been least effective. It is during this exchange that the patient is more likely to accept recommendations and institute them in daily life. Notably, it is also necessary to uncover sources of stress that are not readily apparent. Ask probing questions about preferred forms of stress relief and relaxation techniques. Encourage patients to seek out trusted members of their support network to communicate their needs and ask for help. Overall, a patient's ability to institute the checks and balances required to alleviate stress is crucial.

Self-Care Strategies

The key to addressing and preventing **burnout** is through self-care and building resilience. Self-care requires balancing personal needs with one's responsibilities to others. **Resiliency** is the ability to effectively respond, adapt, and grow in response to adversity. Ways to promote self-care and resilience include development of skills in the areas of emotional regulation, stress management, communication, and boundary setting. Additionally, it requires a holistic approach to preserving and maintaining personal wellness through mental, physical, emotional, and spiritual health activities.

Several evidence-based strategies have been shown to have a positive impact on self-care and resiliency. One way is by building compassion for oneself as well as gratitude. Strategies to achieve this include practicing positive self-talk, accepting that all humans (including oneself) make mistakes, treating oneself like a loved one or friend, writing or voicing things one is thankful for, and practicing mindfulness. Mindfulness refers to accepting reality in the moment without making judgements. Physical strategies for maintaining self-care include taking breaks, eating regularly, moving one's body, being outside, maintaining good sleep habits, maintaining social relationships and support systems, and journaling.

Stress-Related Illnesses

Short periods of stress (e.g., exercise, problem solving) can be beneficial for the mind and body, but prolonged periods of stress are linked to chronic health illnesses. When the body experiences stress, it activates the **sympathetic nervous system** (SNS). The SNS is part of the nervous system and responsible for creating response behaviors relating to fighting or fleeing the stressor. These response behaviors include increased stress hormone production, extended periods of muscle contraction, and heightened inflammatory response. During prolonged periods of stress, the SNS remains activated.

The **parasympathetic nervous system** (PNS), the part of the nervous system that is responsible for rest, recovery, digestion, immunity, and other normal body processes, becomes suppressed. Over time, this can lead to immune system disorders, gastrointestinal disorders, cardiovascular disorders, mood disorders,

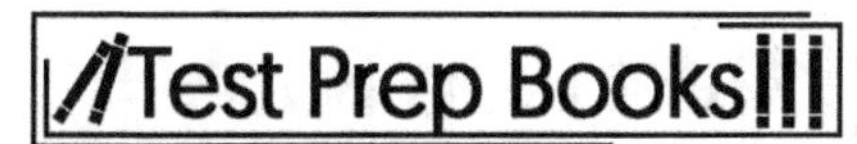

musculoskeletal disorders, and sleep disorders. Illnesses directly linked with chronic stress include autoimmune diseases, depression, anxiety, heart disease, dementia, and ulcers. People who frequently experience stress or are under chronic stress also experience higher incidences of back, neck, and shoulder pain, as well as a higher incidence of acute illnesses like the common cold. They are also less likely to benefit from preventative measures such as vaccinations, simply due to the immune system remaining in a constantly weakened state.

Substance Use

Substance abuse is defined, most simply, as extreme use of a drug. Abuse occurs for many reasons, such as mental health instability, inability to cope with everyday life stressors, the loss of a loved one, or enjoyment of the euphoric state that the overindulgence in a substance causes. Abused substances create some type of intoxication that alters decision-making, awareness, attentiveness, or physical impulses.

Substance abuse results in tolerance, withdrawal, and compulsive drug-taking behavior. **Tolerance** occurs when increased amounts of the substance are needed to achieve the desired effects. **Withdrawal** manifests as physiological and substance-specific cognitive symptoms (e.g., cold sweats, shivering, nausea, vomiting, paranoia, hallucinations). Withdrawal not only happens when an individual stops abusing the substance, but also occurs when he or she attempts to reduce the amount taken to stop using altogether.

Chronic Alcohol Abuse

Considering alcohol is a central nervous system (CNS) depressant, effects of alcohol ingestion tend to include relaxation and lowered inhibitions. However, it also slurs speech and impairs muscle control, coordination, and reflex time. **Alcohol abuse** can cause cirrhosis of the liver; liver, esophagus, and stomach cancers; heart enlargement; chronic inflammation of the pancreas; vitamin deficiencies; certain anemias; and brain damage. Withdrawal from chronic alcohol abuse must be done with caution and in an appropriate timeframe to avoid alcohol withdrawal syndrome.

Chronic Tobacco Abuse

People abuse **tobacco** either in cigarette, cigar, pipe, or snuff form. People report many reasons for tobacco use, including a calming effect, suppression of appetite, and relief of depression. The primary addictive component in tobacco is nicotine, but tobacco smoke also contains about 700 carcinogens (cancer-causing agents) that may result in lung and throat cancers as well as heart disease, emphysema, peptic ulcer disease, and stroke. Withdrawal indicators include insomnia, irritability, overwhelming nicotine craving, anxiety, and depression.

Drug Abuse

Marijuana

Marijuana is considered the most frequently abused illicit drug in the United States. General effects of marijuana use include pleasure, relaxation, and weakened dexterity and memory. The active addictive ingredient in marijuana is tetrahydrocannabinol (THC). It is normally smoked (but can be eaten), and its smoke has more carcinogens than that of tobacco. The individual withdrawing from marijuana will experience increased irritability and anxiety.

Cocaine

Cocaine is a stimulant that can be smoked, injected, snorted, or swallowed. Reported effects include pleasure, enhanced alertness, and increased energy. Both temporary and prolonged use have been known to contribute to damage to the brain, heart, lungs, and kidneys. Withdrawal symptoms include severe depression and reduced energy.

Heroin

Heroin is rapid-acting opioid that is highly addictive. Effects of heroin abuse include pleasure, slower respirations, and drowsiness. Overdose and/or overuse of heroin can cause respiratory depression, resulting in death. Use of heroin as an injectable substance can lead to other complications, such as heart valve damage, tetanus, botulism, hepatitis B, or human immunodeficiency virus (HIV)/AIDS infection from sharing dirty needles. Withdrawal is usually intense and presents as vomiting, abdominal cramps, diarrhea, confusion, body aches, and diaphoresis.

Methamphetamines

Methamphetamine is categorized as a stimulant that produces such effects as pleasure, increased alertness, and decreased appetite. Similar to cocaine, it can be snorted, smoked, or injected, and it can be taken orally as well. Like cocaine, it shares many of the same detrimental effects, such as myocardial infarction, hypertension, and stroke. Other prolonged usage effects include paranoia, hallucinations, damage to and loss of dentition, and heart damage. Withdrawal symptoms involve depression, abdominal cramps, and increased appetite.

Nursing interventions for the individual addicted to tobacco, alcohol, and other drugs centers around the prevention of relapse, and treatment depends on the individual and the substance that is abused. Behavioral treatment assists with recognition of abuse triggers, habits, and drug cravings, as well as providing the tactics to help one cope with these issues. A provider may prescribe nicotine patches for the tobacco abuser and methadone or Suboxone to manage withdrawal symptoms and certain drug yearnings.

Substance Dependence Disorder

When a patient becomes dependent on a substance that causes a disruption in their relationships and physical health, it is called a **substance dependence disorder**. There are several different substances that may cause addiction, including alcohol, tobacco, opioids, hallucinogens, stimulants (e.g., cocaine and amphetamines), and sedatives/hypnotics/anxiolytics (e.g., lorazepam). The patient begins to seek these drugs obsessively, always chasing after the next high. These drug-dependent behaviors, including manipulation, lying, and doing whatever it takes to get the substance, destroy relationships and the patient's ability to function normally.

Intentional Overdose and Ingestions

The definition of an **overdose**, in simplest terms, is a dangerously high amount of something that is generally considered too much. Drug overdoses may be through accidental overuse or intentional misuse. Illicit drugs, which are used to achieve or maintain a euphoric state, may be used hazardously when the body's metabolism cannot detoxify the substance rapidly enough to avoid unplanned side effects. Adolescents and adults are most likely to overdose on one or more substances, either illicit or prescribed, for the purpose of intentionally harming themselves.

Drug overdose symptoms vary with the type of drug taken, but typically they reflect a heightened level of the therapeutic effects seen with prescribed use. In an overdose, the anticipated side effects are more distinct, and other effects that would not normally occur with recommended usage will appear. Vital signs will be erratic (pulse, respirations), mental state will most likely be altered (confusion, intense sleepiness, stupor), angina (chest pain) is possible if overdose caused heart or lung damage, and GI symptoms, such as nausea and vomiting, may be apparent.

Some commonly abused drugs include (but are not limited to) the following:

- Barbiturates: Sedatives like Nembutal® and Seconal®, which are usually prescribed to manage anxiety, panic attacks, and insomnia

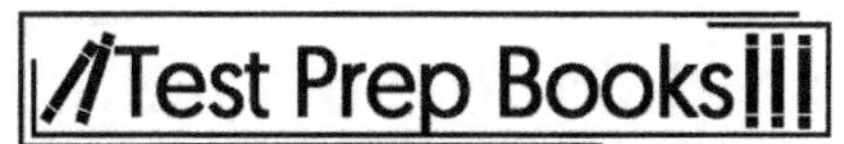

- Benzodiazepines: Sedatives such as Valium® and Xanax®, used to manage anxiety and panic attacks
- Sleep medications: Ambien®, Lunesta®, Sonata®
- Opioids: Pain management drugs such as codeine, morphine, Oxycontin®, Percocet®, and Percodan®
- Opioids plus acetaminophen for pain management: Vicodin®, Lortab®, Lorcet®
- Amphetamines: Stimulants like Adderall® and Dexedrine®; also known as *speed*
- Dextromethorphan (DXM): Common ingredient in OTC medications normally used for cough and other cold symptoms; effective when administered in the correct dosage, but too much causes a euphoric state and hallucinations.
- Pseudoephedrine: Common ingredient in OTC decongestants; it is also a main component of methamphetamine ("meth") and, for this reason, is stored behind the pharmacist's counter

Illicit drug (marijuana, cocaine, heroin) use is at an all-time high, and abuse of one or more of these can lead to detrimental, if not fatal, effects. The youth of America seem especially vulnerable to the risk of overdose of illegal substances, as they are still physically and psychologically developing. Marijuana continues to be the most commonplace prohibited drug used by young people, while cocaine and heroin overdose-related events seem to be chiefly among adults in their mid-to-late thirties.

Withdrawal Syndrome

Withdrawal syndrome refers to the range of physical, mental, and emotional symptoms a patient experiences after ceasing use of an addictive substance, such as alcohol or drugs. Most substances require medically monitored support to effectively stop use if a person has been regularly using the substance; stopping "cold turkey" generally results in highly unpleasant effects. After chronic substance use, the patient's body becomes dependent on the substance and may even require it to function. Often, sudden withdrawal can be dangerous as the patient's body may not be physiologically able to adjust to the substance loss. The intensity of withdrawal syndrome varies based on the type of substance and how long the person was using it. Substances that are known to cause withdrawal symptoms include antidepressants, depressants, opioids, and stimulants.

Withdrawal symptoms may include mood changes, malaise, flu-like symptoms, irritability, sweating, tremors, insomnia, hallucinations, and suicidal ideation. While physical symptoms may only last a few days, psychological symptoms can last for months. These unpleasant feelings can cause people to resume substance use. Therefore, medical monitoring and intervention are especially helpful at first. Medical providers can prescribe non-habit-forming medications that help with the physiological and psychological symptoms. Lifestyle changes during the withdrawal period, such as eating nutritious foods, drinking enough water, increasing physical activity, getting enough sleep, practicing meditation, and utilizing social and family supports can also help reduce symptoms. These changes may also address underlying stressors that perhaps led to the substance abuse in the first place.

Reproductive Life Planning

Reproductive life planning refers to an evidence-based practice of facilitating structured and intentional discussions about a patient's wishes related to current or future pregnancies and incorporating them into her medical care. Practically speaking, practitioners may begin these conversations by asking whether the patient desires any children (or any more children) in the future, and if so, how long she would like to wait until becoming pregnant. This approach empowers individual decision-making and encourages patients to be set up for success if and when they pursue pregnancy. Important points of counseling should include avoiding short intervals between pregnancies (that is, less than 6 months) to reduce the risk of complications to both mother and baby. Additionally, counsel patients to begin taking 400 mcg of folic acid daily at least one month before conceiving. Reproductive life planning also helps both the patient and provider arrange necessary resources to ensure uninterrupted access to prenatal care and addresses any social determinants of health. Although no set structure for these discussions exists, that is to the advantage of each patient engaged in reproductive life planning, as it makes the patient central in her own reproductive healthcare.

Abuse and Violence

Abuse and neglect can take many forms and affect people of various demographics. Children, women, and the elderly tend to be the vulnerable victim populations. Abuse and neglect cases can often put the victim in the emergency room, so medical personnel should be aware that they likely will come across these tragic situations, and intervention may be necessary. It is important to know how to spot abuse and neglect cases for legal and ethical reasons.

Family

In children, abuse and neglect can come from a biological or adoptive parent, guardian, close adult in the child's life, or stranger. Younger children are the most vulnerable individuals in this demographic. This is because they may not be able to speak, defend themselves, or understand that they are being abused, or they may be fearful of reporting a caregiver.

Child abuse can be emotional (such as refusal to provide affection or emotional comfort, criticizing the child in a cruel or unusual manner, or administering humiliation or shame tactics) and may be hard to detect or penalize legally. Physical abuse of a child involves intentional acts of physical violence that could result in injury. Sexual abuse of a child includes sexual acts or interactions by an adult; even if the child provides consent, it is considered abuse, due to the emotional and mental immaturity of the child.

In the United States, legal age of consent varies by state. Signs of abuse in children can include physical indicators, such as cuts, bruises, genital pain or bleeding, and persistent yeast infections. There can also be behavioral indicators, such as slow development, aggression, anxiety, suicidal tendencies, fearful natures, antisocial or awkward behavioral habits, statements describing inappropriate physical or sexual interactions, visibly unusual relationships or interactions with a parent or caregiver, and a lack of desire (or even refusal) to go home.

Child neglect refers to a parent, guardian, or other caretaker's inaction to provide basic care such as food, water, education, medical and dental treatments, safe supervision, and clean and safe living accommodations. Signs of neglect in children can include chronic illness, malnutrition, lack of personal hygiene, above-average school absenteeism, anxiety and depression, and substance abuse.

A single sign may not mean that abuse or neglect is present, but it should be taken seriously by asking further questions and potentially seeking resources, such as social support agencies and legal counsel, to prevent further abuse. Most states require that knowledge of potential abuse or neglect be reported to legal and child protective services. The process of reporting varies by state, and practitioners should familiarize themselves with abuse and neglect reporting practices of the state in which their services will be provided.

Sexual

Sexual assaults are violent, nonconsensual sexual actions against an individual. Common manifestations include the presence of sperm or blood, contusions, local evidence of forceful vaginal penetration, orthopedic injuries, abdominal trauma, and lacerations. The care of a survivor of sexual assault is focused on identifying and treating all injuries; testing and preventive treatment for all possible STDs, HIV, and hepatitis; prescribing preventive antibiotic therapy; and administering interventions aimed at preventing posttraumatic

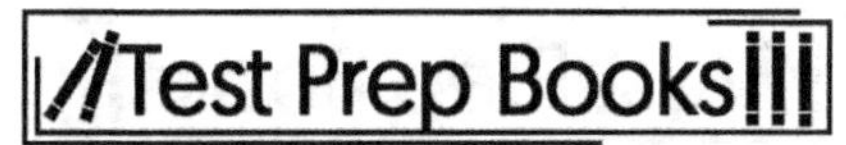

stress disorder (PTSD). Although assault victims might be reluctant or unable to provide a detailed account of the assault, providers are responsible for meticulous and comprehensive documentation to protect the patient's rights. In addition, referrals to appropriate community resources for post-emergency care should be made prior to the patient's discharge from the facility.

Elder

Elder abuse and neglect may occur by family members or other caregivers. Elderly people are vulnerable, as they may be physically weak or have other physical and mental limitations, handicaps, or disabilities. Signs of abuse in elders are similar to those seen in children but can also include the occurrence of adult-minded activities that happen without the elder's consent, such as mishandled financial transactions or healthcare fraud. Physical indicators of abuse in the elderly include bruises, broken bones, and signs of physical restraint. Behavioral indicators include poor relationships with caregivers, anxiety, depression, and a fearful nature. Indicators of neglect in the elderly include missed or improper medication administration, signs of poor hygiene, genital or anal rashes, and malnutrition.

Unfortunately, many signs of elder abuse and neglect are similar to signs of dementia, a natural reaction to ailing health, and other behaviors commonly exhibited by this age demographic. Therefore, due diligence by medical personnel is necessary. All states have elder abuse prevention laws, though procedures for reporting may vary by state, so it is important to know the process for the state in which services will be administered.

Intimate Partner Violence (IPV)

Domestic violence between adult partners, also known as intimate partner violence and abuse, is also a common form of abuse that can require emergency department visits. While this type of abuse can be experienced by partners of either gender or orientation, it is most commonly inflicted by male partners on female victims. Physical indicators of abuse from a partner include marks such as bruises, black eyes, genital or anal damage, scratches, and welts. Behavioral indicators include a fearful nature, low self-esteem, isolation, anxiety, depression, constant excuses for the abusing partner's dangerous actions, and suicidal tendencies. Again, the presence of one sign may not indicate that abuse is occurring, but it can be a call to action to provide resources for the victim's safety.

Human Trafficking

Most trafficking victims are women or young men. Many victims are accompanied by their trafficker, which can complicate the processes of identifying and helping them. They generally show signs of physical and mental abuse. A red flag that warrants further attention is when a patient is accompanied by someone who appears overly involved in the case but does not seem to be genuinely concerned about the patient; this is often the trafficker. Their identification may indicate no relation to the patient, but they will insist that they are a friend or romantic partner. They may control all of the patient's personal identification and insist on paying in cash. The trafficker may be highly resistant to letting the patient go anywhere alone with the healthcare provider, yet this is the best way to identify whether someone is a trafficking victim and help them out of the situation. Many victims are seen for medical issues that do not result from trafficked activities but from delays in receiving routine care. For example, a woman who is being trafficked may become pregnant and not receive prenatal care until she is in an emergency situation.

Most healthcare facilities have specific policies and procedures in place to identify and screen trafficking victims. Screening processes should be age appropriate and sensitive in order to help the victim in the most dignified and compassionate manner possible. In most states, adult victims must choose whether they want an intervention. However, all healthcare providers can anonymously and safely report any suspicions of possibly trafficked individuals to the necessary authorities. Intervention can be a traumatic event for the patient and must be handled cautiously, while also ensuring that it is performed quickly and that the trafficker is restrained. Social services, legal services, and law enforcement are often a part of any intervention, making it a highly complex and collaborative initiative.

Parenting

There are four primary types of **parenting styles**. Each of these styles involve parenting in a particular way, which can have different effects on children.

- Authoritarian: This type of parenting is all about control. Parents who use this style are mostly concerned with setting rules and ensuring their children abide by the rules. Typically, there is a strict and set punishment procedure as well. Children who are raised under this type of parenting style often have issues with social development and communication. These children often go on to use this type of interactions in their relationships outside of their family.
- Uninvolved/Neglectful: This type of parenting style is essentially the opposite of the authoritarian style. These parents hardly parent their children and delegate control and care to secondary caregivers or to the children themselves. Children raised in these type environments often have issues with impulse control, authority, and rule following outside of their homes.
- Indulgent/Permissive: This type of parenting style is very loving and involved with the child. However, this approach to parenting does not typically use rules appropriately or set healthy boundaries. Parents using this style are often more concerned with being a friend figure to their children rather than a traditional parent. Children raised in this manner are often very creative; however, they also tend to be entitled with little self-control and act selfishly in their relationships.
- Authoritative: This type of parenting style is generally regarded as the most desirable type. Parents using this style of parenting will allow their children increasing levels of independence appropriate for their age. Parents will also have clear cut rules and linked consequences. Children who grow up in these type of households are usually seen with increased self-sufficiency and better social skills and self-control.

Sexuality

Sexual dysfunction can be caused by multiple influences, including erectile dysfunction (ED) in men and painful vaginal conditions in women. A physical examination is necessary to detect and treat conditions. Detection of lumps, discharge, or abnormal odors can be assessed during a pelvic examination in the female patient. The frequency of performing a cervical cancer screening for female patients via a Papanicolaou (Pap) smear varies depending on their age and previous results. According to the American Cancer Society, cervical screening should begin at 21 years of age and be repeated every 3 years. Beginning at age 30, a Pap smear, combined with HPV screening, is recommended until the age of 65. Follow-up screening is required for patients with abnormal results within a 6-month to 1-year time frame.

Sexually transmitted infections (**STIs**) are a common diagnosis in the United States. It is important to assess the patient's health practices during the patient history. Unsafe sex practices and the number of sexual partners can be a determinant for further STI screening, which can be performed via urine, blood, or genital swab tests. Treatment of STIs is dependent on the type of disease and includes oral medications, injections, and topical creams. Pregnancy planning and prevention are important topics for female patients. There are numerous contraception methods that can be discussed. The expected outcomes are for patients to understand the adverse effects, effectiveness, affordability, and convenience of the chosen method. Backup methods should also be discussed, particularly concerning the prevention of STIs.

Gender Identity

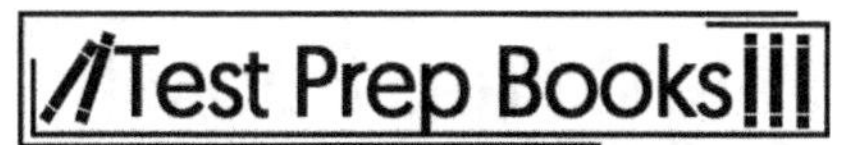

Gender refers to a person's subjective experience of being male or female. **Sexual orientation** has to do with sexual attraction, and includes those who identify as homosexual, heterosexual, asexual, or bisexual.

Gender identity is a person's understanding of their own gender, especially as it relates to being male or female (or something else). **Gender expression** is one's outward presentation (e.g., clothing, hair style, physical appearance) and behaviors that communicate or show their gender identity. Sexual orientation is a more complex concept as it refers to the sexual attraction one feels toward others.

Types of Gender Identity

- Bi-gender: An individual who fluctuates between the self-image of traditionally male and female stereotypes and identifies with both genders.
- Gender Nonconforming: An individual who has a gender identity or expression that is different than the norms associated with the gender they were assigned at birth.
- Genderqueer: A term for an individual who may think of themselves as both male and female, a third or other gender, or moving between the two binary genders.
- Transgender: A generalized term referring to a variety of sexual identities that do not fit under more traditional categories, a person who feels to be of a different gender than was assigned at birth.
- Transsexual: A person who identifies emotionally and psychologically, and sometimes physically, with the gender other than that assigned at birth; lives as a person of the opposite gender.

Those who are transgender or transsexual may be homosexual, heterosexual, or asexual. Sexual identity and sexual attraction are independent.

Gender Dysphoria

Gender dysphoria occurs when distress develops from a conflict between a patient's assigned sex at birth and their gender identity. This internal conflict leads to emotional distress, discomfort with sex characteristics, and a desire to transition to the identified gender. Diagnostic criteria from the DSM-5 include notable incongruences between sex assigned at birth and expressed gender for six or more months, with significant distress in important functioning areas and at least two of the following: strong desire to change/remove sex characteristics, strong desire to be of opposite gender, strong desire to be treated as the opposite gender, and strong conviction of possessing the typical feelings of the opposite gender.

Psychotherapy, including gender-affirming therapy and cognitive behavioral therapy, is used to manage gender incongruence and develop coping strategies. Medical management includes puberty suppressants for adolescents with early-onset gender dysphoria, hormone replacement therapy, and gender-affirming surgeries. Antidepressants and anxiolytics may be used when depression and anxiety are present. Gender-affirming social transitions, such as name and pronoun changes, may also help to reduce gender incongruence.

Preconception Counseling

Preconception care begins with asking patients of reproductive age whether they desire pregnancy in the near future. For those who do, care should focus on health optimization, such as screening for STIs, cervical cancer, diabetes, hypertension, thyroid disease, and intimate partner violence. Appropriate advice on nutrition and immunizations is important, and clinicians should encourage patients to begin prenatal vitamins containing folic acid.

Immunizations

Part of preventive care is promotion of immunity. **Immunization** records should be obtained from patients during their visit. Education regarding immunization schedules and the need for disease prevention should be shared with patients and/or caregivers. The vast majority of immunizations are administered during the first 15 months of life. Remaining doses of immunization series are given throughout childhood and adolescence. Disease-specific immunizations are given initially or as a booster throughout adulthood. The hepatitis B vaccine is administered initially at birth. The second dose is given a month or two later. The third dose can be administered from the age of 6 to 18 months. The hepatitis A vaccine is a two-dose series that requires a 6-month interval and can be administered beginning at the age of 12 months. The first dose of the RV, DTaP, Hib, PCV13, and IPV should be administered at 2 months of age. The second and third doses may be given in 2-month intervals. DTaP, Hib, and PCV13 require additional doses and can be given after 12 months of age.

The MMR and varicella vaccines are two-dose series that are given at 1 year of age and a second dose between the ages of 4 and 6. The meningococcal vaccine is a two-dose series administered at the age of 11 and a second dose at the age of 16. The HPV vaccine is recommended at the age of 11 or 12. The HPV vaccine can be administered at the age of 9. Past the age of 26, the HPV vaccine can be discussed and administered through the age of 45. The influenza vaccine is an annual vaccine that can be administered beginning at the age of 6 months. In adulthood, a DTaP booster should be administered every 10 years. The zoster recombinant vaccine (RZV) is recommended for older adults beginning at 50 years of age. The Shingrix vaccine is a two-dose series with a minimal interval of 4 weeks. The pneumococcal polysaccharide vaccine (PPSV23) is recommended for adults over the age of 65. Adults with chronic medical conditions, such as diabetes, liver disease, or alcoholism, should be encouraged to receive the vaccine as early as 19 years of age.

Vaccine Information Statement (VIS)

The Centers for Disease Control and Prevention (CDC) issues a **Vaccine Information Statement** that documents the benefits and risks associated with an individual vaccine.

The provider must supply the Vaccine Information Statement to the patient or the patient's legal representative before the vaccine is administered.

Vaccine Adverse Event Reporting System (VAERS)

Patients may develop an adverse effect when they receive a vaccine. Should injury be caused by the vaccine administration, healthcare providers are required by law to report adverse effects such as anaphylaxis and skin reactions to the toxoid that occur shortly after a vaccine is administered. The **Vaccine Adverse Event Reporting System** (**VAERS**) is a program analyzed by the Centers for Disease Control and Prevention (CDC) and the FDA. The report should include information on the patient, reporter, facility, vaccine, and accompanying details. All reports filed on the VAERS system are analyzed to determine whether the adverse events were directly caused by the vaccine or resulted from a medical condition or other occurrence.

Practice Quiz

1. Which item in the family history assessment performed by women's health nurse practitioner is a red flag for hypertrophic cardiomyopathy and should be investigated further?
   a. Heart disease of the father
   b. Diabetes mellitus of the mother
   c. Sudden death of a grandmother
   d. Stroke of a grandfather

2. Which of the following anemia categories, in which heme and globin do not synthesize appropriately, does thalassemia fall into?
   a. Thrombocytic
   b. Macrocytic
   c. Normocytic
   d. Microcytic

3. Which of the following metabolic components involved in diabetic ketoacidosis is responsible for the "fruity" smell that a person with DKA gives off when they breathe?
   a. Alanine
   b. Triglycerides
   c. Acetone
   d. Glycerol

4. Which of the following statements correctly identifies the relationship between hypokalemia and the development and duration of an ileus?
   a. K level of 6.0 mEq/L causes metabolic alkalosis, which affects the bowel wall motility.
   b. K level of 2.6 mEq/L causes muscle weakness that can progress to paralysis of the intestinal musculature.
   c. K level of 4.5 mEq/L decreases the capillary permeability of the bowel wall, which decreases the amount of gastric fluid in the bowel.
   d. K level of 3.7 mEq/L increases the incidence of vomiting, which further decreases the bowel contents.

5. Which of the following is the *best* example of a patient-centered health goal statement?
   a. Patient will demonstrate safe and effective self-administration of insulin.
   b. Patient will complete IV antibiotic therapy in two days.
   c. Patient will be able to walk for ten minutes, twice daily, before discharge.
   d. Patient will verbalize pain level of five out of ten or less throughout day shift.

See answers on the next page

Answer Explanations

1. C: The sudden death of a grandmother needs to be probed for if a cause was determined. If she passed away suddenly because of hypertrophic cardiomyopathy that had been previously undiagnosed before autopsy, the patient should be screened for this condition as well, as it often may be asymptomatic until syncope or sudden death occurs. The other three items listed are of value, but do not point toward hypertrophic cardiomyopathy specifically.

2. D: Thalassemia is considered a microcytic anemia, in which heme and globin do not synthesize appropriately, and oxygen-carrying capacity is compromised. Normocytic anemias are those that include normally sized red blood cells that are deficient in number. Aplastic anemia is an example of a normocytic anemia. Macrocytic anemias are defined as red blood cells that are quite large in shape, leading to abnormalities in oxygen-carrying ability and oxygen delivery. Thrombocytic refers to a platelet, a different component of the blood, and is thus irrelevant in this scenario.

3. C: Acetone, a ketoacid produced during the breakdown of fatty acids during diabetic ketoacidosis, is expelled through respiration, thus giving a person in DKA a "fruity" smell to the breath. Glycerol and alanine are byproducts of fat and muscle breakdown as alternative energy sources convert to glucose. Triglycerides are broken down into free fatty acids as another alternative to glucose as energy for metabolism in the body.

4. B: Serum potassium levels less than 3 mEq/L are associated with generalized muscle weakness, which includes the intestinal musculature. If hypokalemia is present in post-operative patients, the potential for the development of an ileus increases, and the duration of an existing ileus also increases. A potassium level of 6.0 mEq/L (Choice *A*) is associated with metabolic acidosis, rather than alkalosis, and there is no relationship between this potassium level and the motility of the bowel wall. The remaining potassium levels (Choices *C* and *D*) are normal and not associated with any alteration of the intestine.

5. C: "Patient will be able to walk for ten minutes, twice daily, prior to discharge." is the *best* example of a patient-centered goal statement. Effective goal statements can be formulated using the *SMART* goal criteria: specific, measurable, achievable, relevant, and time-bound. Choice *A* is not the best example of a patient-centered goal statement, as the statement could be more specific and is not measurable or time-bound. Choice *B* is also not the best example of a patient-centered goal because this is not patient-driven and is not specific or measurable. Choice *D* is also not the best choice because this goal does not provide a specific means to achieve the pain level of five out of ten or less.

Gynecologic and Reproductive Health

Reproductive Anatomy and Physiology

Anatomy and Physiology of Reproduction Throughout the Life Cycle

The major organs of the female reproductive organs include the uterus, cervix, vagina, ovaries, and fallopian tubes.

The **uterus** is a hollow, pear-shaped organ with a muscular layer that is positioned between the bladder and the rectum. The uterus terminates at the **cervix**, which opens into the **vagina**, which is open to the outside of the body. The **ovaries**, supported by several ligaments, are oval organs one to two inches long that are positioned on either side of the uterus in the pelvic cavity. The **fallopian tubes**, which are four inches long and half an inch in diameter, connect the uterus with the ovaries.

The male reproductive organs include the penis, scrotum, testicles, vas deferens, seminal vesicles, and the prostate gland. In addition to the urethra, the **penis** contains three sections of erectile tissue. The **scrotum** is a fibromuscular pouch that contains the testes, the spermatic cord, and the epididymis. The pair of **testes** is suspended in the scrotum and each one is approximately two inches by one inch long. The **vas deferens** is a tubular pathway between the testes and the penis, and the **seminal vesicles** are small organs located between the bladder and the bowel. The **prostate gland** surrounds the proximal end of the urethra within the pelvic cavity.

The main function of the male reproductive system is the production of **sperm**. Unlike the female, beginning at puberty, several million immature sperm are produced every day in the testes. The sperm are transported through the vas deferens to the penis, and the prostate gland and seminal vesicles contribute fluids that support the activity of the sperm after ejaculation.

At puberty, **egg** maturation, menses, and sperm production begin, and the secondary sex characteristics appear. Female fertility declines at thirty years of age, and the maturation of eggs in the ovaries ceases at menopause, which occurs at fifty years of age. Sperm production continues from puberty until death; however, after sixty years of age the ability of the sperm to travel to the fallopian tube to fertilize an egg is decreased.

Hypogonadism

Hypogonadism is characterized by the malfunction of the ovaries in women or testes in men, which results in low estrogen and testosterone levels, respectively. If hypogonadism is diagnosed prior to puberty, women may experience a decrease in breast development and absence in menstruation, while men exhibit a delay in voice and facial hair development. When hypogonadism presents after puberty, issues with low libido, hot flashes, decreased muscle mass, infertility, and low energy may appear. Hypogonadism can be primary or secondary. Primary hypogonadism is characterized by low testosterone levels with high luteinizing hormone (LH) levels and is associated with testicular malfunction. Secondary hypogonadism involves low testosterone levels as well as low LH levels due to pituitary or hypothalamus dysfunction. Men over forty-five years of age are at the highest risk of developing hypogonadism. Diagnosis is made with laboratory testing of estrogen levels in women and testosterone levels in men, along with follicle-stimulating hormone (FSH) and LH levels. **Testosterone** tests must be taken in the morning and result in less than 300 nanograms per deciliter twice to confirm the diagnosis. Treatment includes testosterone replacement therapy for men and estrogen or progesterone replacement therapy for women.

Menarche

Menarche refers to the onset of menstruation in adolescent female patients, which normally occurs between 10 and 16 years of age. Physiologic development leads to pulsatile secretion of gonadotropin-releasing hormone (GnRH) by the hypothalamus and, in turn, FSH and LH by the anterior pituitary gland. Proper adrenal, thyroid, and ovarian function is also necessary for regular menses. Menarche should occur 2 to 3 years after thelarche (the appearance of breast buds). At least the first several menstrual cycles after menarche are often irregular; in most patients, menses become more regular by 3 years after menarche, with cycles ranging from every 21 to every 35 days. Importantly, menarche is considered early if it occurs before age 10 and late if it is delayed past age 15. Primary amenorrhea refers to the absence of menses by age 15 in the presence of secondary sexual characteristics or by 13 in the absence of secondary characteristics. Conversely, secondary amenorrhea refers to the absence of menses for over 6 months in a previously menstruating patient. The most common cause of secondary amenorrhea is pregnancy.

Menopause

Menopause refers to the permanent cessation of estrogen release by the ovaries; it is diagnosed after twelve consecutive months of amenorrhea. The median age of occurrence is fifty-one, and menopause is preceded by perimenopause, which involves fluctuations in estrogen production leading to irregular menses. Though menopause is a normal process, it causes multiple symptoms that may diminish quality of life. Vasomotor symptoms ("hot flashes") are the most common—and disruptive—manifestation of menopause and may be the first signal of its approach. Patients report sudden waves of heat accompanied by flushing and sweating; these commonly occur at night. Patients may experience mood swings, sleep disturbances, and dyspareunia due to vulvovaginal atrophy, dryness, and itching. Though unnecessary, a serum FSH test will return elevated.

Treatment of vasomotor symptoms includes avoidance of caffeine, spicy foods, and alcohol; the administration of certain medications such as duloxetine or clonidine; and, for eligible patients, estrogen replacement therapy. For patients with an intact uterus, this must be given as combined estrogen-progesterone to offset the risk of endometrial hyperplasia. Patients must also be counseled on multiple other risks, including breast cancer and venous thromboembolism.

Gynecologic – Disorders

Bartholin Gland Abscess/Cyst

The **Bartholin glands** are two mucus-producing glands that aid in vaginal lubrication. They are located at the lower right and left aspects of the introitus. If a gland becomes blocked, accumulation of fluid produces a cyst. These are frequently asymptomatic, but patients may experience pelvic pain, dysuria, or dyspareunia. Physical exam typically shows an asymmetric vaginal introitus with a unilateral protuberance in the four- or eight o'clock positions. Clinicians should ask patients about excessive tenderness, purulent drainage, or erythema given the possibility of abscess formation. In the absence of symptoms or exam findings suspicious for abscess formation (e.g., erythema, induration, severe tenderness, or fluctuance), abscess is very unlikely. Conservative treatment is sufficient for **Bartholin cysts**; if painful, patients may use over-the-counter analgesics and sitz baths. Otherwise, most cysts drain spontaneously. If abscess is suspected, incision and drainage with Word catheter placement is the treatment of choice.

Menstrual Disorders

Premenstrual Syndrome (PMS)

Premenstrual syndrome (**PMS**) refers to a wide range of somatic, emotional, and psychological symptoms experienced by some patients in the luteal phase, or second half, of the menstrual cycle. The exact

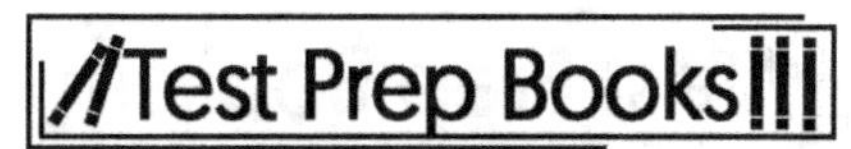

pathophysiology remains unclear; most hypotheses center around the estrogen deficiency and progesterone surge that characterize the luteal cycle, though dysregulation of serotonin has also been theorized. Patients may experience appetite or weight changes, abdominal or back pain, headache, breast swelling or pain, constipation, irritability, mood swings, fatigue, insomnia, and/or restlessness. PMS is distinct from the more severe premenstrual dysphoric disorder (PMDD), which is an established Diagnostic and Statistical Manual of Mental Disorders, 5th Edition (DSM-5), diagnosis often treated with SSRIs. Importantly, treatment should begin with a conversation with the patient about her experience and symptoms. Depending on which symptoms predominate, treatment may include any combination of the following: lifestyle modifications such as sleep hygiene and regular exercise; cognitive behavioral therapy; medications such as NSAIDs, SSRIs, or hormonal therapy such as contraceptives; and other modalities, such as massage or light therapy. Consider encouraging patients to maintain a journal of symptoms to assess for variability between cycles.

Premenstrual Dysphoric Disorder (PMDD)

Premenstrual dysphoric disorder is a severe form of premenstrual syndrome that results in significant mood and behavior changes as well as physical symptoms that impair daily functioning. The exact cause is unknown; however, contributing factors include hormonal fluctuations (causing serotonin dysregulation), stress, history of trauma/abuse, family history of mood disorders, and abnormal hypothalamic-pituitary-adrenal axis or thyroid functioning.

Diagnostic criteria from the DSM-5 include at least five mood and physical symptoms that cause notable distress to daily function (e.g., depressed mood, irritability, mood swings, anxiety, fatigue, sleep trouble, appetite changes, joint/muscle pain, and bloating). These symptoms occur in the luteal phase of the menstrual cycle, improve within a few days of beginning menstruation, and subside by the end of the menstrual period. Tracking of at least two menstrual cycles with timing and severity of symptoms is also helpful to confirm diagnosis. Differential diagnoses to rule out include major depressive disorder, generalized anxiety disorder, thyroid disorders, anemia, sleep disorders, and chronic fatigue syndrome.

Nonpharmacological interventions include lifestyle adjustments, dietary changes (e.g., limitations on caffeine, sugar, and alcohol), regular exercise, stress reduction, and good sleep hygiene. For severe cases or when lifestyle adjustments are not successful in managing symptoms, medications such as SSRIs, SNRIs, and oral contraceptives may be prescribed. Anxiolytics, NSAIDs, and diuretics may also be used to manage physical symptoms like pain and anxiety.

Primary and Secondary Amenorrhea

Menstruation is vaginal bleeding that occurs when the uterus sheds its lining if an ovum is not implanted. Female menstrual cycles vary, and a health history should be taken to determine the cycle length. The lack of menstruation is known as **amenorrhea**. Amenorrhea can result from primary and secondary causes. **Primary amenorrhea** is the absence of menarche by the age of 16. Pubertal growth and development should be assessed. **Secondary amenorrhea** occurs when menstruation is absent for at least three cycles in women who menstruate regularly.

For women who have menstrual periods in intervals that are more than 35 days, 9 months without a period is a form of secondary amenorrhea. The first condition to rule out is pregnancy. Discontinuation of contraceptive use may cause amenorrhea. Patients with weight extremes, such as anorexia or obesity, may also experience an absence of menstruation. A disorder with a classic sign of amenorrhea is polycystic ovarian syndrome (PCOS). Female patients with PCOS are usually obese and show large cystic ovaries in an ultrasound. Excess production of testosterone leads to overgrowth of facial, chest, and back hair, termed hirsutism.

Dysmenorrhea

Dysmenorrhea refers to painful menstruation and is divided into primary (not associated with underlying pathology) or secondary (resulting from underlying pathology) types. Dysmenorrhea occurs in up to 90 percent of menstruating women, with at least 30 percent experiencing severe pain. Primary dysmenorrhea is considered related to over-secretion of prostaglandins from the uterine lining. Prostaglandins then increase uterine contraction and pressure during menses, accounting for pain. This process, combined with high levels of COX-2 during menses, has made NSAIDs a first-line treatment for primary dysmenorrhea. Secondary dysmenorrhea, conversely, is most often caused by endometriosis or adenomyosis; these should be considered in every patient complaining of dysmenorrhea, and it is crucial to take these complaints seriously, as they can greatly affect patients' quality of life. In addition to pain, dysmenorrhea may cause fatigue, headache, nausea, vomiting, and even diarrhea. In addition to NSAIDs, heat application to the lower abdomen has been shown to be highly effective in some patients. Moderate exercise and a well-balanced diet are also recommended as patients are able. Hormonal contraceptives may be necessary in some patients as well. Crucially, maintain a low threshold for further evaluation in any patient whose symptoms do not improve, as a pelvic exam and/or ultrasound may suggest underlying pathology, such as endometriosis or adenomyosis.

Vaginitis/Vaginosis

Vaginitis is inflammation of the vaginal canal, and is has multiple possible causes, including **bacterial vaginosis** (**BV**), candidiasis, and trichomoniasis. BV is caused by dysregulation of normal vaginal flora; predisposing factors include sexual activity with multiple partners, low socioeconomic status, and insufficient hydrogen peroxide-secreting lactobacilli. Infectious causes include candidiasis (fungal), which is caused by vaginal pH changes, diabetes, and antibiotic use, and trichomoniasis (protozoan), an STI.

Diagnosis of BV uses Amsel's four criteria: thin clear-white discharge; vaginal pH over 4.5; more than twenty percent clue cells on wet mount; and a positive "whiff" test, wherein application of potassium hydroxide to discharge produces a fishy amine odor. BV is diagnosed when three of four criteria are met, and metronidazole is the treatment of choice.

Candidiasis presents with vaginal redness, itching, and burning accompanied by thick, white, cheese-like discharge. Vaginal pH is typically less than 4.5, and wet mount reveals spores or budding hyphae. Treatment consists of either one-time oral fluconazole or vaginal application of an -azole antifungal.

Finally, **trichomoniasis** features malodorous, frothy white, yellow, or green discharge along with marked erythema and severe itching. Wet mount reveals flagellated trichomonads; vaginal pH over 4.5 also supports diagnosis. Like BV, trichomoniasis is best treated with metronidazole for both patient and partner(s). Patients with trichomoniasis should also be screened for other STIs.

Sexually Transmitted Infections

Chancroid

Chancroid is a type of sexually transmitted infection caused by a highly contagious bacterium, *H. ducreyi*. Patients present with deep, painful ulcers on the genitalia. Laboratory diagnosis is not needed; instead, clinical criteria can be met to confirm diagnosis. These include one or more painful ulcers, swollen lymph nodes in the groin, no evidence of *Treponema pallidum* infection confirmed by microscopy of exudate, and negative herpes simplex virus. Patients should be treated with antibiotics, typically azithromycin, ceftriaxone, ciprofloxacin, or erythromycin. After three to seven days of antibiotic therapy, patients should be reassessed to ensure clinical improvement. Patients should be advised to avoid sexual activity until the infection has completely cleared.

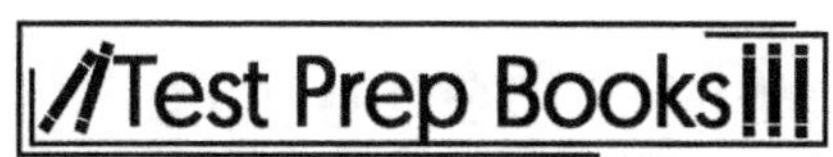

Chlamydia

The most common sexually transmitted infective agent in the United States is **chlamydia**, which is spread by unprotected vaginal, oral, or anal sexual activity. The organism can also be transmitted to an infant delivered vaginally by an infected mother. Risk factors common to all sexually transmitted diseases (STDs) include a history of multiple sexual partners, unprotected sexual intercourse, coinfection with other infective agents, and young age, with most infections occurring in women from fifteen to twenty-four years old. Chlamydial infections may be asymptomatic, which has prompted the U.S. Preventive Services Task Force to recommend routine screening of all females fifteen to twenty-four years of age and all females older than twenty-four who have identifiable risk factors for chlamydia.

Manifestations are specific to the involved organs, as either contained to the vagina and cervix or affecting the uterus, and fallopian tubes and include abnormal vaginal bleeding, rectal and vaginal discharge, and possible infection of the conjunctiva if the patient is pregnant. Diagnostic tests for lower tract infections include Pap smear, pregnancy tests, cultures, and HIV tests, while the diagnosis of infection of the upper GYN tract includes ultrasonography and CT scanning. Untreated infections often result in pelvic inflammatory disease (PID), infertility, and chronic pelvic pain. The treatment of lower tract infection is the administration of a single dose of azithromycin that is witnessed and confirmed by a health care provider to decrease costs of noncompliance. More complicated infections require extended antibiotic therapy to avoid long-term complications.

Gonorrhea

Gonorrhea infections are associated with risk factors, manifestations, complications, and diagnostic studies, similar to chlamydia infections. Newborns are treated prophylactically for gonorrhea infections; however, care of a child with a gonorrheal infection involves collection of appropriate samples for possible forensic investigation. Untreated gonorrhea can progress to PID, and rarely, to gonococcemia or fatal systemic shock. Typical treatment includes ceftriaxone and azithromycin.

Syphilis

Syphilis can progress through four stages if left untreated, with manifestations ranging from the initial chancre at the point of contact to systemic neurological effects, including dementia. Penicillin is the treatment of choice, and the dosage protocol is specific to the stage of the infection when diagnosed.

Trichomoniasis

Trichomoniasis is a parasitic infection caused by *Trichomonas vaginalis*. It is spread through sexual contact, including vaginal, oral, and anal sex. Many patients will not have symptoms. Males may experience frothy penile discharge, burning or painful ejaculation or urination, or itching inside the penis. Females may experience vaginal discharge that is white, green, or yellow, malodourous, and thin or foamy; irritation of the vagina; and pain or discomfort during urination and sex. Trichomoniasis is a very common non-viral infection, and people with greater risk factors include those who have had multiple unprotected sexual encounters, incarcerated individuals, and African American women. For diagnosis, a physical exam of the genitals or a pelvic exam should be completed. In addition, a vaginal swab and urine sample should be obtained. Nucleic acid amplification test (NAAT) should be completed on the sample to confirm diagnosis. Trichomoniasis is treated with a course of antibiotics, such as metronidazole and tinidazole.

Cervicitis

Cervicitis is an inflammation of the cervix most often caused by infection. The most common culprit is *Chlamydia trachomatis*, followed by *Neisseria gonorrhoeae* and *Trichomonas vaginalis*. All three are sexually transmitted infections (STIs). As such, risk factors for cervicitis include multiple sexual partners, inconsistent use of protection, and illicit sexual contact. Patients typically complain of vaginal discharge that is readily visible on physical exam. Purulent discharge indicates chlamydia or gonorrhea, while frothy clear to green discharge from a deep red "strawberry cervix" denotes trichomoniasis. Conversely, vesicular cervical lesions suggest infection with herpes simplex virus.

An exam revealing pelvic pain or cervical motion tenderness is concerning for **pelvic inflammatory disease** (**PID**). Appropriate testing includes nucleic acid amplification testing (NAAT) for chlamydia and gonorrhea; wet mount to identify motile trichomonads; and urine sample for pregnancy and UTI testing. The patient and all partner(s) must be treated and advised to abstain from sexual contact during treatment. Doxycycline and ceftriaxone are typically given together to cover chlamydia and gonorrhea, respectively. Trichomoniasis is best treated with metronidazole. Full treatment is essential to prevent serious complications such as PID, infertility, ectopic pregnancy, and tubo-ovarian abscess.

Pelvic Inflammatory Disease (PID)

PID is a potential complication of untreated or recurrent infection by any of the organisms that are sexually transmitted; however, PID most commonly results from chlamydial infection. The infection and inflammation proceed from the vagina through the cervix to the uterus and fallopian tube, with eventual progression to the abdominal cavity. The most common presenting manifestations include lower abdominal pain and possible abnormal vaginal discharge.

Untreated, the condition leads to systemic manifestations that include fever and elevated sedimentation rate. Complaints of upper right quadrant pain may be associated with Fitz-Hugh–Curtis syndrome (perihepatitis), which may present with jaundice and altered liver function studies. Diagnosis is made by the patient's history and physical and the exclusion of pregnancy or other pelvic pathology as the cause of the patient's pain. Treatment is focused on the relief of pain, resolution of the infection, decreasing the risk of long-term effects including sterility and the risk for obstetrical failure, and preventing further transmission of the infective agent. Antibiotic therapy is the treatment of choice and is generally effective in up to 75 percent of cases of PID, with surgery indicated for patients who do not respond to antibiotics.

Pelvic Pain

The differential diagnosis of **pelvic pain** is broad, and workup should begin with a thorough history. Ask about the onset, location, duration, frequency, timing, severity, and quality of the pain. Overall, dysmenorrhea is the most common cause of pelvic pain and is defined by its cyclical nature and concomitant menstrual bleeding. Irritative voiding symptoms suggest cystitis and warrant evaluation with a urinalysis and urine culture. The presence of systemic symptoms like fever and chills is concerning for pyelonephritis or pelvic inflammatory disease; depending on age and risk factors, patients may need evaluation in the emergency department with advanced imaging. The combination of dysmenorrhea, dysuria, dyschezia, and dyspareunia is suspicious for endometriosis. Additional possible causes of intermittent pelvic pain include uterine fibroids, functional ovarian cysts, or irritable bowel syndrome. Acute, severe, and unilateral pelvic pain may represent a medical or even surgical emergency; serious conditions that must not be missed include appendicitis, ovarian torsion, and ectopic pregnancy. Diagnostic testing may include any combination of the following: pelvic exam, urinalysis, STI testing, pregnancy test, pelvic or transvaginal ultrasound, and/or CT scan. Treatment depends on the identified cause.

Endometriosis

Endometriosis is a difficult diagnosis but one that is painful and disruptive to many women. It involves growth of endometrial tissue outside the uterus, most often on the ovary or elsewhere in the pelvis. Risk factors include early menarche, short menstrual cycles, heavy flow, and family history. Pain is often cyclical as ectopic endometrium is hormone-sensitive; as such, it thickens and bleeds along with the menstrual cycle.

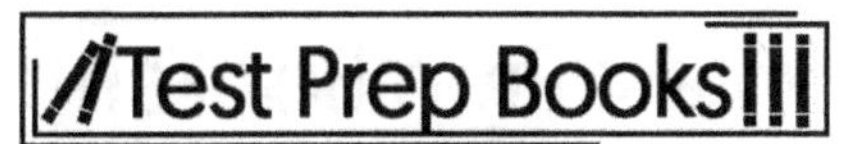

Unfortunately, endometriosis is often misdiagnosed as normal menstrual pain. Patient concerns must be taken seriously and never dismissed. Symptoms include dysuria, dyschezia, dyspareunia, dysmenorrhea, and/or infertility.

Physical exam may reveal an immobile and/or retroverted uterus, palpable pelvic masses, or cervical motion tenderness. Masses may be visible on the ovaries or bladder via ultrasound, but diagnosis can only be confirmed by laparoscopy for direct visual assessment. Treatment is targeted toward pain control and maintenance of fertility. Symptoms may be improved with acetaminophen, NSAIDs, and combined or progesterone-only contraceptives. Ectopic endometrial tissue may be surgically removed; however, it is known to grow back and produce recurrent symptoms.

Adenomyosis

Adenomyosis refers to the abnormal presence of endometrial tissue located within the myometrium, or the thick muscular layer of the uterine wall. The most plausible hypothesis for its cause involves disruption of the boundary between the endometrium and myometrium, allowing for infiltration of endometrial tissue followed by angiogenesis and hypertrophy of the adjacent myometrial tissue. Patients typically describe heavy and/or painful menses but may also report chronic pain or dyspareunia. A fair portion of patients, though, deny any symptoms. Classically, a large "boggy" uterus is described on physical exam, though uterine tenderness may be the only finding. Transvaginal ultrasound is the first-line diagnostic study and may reveal increased vascularity of the myometrium, smooth muscle hypertrophy, and/or endometrial proliferation. If the ultrasound is nondiagnostic and other causes of pelvic pain have been ruled out, magnetic resonance imaging (MRI) may be considered. Once diagnosed, treatment typically starts with NSAIDs or contraceptive therapies, the latter of which alleviate symptoms by reducing the effects of estrogen, which promotes endometrial growth. Patients in whom symptoms persist and significantly affect quality of life may be considered for a variety of surgical treatments.

Adnexal Masses

Ovarian Disorders

Cyst

An **ovarian cyst** is defined as a discrete accumulation of fluid in an ovary resulting from an alteration in hormonal function. It can form at any point in a female's lifetime. Risk factors for benign ovarian cysts include a history of breast cancer, infertility treatment, smoking, hypothyroidism, and tubal ligation, while malignant cysts are associated with a positive family history, advancing age, Caucasian ethnicity, infertility, nulliparity, early menarche, delayed menopause, and a history of breast cancer. Most cysts are asymptomatic but may be associated with abdominal bloating, early satiety, change in bowel habits, and weight loss and severe abdominal pain if the cysts rupture. Diagnosis is made by the patient's history and physical examination in addition to pelvic ultrasonography, CA-125 measurement, and pregnancy testing. Initial treatment of simple cysts is observation and/or the use of oral contraceptive medications. If cysts grow in size or are associated with increasingly severe manifestations, laparoscopic removal of the cyst and/or the ovary is indicated.

Torsion

Ovarian torsion is a condition in which the ovary twists around adjacent, supportive vascular tissues. It is characterized by sudden abdominal pain, period-like cramps, and nausea. Women who have a history of polycystic ovarian syndrome, tubal ligation, or are experiencing hormonal shifts (e.g., during the in vitro fertilization process) are at a higher risk of developing ovarian torsion. While this is a rare condition, it is most commonly seen in young, pregnant women or women experiencing menopause. Treatment involves surgery to release the twisted ovary manually; however, even with prompt medical intervention, there is a high risk of the ovarian tissue necrotizing because torsion typically results in reduced blood flow to the ovary. Patients often have to undergo removal of the affected ovary and respective fallopian tube.

Rupture

Ovarian ruptures occur when a cyst on the ovary bursts. The severity of ruptures can vary; some situations are asymptomatic while others may require emergency surgery. In more critical instances, patients may experience severe cramping, pain, and heavy vaginal bleeding. When bleeding is involved, the case becomes more critical, as patients can potentially hemorrhage or lose vital blood supply to other organs. Such cases require immediate medical monitoring and may need surgical intervention. Medical monitoring focuses on managing bleeding from the ruptured cyst, while surgery involves removing clots, other extra fluids, and potentially the cyst itself. In addition, the healthcare team may assess any other cysts that are present and determine if they should also be removed. If surgery is not required, patients may be discharged when bleeding stops. If surgery is required, patients will need to be mindful of movement and physical activity until the wound is fully healed.

Abnormal Uterine Bleeding

Abnormal or irregular uterine bleeding is defined as episodes of bleeding that are not caused by any specific pathology, systemic illness, or normal pregnancy. It is most often due to alterations in the hormonal stimulation of the endometrium by some source. The bleeding episodes vary widely as to the amount of blood loss and the duration and frequency of the episodes in the same individual. The most common cause of this anovulatory cycle is the presence of an abnormal pregnancy, which may be a threatened or incomplete abortion or an ectopic pregnancy. There are several additional conditions associated with abnormal uterine bleeding, including polycystic ovarian including polycystic ovarian syndrome, thyroid dysfunction, liver dysfunction, that affect estrogen metabolism. Endometrial fibroids, polyps, hyperplasia, or cancer can also cause abnormal uterine bleeding. The condition is more common in adolescent women and women over the age of forty.

Once an abnormal pregnancy has been excluded, common diagnostic studies include CBC, Pap smear, thyroid and liver function tests, coagulation studies, and hormonal assays. Routine imaging studies are recommended only if the pelvic examination is unacceptable, as might occur in a patient with morbid obesity. However, pelvic ultrasonography is recommended in all patients who present with abnormal bleeding and are at high risk for cancer. Any identified pathology will be treated first; however, there are general guidelines for idiopathic ovulatory dysfunction, which include age-specific treatment protocols for the use of oral contraceptives as the initial treatment. Oral contraceptives suppress the thickening of the endometrial lining, regulate the menstrual cycle, and decrease menstrual flow, which reduces the risk of iron-deficiency anemia. In the event of the failure of medical treatment, hysterectomy may be recommended. The emergency care of the patient with abnormal bleeding is focused on hemostasis, aggressive fluid replacement, and treatment of the cause, which may require surgical intervention.

Cervical and Endometrial Polyps

Cervical polyps occur in up to 5 percent of female patients and are benign the vast majority of the time. They vary in size but typically appear as a red or purple nodular growth on the cervix. Most are asymptomatic, but some may cause postcoital bleeding or abnormal uterine bleeding. Cervical polyps are thought to arise from congestion of cervical vasculature or possibly from infections or chronic inflammation. Though malignancy is extremely rare (only 0.1 to 0.2 percent of cases), histological evaluation remains essential for both diagnosis of the polyp and exclusion of cancer. Polypectomy is the most common method for removal and analysis. After removal, the clinician should cauterize the base or apply silver nitrate to reduce the likelihood of recurrence.

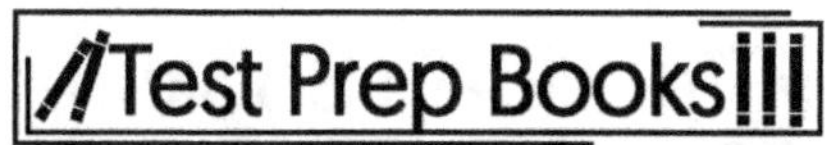

Endometrial polyps are overgrowths of glandular or stromal tissue and may grow up to several centimeters in diameter. Similar to cervical polyps, most are benign, but they carry a risk of malignant transformation. The best-known contributor to endometrial polyps is unopposed estrogen influence, which promotes endometrial hyperplasia. Patients typically report abnormal uterine bleeding, pelvic pain or pressure, and even infertility; however, others deny any symptoms. The presence of abnormal uterine bleeding, especially in postmenopausal women, absolutely merits evaluation with transvaginal ultrasound. This imaging typically reveals endometrial thickening greater than 4 millimeters. After identification of this thickening, the tissue must be biopsied to ensure this is a polyp rather than endometrial carcinoma. Asymptomatic polyps may be observed without treatment, and many spontaneously resolve. Symptomatic and/or persistent polyps warrant removal, most often via hysteroscopic polypectomy.

Leiomyomata Uteri

Leiomyomas, commonly known as **fibroids**, are smooth muscle tumors that are benign. Fibroids can increase significantly in size and cause the uterus to be asymmetrical. An ultrasound can confirm the presence of uterine fibroids. If fibroids cause compression of other organs, surgical removal may be implemented.

Malignant Disorders

Endometrium

Endometrial cancer is the most common gynecologic malignancy in the US; adenocarcinoma is the most frequent subtype. Its pathophysiology stems from high estrogen levels that promote endometrial thickening. Thus, patients with increased cumulative estrogen exposure face higher risk, such as those with early menarche, late menopause, nulliparity, obesity, and PCOS. Conversely, progesterone-containing contraceptives protect against endometrial cancer by opposing estrogen's influence on the endometrium. Symptoms may be subtle, but the most common manifestation is abnormal uterine bleeding. This complaint must always be taken seriously, especially in post-menopausal women.

Diagnosis is established with endometrial biopsy, and CT or PET scans are useful in assessing for metastasis. Treatment typically entails total hysterectomy with lymph node dissection, possibly with bilateral salpingo-oophorectomy, as well as radiation and chemotherapy where indicated. Fortunately, endometrial adenocarcinoma typically carries a good prognosis; patients should be monitored with regular pelvic examinations after treatment.

Cervix

Cervical intraepithelial neoplasia (**CIN**) involves a spectrum of abnormal cell growth ranging from benign to cancerous; dysplasia is screened for by Papanicolaou tests, or pap smears. The leading risk factor for CIN is **human papillomavirus** (**HPV**)—specifically, HPV types 16 and 18. More than seventy-five percent of Americans are estimated to have some type of HPV, though the highest-risk types are much less common. Risk factors for HPV include early sexual activity, multiple partners, immunosuppression, and low socioeconomic status. Current guidelines advise screening for CIN from ages twenty-one to sixty-five. This usually involves cervical cytology via pap smear every three years, but screenings can be extended to every five years if HPV co-testing is performed. Testing is essential because a physical exam cannot identify dysplasia.

Abnormal pap smear results include ASCUS (atypical squamous cells of undetermined significance), LSIL (low-grade squamous intraepithelial lesions), HSIL (high-grade squamous intraepithelial lesions), and atypical glandular cells. LSIL refers to mild dysplasia (CIN1), while HSIL involves moderate or severe dysplasia (CIN2-3). Colposcopy with biopsy is indicated for HSIL. For limited dysplasia, the lesion can be excised via conization or trachelectomy (cervical removal), which can preserve fertility. Advanced dysplasia and cancer may require hysterectomy and possible oophorectomy with or without chemotherapy and radiation.

Cervical and uterine cancers have similar 5-year survival rates. For localized disease, the 5-year survival rate is nearly 100 percent, but it drops to less than 60 percent if there is localized lymph node involvement and less than 15 percent for metastatic disease. In cervical cancer, adenocarcinomas have a worse prognosis than squamous cell. Poor prognostic factors for uterine cancer include older age, lymph node involvement, large tumors, and non-endometrioid histology. High estrogen receptor levels have a positive impact on prognosis.

Ovarian

Unfortunately, **ovarian cancer** represents the deadliest gynecologic malignancy due to its subtle presentation and a lack of adequate screening. The most prevalent histologic subtype is epithelial ovarian cancer; risk factors resemble those of breast and endometrial cancer. Symptoms are frequently non-specific, such as pelvic pain or pressure, bloating, early satiety, unexpected weight loss, urinary or fecal incontinence, dyspareunia, or abnormal uterine bleeding. Large tumors may be palpable and tender.

Labs may show elevated CA-125, which is relatively specific to ovarian cancer. However, it is not highly sensitive; that is, a normal level does not rule out cancer. Consider drawing serum alpha-fetoprotein (AFP), human chorionic gonadotropin (hCG), and lactate dehydrogenase (LDH) to evaluate for less-common germ cell tumors. Ultrasound is first-line imaging, with concerning findings including large or expanding masses, especially those over eight centimeters in diameter. Any concern for malignancy should be referred for mass resection; treatment may also include hysterectomy, salpingo-oophorectomy, and chemotherapy and/or radiation.

Ovarian cancer prognosis has a 5-year survival rate of 48 percent. Localized disease has a 93 percent survival rate; however, it is usually diagnosed in an advanced state. Prognosis is determined by stage, histologic type and grade, and residual bulk of tumor after surgery. Positive prognostic factors include younger age, good performance status, absence of ascites, and a cell type other than mucinous or clear cell carcinoma.

Vagina

Most **vaginal malignancies** occur as metastases from other primary tumors, especially cervical, vulvar, bladder, or ovarian cancer. In fact, primary vaginal cancers comprise only 2 percent of all vaginal malignancies. Crucially, they are defined as tumors without current or past history of vulvar or cervical cancer. SCC accounts for the vast majority of vaginal cancers, and the most commonly reported symptom is abnormal bleeding or discharge. As with most cancers, biopsy remains the gold standard for diagnosis, and subsequent imaging involving MRI, CT, and/or PET is crucial in evaluation for spread. Surgical excision is the preferred treatment for primary tumors, while radiation, chemotherapy, and/or immunotherapy may be required for metastatic disease.

Vulva

Vulvar cancer is almost always caused by SCC. Risk factors include HPV infection, smoking, radiation exposure, and immunosuppression. Fortunately, the 5-year survival rate for SCC remains quite high, but the prognosis is less encouraging for the lower percentage of vulvar cancers involving melanoma. Patients may describe itching, irritation, or pain and may even present initially with a visible mass that may be friable or bleed with contact. Lesions related to HPV infection may take a verrucous or cauliflower-like appearance. The lesion may also appear red, scaly, or ulcerated. Biopsy is required for diagnosis, and providers should carefully denote the exact location and dimensions of the lesion to assist in surgical planning. Surgical excision is the gold standard treatment, but advanced imaging may be indicated with subsequent systemic treatment for metastases.

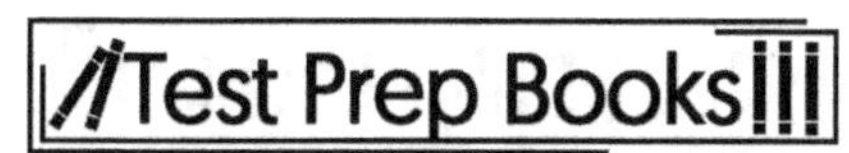

Breast Disorders

Breast Cancer

Breast neoplasms are frequently benign in patients under forty years of age; fibroadenomas are a common example. However, unilateral masses must always be taken seriously and be evaluated for possible malignancy. Risk increases with age, early menarche, late menopause, nulliparity, hormonal medications, BRCA genetic mutation, and tobacco and alcohol use. The most common type of **breast cancer** is infiltrating ductal carcinoma; inflammatory breast cancer, or Paget's disease of the breast, is rare but also the most aggressive. The latter may resemble mastitis with erythema and itching.

Alarming features include dimpling, skin retractions, fluid discharge, and a classic orange-skin appearance. Additional concerning signs for breast cancer include a fixed, immobile mass, skin discoloration, and axillary lymphadenopathy. If breast cancer is suspected, initial imaging involves ultrasound and mammography. The presence of spiculations, irregular shape, and posterior shadowing are particularly concerning. Diagnosis is confirmed via core needle biopsy. Treatment involves lumpectomy or mastectomy, possibly with chemotherapy and/or radiation depending on stage. For prevention, screening mammograms should be strongly encouraged at least every two years starting at forty years of age.

The breast cancer 5-year survival rate for all stages is 90 percent, with localized disease being 99 percent, regional 86 percent, and metastatic 29 percent. Poor prognostic factors include lymph node involvement, larger tumors, higher-grade tumors, hormone receptor-negative cancer, and invasive tumors.

Fibroadenoma

Fibroadenomas represent the most common benign breast mass. They are usually unilateral and most often occur in young women between fifteen and thirty-five years of age. They are hormone-sensitive and thus typically wax and wane throughout the menstrual cycle as fluctuations in estrogen and progesterone cause buildup of epithelial and stromal breast tissue. Patients may present with concerns about breast cancer after finding a painless lump in one breast. Physical examination reveals a smooth, freely mobile mass with well-delineated borders; the presence of these features is reassuring for a benign lesion. Fluctuation in size throughout the menstrual cycle provides further assurance.

Breast ultrasound is first-line imaging for patients under thirty years of age; above age thirty, mammogram is typically indicated. If the diagnosis remains in doubt, the lesion can be biopsied via core needle aspiration. If the fibroadenoma is asymptomatic, the patient can be reassured without treatment. However, if the mass causes discomfort or is concerning for malignancy, providers may consider excision.

Fibrocystic Breast Changes

Fibrocystic breast changes involve the overgrowth of connective tissue and development of cysts in both breasts. Like fibroadenomas, fibrocystic breast changes are benign lesions. However, they are distinct in that they occur bilaterally and at an older patient age than fibroadenomas, usually arising in the fifth decade of life and persisting until menopause. Signs and symptoms include intermittent or continuous bilateral breast pain, symmetric increase in breast size leading up to menses, and an irregular cord-like texture on palpation.

Breast ultrasound is usually sufficient for diagnosis; however, given the age at which fibrocystic changes most often occur, patients should be counseled on regular screening mammograms per United States Preventive Services Task Force (USPSTF) or American College of Obstetricians and Gynecologists (ACOG) guidelines. Simple cysts can be drained via fine needle aspiration. Complex cysts, such as those with septations or solid contents, require a core needle biopsy for drainage and evaluation. Otherwise, treatment includes reassurance, well-fitting bras for improved ligament support, and topical diclofenac for symptom relief. Nearly ninety percent of patients enjoy symptom relief with these conservative measures.

Other Benign Breast Disorders

Breast Abscess

Breast abscesses can develop as an uncommon complication of mastitis, or inflammation of the breast tissue. Because mastitis is typically caused by mechanical trauma during breastfeeding, lactation is a leading risk factor for **breast abscess**. The primary causative organism is *Staphylococcus aureus*, with *Escherichia coli* and *Streptococcus pyogenes* as less common culprits. Signs and symptoms include unilateral pain, warmth, and swelling of the breast, and patients may also report constitutional symptoms, such as fever, chills, and malaise. Importantly, physical exam will reveal a tender, fluctuant mass, which is the distinguishing feature of breast abscess. Diagnosis is made clinically; there is usually no need for lab studies or imaging. Breast abscess is treated with incision and drainage (I&D), followed by antibiotics against *S. aureus*, such as dicloxacillin. Warm compresses, antipyretics, and regular cleaning should also be encouraged. Patients may continue lactation if the I&D site is not reachable by the infant and if lactation is not excessively painful.

Gynecomastia

Gynecomastia occurs in male patients and involves bilateral breast enlargement due to hormonal changes. Anything that increases estrogen's influence or decreases that of androgen can produce gynecomastia. As such, this condition occurs frequently with advancing age. Other common causes include cirrhosis, prolactinomas, hypogonadism, hyperthyroidism, and malnutrition. Additionally, certain medications promote gynecomastia, including spironolactone, statins, and 5α-reductase inhibitors like finasteride. Though the diagnosis is clinical, the underlying cause should be investigated. Appropriate tests include serum testosterone, TSH, follicle-stimulating hormone (FSH), luteinizing hormone (LH), and estradiol.

Unilateral gynecomastia is concerning for malignancy, especially when associated with unilateral nipple discharge, rash, retraction, axillary lymphadenopathy, or palpable mass. Otherwise, patients can be reassured and the root cause treated. This may involve antithyroid medications for hyperthyroidism, cessation of causative medications if safe for the patient, or careful supplementation of testosterone in eligible patients. Importantly, medications should not be added or discontinued for treatment without careful evaluation of risks and benefits, given that bilateral gynecomastia itself is physiologic and benign.

Nipple Discharge

Galactorrhea refers to bilateral discharge of fluid from the nipple. Although the fluid often resembles breast milk, this condition occurs in patients who are not actively breastfeeding. Galactorrhea is most commonly caused by endocrine pathologies—usually hyperprolactinemia due to a prolactinoma. It can also occur during menarche and menopause due to significant hormonal changes. Medications such as hormone replacement therapy and risperidone, an atypical antipsychotic associated with hyperprolactinemia, can also promote galactorrhea.

Diagnosis is clinical based on the bilateral spontaneous expression of thin, milky discharge. However, patients should be evaluated for a root cause, including a urine pregnancy test as well as thyroid stimulating hormone (TSH) and serum prolactin levels. If labs show hyperprolactinemia, MRI is indicated to evaluate for a prolactinoma. Treatment is based on the root cause. Examples include dopamine agonists such as bromocriptine for a prolactinoma of less than one centimeter in diameter, surgical resection of a pituitary macroadenoma (defined as greater than one centimeter in diameter), and—if safe—withdrawal of any causative medications.

Breast Augmentation/Reduction

Breast augmentation involves enhancing the size of the breasts typically with a silicone implant or, occasionally, via fat transfer. This is a common cosmetic procedure that may be performed electively or

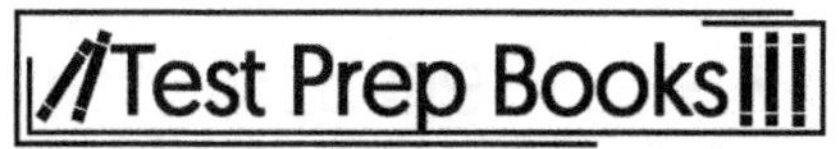

restoratively, such as in patients who undergo mastectomy for breast cancer. Additionally, patients whose breasts do not develop appropriately during adolescence may seek augmentation. Contraindications are rare but include active infection or cancer, radiation treatment, history of autoimmunity, silicone hypersensitivity, and unrealistic expectations or untreated behavioral conditions. Other potential complications include infection, asymmetry, pain, disrupted sensation, hematoma, or implant rupture.

Conversely, **breast reduction** removes excess tissue, such as in patients with disproportionately pendulous breasts, which may cause poor posture as well as chronic back, shoulder, and/or neck pain. Breast reduction may also be indicated for symmetry after reconstruction of the contralateral breast or due to unilateral hyperplasia. Patients should control other medical conditions, such as diabetes and hypertension, to reduce risk of complications. If over age 40, patients should first undergo a screening mammogram. Additionally, they should be counseled on postoperative expectations, including a noticeable cosmetic difference. Complications to explain include dehiscence, asymmetry, infection, and scarring. Still, most patients describe satisfaction with this procedure and enjoy significant improvement in their chronic symptoms thereafter.

Pelvic Organ Relaxation & Prolapse

Pelvic organ prolapse (**POP**) is an umbrella term encompassing protrusion of the uterus, bladder, or rectum into the vaginal introitus, producing a visible mass. Although locations vary depending on the specific organ involved, risk factors and presentations are similar across all types. POP typically results from pelvic muscle weakness, possibly along with increased intra-abdominal pressure. For example, multiple childbirths, past pelvic or gynecological surgery, constipation, connective tissue disease, obesity, or even chronic cough or heavy lifting can precipitate POP.

Symptoms depend upon severity of prolapse, which is graded using the **POP-Q scale** based on physical examination. Patients often describe intravaginal pressure, possibly urinary or defecatory dysfunction, and dyspareunia. POP is diagnosed on pelvic examination, during which patients should perform the Valsalva maneuver to allow assessment of any protrusions. Treatment is based upon symptom severity and patient wishes regarding relief, fertility, and sexual function. Pelvic floor muscle strengthening and pessary placement are mainstays of treatment for any form of POP. Patients with constipation should also increase fiber and fluid intake. For severe POP, surgical reduction with mesh placement should be strongly considered.

Cystocele

Cystocele is a form of pelvic organ prolapse (POP) involving herniation of the bladder through the anterior vaginal wall. Risk factors include pelvic floor weakness, chronic constipation, obesity, multiparity, and advanced age. Patients with cystocele complain of vague intravaginal pressure and often urinary frequency, urgency, or incontinence accompanying a soft, palpable vaginal mass. They may report improvement of urinary symptoms with manual reduction of the mass. Sexual dysfunction may also occur due to either dyspareunia or urinary incontinence during intercourse. Diagnosis is clinical and described with the POP-Q scale. However, a focused neurological exam is indicated if patients report urinary incontinence. Observation is appropriate for patients with few or no symptoms. Otherwise, treatment begins with physical therapy for pelvic floor strengthening, and pessary placement splints the bladder in place to improve urination. For those with severe cystocele or who fail conservative management, surgical evaluation by urogynecology is appropriate; procedures include anterior colporrhaphy or sacral colpopexy. Although vaginal atrophy may coincide with any form of POP, hormone replacement therapy as treatment for atrophy does not improve cystocele.

Rectocele

Rectocele is a form of POP involving a posterior vaginal mass due to rectal tissue herniation. Risk factors resemble those of other varieties of POP. Rectocele produces similar presentations, as well, including intravaginal pressure and possibly constipation, dyschezia, and dyspareunia. Patients may report a palpable mass, of which manual reduction improves defecation. Patients should be evaluated with a gastrointestinal and neurological exam to ensure no other causes of constipation. Otherwise, diagnosis is usually clinical based on the presence of a posterior wall mass; it is quantified with the POP-Q scale. All patients should be recommended to follow a high-fiber diet and increase water consumption. At-home exercises, such as Kegel maneuvers, may improve strength in the weakened pelvic muscles. Like other forms of POP, treatment may range from observation, physical therapy for pelvic floor strengthening, or pessary placement to surgical repair for severe or refractory symptoms. Patients may continue sexual activity as tolerated.

Urethrocele

Urethral prolapse occurs when there is external protrusion of the urethra. Symptoms include pain at the urethra, pain with urination, bleeding, and visible urethra. Risk factors include low estrogen levels (making the condition more common in pre-pubescent girls), history of pelvic surgery, and history of childbirth. The condition is also more common in African American and Hispanic females. Diagnosis is completed through a pelvic examination. Topical estrogen cream is typically sufficient for treatment; however, supportive care measures should also be recommended, such as sitz baths to maintain cleanliness of the area and petroleum jelly to soothe irritation.

Uterine Prolapse

Uterine prolapse involves protrusion of the uterus into—and, rarely, completely through—the vaginal introitus. Risk factors include connective tissue disorders (especially those involving uterosacral or cardinal ligament dysfunction) and conditions that increase intra-abdominal pressure, such as obesity, chronic cough, and constipation. Prolapse may be asymptomatic, or patients may describe vague feelings of pelvic or vaginal pressure. Pressure may increase with straining during urination or defecation. However, prolapse is rarely painful. Patients may also complain of urinary frequency, urgency, incompletion, or painful intercourse. Diagnosis is made clinically with no need for imaging and prolapse is often quantified and documented with the POP-Q score.

First-line treatment involves pelvic floor strengthening with a physical therapist, with or without pessary placement. Severe prolapse merits referral to a urogynecologist for surgical consultation. Total hysterectomy may also be considered depending on the patient's wishes or concomitant conditions. Patients can be advised that sexual activity is safe as long as prolapse does not cause excessive discomfort.

Polycystic Ovarian Syndrome (PCOS)

A disorder with a classic sign of amenorrhea is **polycystic ovarian syndrome** (**PCOS**). Female patients with PCOS are usually obese and show large cystic ovaries in an ultrasound. Excess production of testosterone leads to overgrowth of facial, chest, and back hair, termed hirsutism. If PCOS is suspected, the provider should expect to see a three-to-one ratio for the luteinizing hormone (LH) to follicle-stimulating hormone (FSH). The dehydroepiandrosterone sulfate (DHEAS) level will also be elevated.

Treatment for PCOS includes contraceptive medication to lower androgen production and regulate estrogen levels. Excess insulin is a possible factor for PCOS development. Increased insulin levels can lead to an increase in androgen production. **Metformin** (Glucophage) is often used to treat PCOS. Glucophage decreases insulin resistance and can assist with weight loss and prevent the development of type 2 diabetes. Obesity is part of the metabolic syndrome that often accompanies PCOS. Common side effects of metformin include diarrhea, nausea, vomiting, and loss of appetite. Excessive hair growth on the face and chest is a manifestation of PCOS. Medications such as spironolactone (Aldactone) help block the effects of androgen hormones on the skin. Aldactone is a potassium-sparing diuretic that prevents the loss of potassium from the

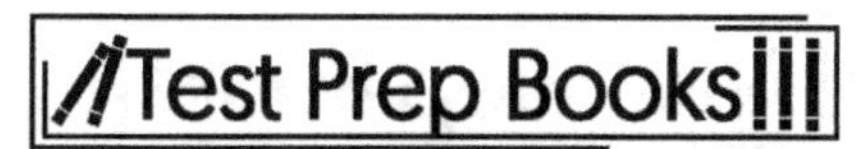

body. Patients should be educated on avoiding potassium supplements and excessive ingestion of potassium-rich foods. Common side effects are fatigue, headaches, nausea and vomiting.

Urinary Incontinence

The inability of the body to control voluntary sphincters is known as incontinence. One form of incontinence is the inability to control urine excretion, or urinary incontinence. An acute form of incontinence is known as transient incontinence, which lasts 6 months or less. Intra-abdominal pressure causes another form of urinary incontinence known as stress incontinence. Overflow incontinence occurs when the bladder is filled and can no longer hold urine. Functional incontinence is the lack of proper toileting. Reflex incontinence occurs when the body cannot feel the release of urine. Total incontinence happens when the urine loss is continuous and the patient does not have the ability to stop its flow.

Mixed incontinence occurs when a patient experiences one or more types of incontinence. Many factors can contribute to urinary incontinence. Some are medically induced, others are due to illness or an acute change in health status, and some are psychologically driven. Patients who are dehydrated may require intravenous fluids that increase fluid volume in the body. Diuretic medications that treat HTN are used to excrete excess fluid from the systemic circulation. This increases urine volume in the bladder. Activities that produce pressure in the intra-abdominal cavity, such as sneezing or coughing, can lead to stress incontinence. Obesity and pregnancy increase the weight that is pressed onto the bladder and can also lead to stress incontinence. The bladder empties when the stretch receptors along the bladder wall are activated by urine. The stretch receptors are controlled by the nervous system.

Patients who have spinal cord injuries or nerve damage do not have an intact nervous system, leading to overflow, or reflex incontinence. Patients who have conditions affecting orientation can have functional incontinence. Dementia, Alzheimer's, acute psychotic episodes, or confusion may lead to decreased toileting. Patients may not utilize the restroom appropriately and suffer incontinence in inappropriate places. Patients who suffer trauma or develop cancers in the pelvic area may have a urostomy. Artificial openings do not have sphincters. A urostomy does not provide control over urine excretion and is a form of total incontinence.

Vulvar Dystrophies and Dermatoses

Vulvar dystrophies and dermatoses include a variety of inflammatory conditions affecting the vulvar tissue. Three of the most common of these include **lichen sclerosus** (LS), **lichen simplex chronicus** (LSC), and **lichen planus** (LP). First, LS is a chronic inflammatory condition arising from a variety of genetic and autoimmune factors that involves skin atrophy and hypopigmentation. LS lesions appear as thin, pale to ivory, porcelain-like plaques and frequently produce severe itching, burning, and even dyschezia. This is treated first with superpotent topical corticosteroids and, if necessary, imiquimod or calcineurin inhibitors. Clinicians should also counsel patients to apply emollients and avoid direct application of soap or other potential irritants. Patients should also be monitored for malignant transformation to SCC, which can occur in up to 5 percent of patients.

LSC is a highly common cause of vulvar itching that is often worsened by cleaning, moisture, warmth, and even tight clothing. It is characterized by short-term relief with scratching followed by recurrence and worsening of symptoms as the tissue thickens, a phenomenon known as the *scratch-itch cycle*. Many patients become aware of this cycle and may try topical medications or cleaning more intentionally, but these measures usually make symptoms worse. Examination reveals skin thickening with or without excoriations or erythema. Treatment involves bland skin care, avoidance of scratching and other irritants, and a course of superpotent topical corticosteroids followed by longer-term use of less potent topical corticosteroids.

LP can occur anywhere on the body, but up to half of women with LP experience it at least in part in the genital region. The physical appearance of LP is characterized by the "6 Ps": purple, pruritic, polygonal, planar, papules, and plaques. Lesions may also feature white lacy patches known as Wickham's striae. Vulvar LP may cause erosion of vulvar tissue, leading to vaginal stenosis and strictures. Like other dermatoses, LP requires superpotent topical corticosteroids and may even require systemic steroids in some cases. Additionally, some specialists may employ immunomodulators or biologic agents, such as monoclonal antibodies, given the immune-mediated nature of this condition.

Müllerian Defects

Müllerian defects refer to a group of congenital malformations affecting the female reproductive tract, ranging from structural changes of the uterus to complete absence of the uterus, ovaries, and fallopian tubes. The most common type of Müllerian defect is that of the **bicornuate uterus**, which occurs when the Müllerian ducts fail to unite during the first trimester, resulting in two endometrial cavities that join at one cervix. Additional Müllerian abnormalities include a unicornuate uterus, which involves one uterine cavity that deviates to one side with an absent ovary and fallopian tube contralaterally; a septated uterus; a septated vagina; and cervical agenesis, among others. Patients with Müllerian defects may experience any combination of pelvic pain, abnormal bleeding, and/or dyspareunia. Furthermore, Müllerian defects pose a very high likelihood of infertility, early pregnancy loss, preterm delivery, fetal malpresentation, and low birth weight. Patients discovered with Müllerian defects should be referred to specialist providers, especially when pregnant or desiring to become pregnant. It is vital that such patients be accurately diagnosed and counseled on the risks associated with their specific type of Müllerian defect.

Fertility Awareness and Contraception

Fertility Awareness

Fertility awareness refers to habits aimed at natural family planning in order to achieve or avoid becoming pregnant. As a contraceptive method, it has no contraindications or negative effects but is unreliable, with a failure rate near 25 percent. Still, fertility awareness confers education and empowerment to couples by determining the days of the menstrual cycle when pregnancy is most likely. This is accomplished by first identifying when the progesterone-driven rise in basal body temperature occurs on the day of ovulation, which should happen on around day 14 of the menstrual cycle. Additionally, cervical secretions of a clear and "stretchy" consistency appear 3 to 4 days before ovulation. After these are observed, they can aid in the timing of efforts to become pregnant or avoid it. A woman is typically fertile from about 5 days before ovulation to 1 day after, owing to the ability of sperm to survive for up to 5 days after ejaculation. Couples who wish to avoid pregnancy during these periods should be educated on options for contraception, as the withdrawal method is not sufficiently effective for pregnancy prevention.

Infertility

Infertility is defined as failure to conceive after twelve months despite properly timed, unprotected intercourse. The timeframe for diagnosis decreases to six months after the patient reaches thirty-five years of age. The most common reasons for male-factor infertility include low sperm count or motility. Abnormal ovulation, endometriosis, and anatomic anomalies (e.g., abnormal fallopian tubes and uterine adhesions) account for most female-factor infertility. Both partners should be asked about prior illnesses and STIs, sexual practices, substance use, and toxic exposures, along with menstrual and contraceptive history for the female partner.

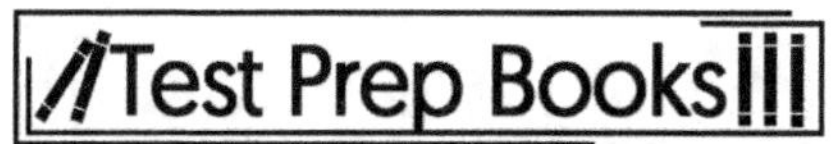

Diagnostic workup for the male partner begins with semen analysis, which, if normal, makes male-factor infertility less likely. Ovulation must be tested via day twenty-one progesterone level. If progesterone level returns normal, patients are evaluated for anatomic abnormalities. Low progesterone suggests abnormal ovulation, and follow-up testing of TSH, FSH, estradiol, and prolactin is indicated. Treatment is multifaceted and starts with counseling patients on appropriate lifestyle modifications, avoidance of substance use, and appropriate timing to maximize chances of conception. Clomiphene can induce ovulation when necessary. If all else fails, referral to a reproductive endocrinologist should be offered.

Barrier Methods

Barrier contraceptives include multiple devices, such as external (male) condoms, internal (female) condoms, cervical caps, diaphragms, sponges, and spermicides. They are common and often preferred by those who favor event-specific contraception rather than long-acting contraception. Importantly, though, their failure rates with typical use reach as high as 20 percent, depending on the method. Overall, the external condom is the most effective form of barrier contraception, but even with perfect use, its failure rate remains approximately 3 percent. In terms of STI protection, external and internal condoms are the only reliable methods for prevention of transmission of diseases like HIV, hepatitis B, gonorrhea, chlamydia, trichomoniasis, HSV, HPV, and syphilis. It is essential that sexually active patients be educated on the vital importance of these two barriers for protection against STIs and especially so in patients who are not monogamous or have partners who are not. Similarly, patients should receive realistic counseling that pregnancy may still occur even with barrier protection and that the fertile window surrounding ovulation is when pregnancy is most likely.

Emergency Contraception

Emergency contraception acts as a backup for patients whose primary contraception fails or who have unprotected intercourse without the desire to become pregnant. It is also vitally important to prevent pregnancy in victims of sexual assault. Without emergency contraception, the chance of pregnancy after unprotected sex is about 5 percent but rises to near 30 percent during the period surrounding ovulation when a woman is fertile. The two main emergency contraceptive methods include the **copper intrauterine device (Cu-IUD)** and the oral hormonal method. The Cu-IUD is the most effective method and works by releasing a copper ion that is cytotoxic to gametes and also promotes localized inflammation to prevent implantation of an already fertilized egg. Conversely, levonorgestrel is the most common oral hormonal contraceptive and works by inhibiting the LH surge that promotes ovulation. Ulipristal acetate is another option with a similar mechanism. Treatment is most effective when initiated as soon as possible after unprotected intercourse; if possible, patients should be treated within 3 days. The Cu-IUD is preferred for patients who present after this time frame.

Pharmacologic Methods

Oral

Oral contraceptives can provide hormones (estrogen and/or progestin), which suppress the egg maturation and ovulation process. Additionally, hormonal contraceptives prevent the endometrium from thickening in preparation to hold the fertilized egg. A mucus barrier is created by progestin, which stops the sperm from migrating to the fallopian tubes and fertilizing the egg.

There are many side effects associated with oral contraceptives, including increasing the risk of fatal blood clots, especially in women older than 35 or in women who smoke. More common and less severe side effects include:

- Nausea and stomach upset
- Headache
- Weight gain
- Spotting between periods
- Mood changes
- Lighter periods
- Aching or swollen breasts

More serious side effects that need immediate emergency care include:

- Chest pain
- Blurred vision
- Stomach pain
- Severe headaches

Examples of some commercially available brands of contraceptive include:

- Yasmin
- Ortho Tri-Cyclen
- TriNessa
- Sprintec
- Ovcon
- Plan B (emergency contraceptive)

Injection

Injectable contraceptives are highly effective and usually involve intramuscular administration of **medroxyprogesterone acetate** (**DMPA**), a progesterone-only medication. This injection is given once every three months. Compared to implants and intrauterine devices (IUDs), the removal of which may rarely be difficult, injectable contraception carries minimal risk of mechanical complications. Despite a failure rate of less than one percent, it is considered slightly less effective than implants and IUDs because of the frequent need for return and re-injection.

Adverse effects include amenorrhea and weight gain. Patients should be counseled that after discontinuation of injections, menses may be irregular or remain absent for up to eighteen months. As with other hormonal contraceptives, DMPA should be avoided in patients with a history of breast cancer and should be used cautiously in those with abnormal uterine bleeding. Providers must remind patients of the importance of on-time follow-up. Although menses and fertility may not return for months after the last injection, pregnancy remains possible after a three-month window.

Implants

Implantable contraceptives are progesterone-secreting rods typically placed in the medial upper arm for up to three years. Along with IUDs, they are considered long-acting reversible contraception and are the single most effective form of reversible contraception. Their failure rate of less than one percent is attributed to their self-sustaining nature; patients need not manage dosing or change any habits to ensure their efficacy. Implants also feature fewer contraindications compared to other contraceptives. While all hormonal contraceptives are contraindicated for patients with current or past breast cancer, implants are generally safer than estrogen-containing medications for patients who are breastfeeding and for those with diabetes,

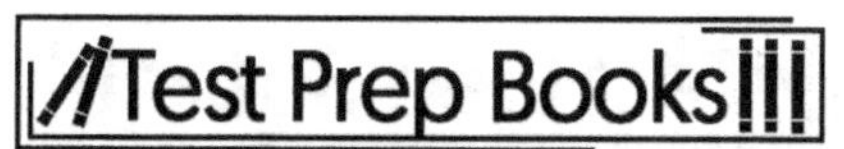

migraine with aura, smoking history, and risk of clotting. Implants are associated with irregular menstrual bleeding, and removal can be difficult after three years. Progesterone-based contraceptives may also cause headache, depression, and breast tenderness. As always, patients should be counseled on all risks and benefits of implants and other forms of contraception in order to make an informed decision.

Transdermal

Transdermal contraception utilizes a patch containing both estrogen and progesterone that is absorbed through the skin and acts with similar efficacy to combined oral contraceptives. A typical regimen involves weekly application to the arm, torso, abdomen, or buttocks for 3 weeks, followed by a patch-free week to allow for withdrawal bleeding. Adherence is often better than for oral therapy due to less frequent dosing, but a failure rate of 7 percent is still observed with typical use. Transdermal contraception is generally well-tolerated, but providers should counsel patients about the failure rate and adverse effects, such as skin irritation and breast tenderness.

Vaginal Rings

Vaginal rings are another form of combined contraception that acts similarly to oral and transdermal therapy by suppressing ovulation, thickening cervical mucus, and altering endometrial composition and structure to prevent implantation. Most rings are inserted for three weeks and then removed for a ring-free week to allow for withdrawal bleeding. A new ring is then inserted to start the new cycle. However, some rings allow for long-term use, following the same "3-weeks-in/1-week-out" pattern but with the same ring washed and reinserted each time the cycle restarts. They share similar efficacy and failure rates as other forms of combined contraception and need not be removed for intercourse or tampon insertion.

Vaginal Gel

Vaginal gel refers to nonhormonal topical solutions that alter vaginal pH or contain spermicide. Nonoxynol-9 is widely available over the counter as a gel or several other formulations; its mechanism of action involves disrupting the cell membranes of sperm, inhibiting their motility and reducing their lifespan. Crucially, nonoxynol-9 does not protect against STIs and carries a failure rate of about 20 percent, so providers must counsel patients regarding these drawbacks. Phexxi® is a newer product composed of citric acid, lactic acid, and sodium bitartrate that can be applied immediately before or after intercourse. It reduces vaginal pH, which hinders spermatic motility. Unfortunately, its failure rate is near 15 percent. However, patients may combine either of these contraceptives with other methods, except the vaginal ring, for increased total efficacy.

Intrauterine Contraception

Intrauterine devices (**IUDs**) are one of the most popular contraceptive options, with both progesterone-based and non-hormonal (copper) devices. IUDs also boast the longest duration of any contraceptive: progesterone IUDs now last from three (Skyla) to eight (Liletta and Mirena) years, and copper IUDs can now remain in place for up to twelve years. An additional advantage of the copper IUD is that it functions as emergency contraception if placed up to five days after intercourse. No IUD prevents ovulation; however, progesterone IUDs work by thickening cervical mucus and thinning the uterine lining, and copper devices produce localized inflammation that inhibits spermatic motility. Additional advantages include substantial reduction in menstrual blood loss and lower risk of endometrial cancer. Contraindications to IUDs include active PID, suspected pregnancy, or unexplained abnormal uterine bleeding. If a patient develops a sexually transmitted infection (STI) when an IUD is in place, the device does not need to be removed unless the patient first fails antibiotic therapy.

Permanent Methods

Tubal Ligation

Tubal ligation involves surgically separating both fallopian tubes and tying the free ends. Its goal is the inhibition of sperm traveling into the tube to fertilize an egg. Though this procedure can be reversed with a subsequent surgery, tubal ligation is still considered a permanent contraceptive option. Successful reversal is less likely in patients over thirty-five years of age; this is significant as tubal ligation is associated with high rates of regret, particularly for patients younger than thirty years of age. Despite a failure rate of less than one percent, the risk of ectopic pregnancy is somewhat higher than with other contraceptives due to the remote possibility of fertilization occurring in a ligated tube followed by obstructed travel to the uterus for implantation. Additionally, providers should advise patients that tubal ligation carries the usual risks of surgery, including intraoperative complications, blood loss, and surgical site infection. Nevertheless, successful procedures are typically highly protective against unwanted pregnancy.

Tubal Occlusion

Tubal occlusion, along with tubal ligation or removal, represents permanent contraception and the most common such method worldwide. It usually involves interruption of the isthmus of the fallopian tube. Though reversal is sometimes possible, clinicians must inform patients that tubal sterilization is meant to be permanent and that short-acting or long-acting reversible options are available. Still, for patients who express understanding of this information and consent to the procedure, no absolute contraindications exist, and clinicians should take patients' wishes and concerns seriously. The procedure can be performed at any time but is often carried out during a cesarean delivery or in the immediate postpartum period. Another key piece of counseling is that, while tubal occlusion is highly effective at preventing pregnancy, even it is imperfect. Though extremely rare, pregnancy remains theoretically possible, with a higher risk of ectopic pregnancy in particular.

Vasectomy

Vasectomy is similar to tubal ligation in that it involves surgical disruption of a reproductive pathway. Specifically, a urologist separates and ligates the vas deferens, the pathway through which sperm travels from the testes to the ejaculatory duct. Like tubal ligation, this procedure is reversible, though successful reversal wanes with age and the amount of time passed since separation. Still, a vasectomy is considered a highly effective permanent contraceptive, with a failure rate of less than one-fourth of one percent. Risks include intraoperative complications, infection, pain, and even psychiatric issues such as depression. Patients must continue using condoms for at least six weeks to allow for discharge of all sperm already present in the vas deferens. Furthermore, a vasectomy does not prevent infection with or transmission of any STI, so condoms should still be encouraged for patients at risk of exposure.

Unintended Pregnancy

Options Counseling

Just as providers must communicate in a nonjudgmental and supportive manner about reproductive life planning, so too they must counsel patients experiencing unplanned pregnancy. Indeed, this counseling must remain unbiased and patient-centered, setting aside any personal beliefs. Patients must be informed of each option available to them, including continuing the pregnancy and parenting or seeking adoption or foster care. Alternatively, patients should be informed of the option of terminating the pregnancy, though this option currently depends on individual state law. As with any other pregnancy, a thorough understanding of the patient's medical history and social determinants of health is essential. Patients with limited access to care should be informed of available resources either in clinic or other organizations. Additionally, screen patients early for intimate partner violence, which is most prevalent in the peripartum period. Finally,

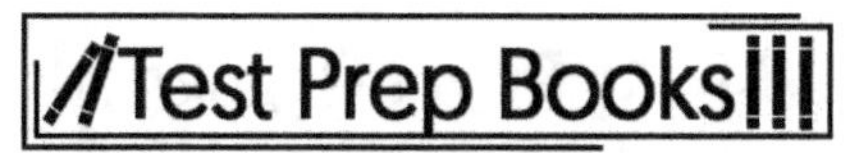

patients with history of diabetes, preeclampsia, spontaneous abortion, and other high-risk conditions merit referral to maternal-fetal medicine for more frequent monitoring, regardless of the ultimate choice the patient makes regarding her pregnancy.

Pregnancy Termination

Counseling on **pregnancy termination** must be tailored to the patient's personal and gestational age, medical history, and social situation. Conversations should begin with quietly and attentively allowing the patient to process life-changing news about an unplanned pregnancy. Use open-ended questions to determine whether the patient has initial concerns or preferences on how to proceed. Patients who do wish to terminate the pregnancy should be met with compassion and open-mindedness but never with judgment. Options for termination include procedures such as dilation and curettage and vacuum extraction, among others. Medication-induced abortion involves mifepristone and misoprostol, which antagonize progesterone and cause uterine contractions, respectively, to promote gestational sac expulsion. Medication abortion has become more favorable due to its availability, effectiveness, and flexibility. Providers must also stay abreast of the evolving social and political climate surrounding abortions to avoid endangering themselves or their patients' rights.

Sexual and Reproductive Health for Males, LGBTQ+, and Gender Non-Conforming Individuals

Male Reproductive System Disorders

Congenital and Acquired Abnormalities

Cryptorchidism

Cryptorchidism is a congenital condition where one or both testicles do not descend into the scrotum within the first few months after birth. The patient will present with one or no palpable testicle within the scrotum. Undescended testicles can sometimes be palpated in the abdomen. Cryptorchidism does not typically have any other associated symptoms and the cause is unknown. If the testicles do not descend on their own within the first six months, a referral to a urologist is warranted for an orchiopexy. An **orchiopexy** is typically performed between twelve and twenty-four months of age and surgically moves the testicle(s) to the scrotum. It is important to address cryptorchidism, as failure to do so puts the patient at an increased risk of infertility and testicular cancer later in life.

Peyronie Disease

Peyronie disease is a condition that occurs due to scar tissue development under the skin of the penis, which causes an abnormal curvature during erection. The scar tissue that develops can harden to the thickness of bone. Primary presenting symptoms include palpable scar tissue, painful erections and intercourse, curved erections, and erectile dysfunction. While the exact cause is unknown, there is thought to be a link between genetics and trauma, such as penile fracture or microtrauma from sexual activity. A physical exam is often sufficient for diagnosis; however, an ultrasound can also be used to better visualize the scar tissue and blood flow. Resolution can be spontaneous. Other treatment options include injections of Xiaflex, verapamil, and interferon into the scar tissues to break the tissue down. Stretching of the penis, or traction therapy, may be recommended for early phases and in combination with other therapies. In severe cases, surgery may be required.

Penile Disorders

Erectile Dysfunction

Erectile dysfunction (ED) is a condition in male patients that prevents them from achieving or sustaining an erection during sexual intercourse. Many factors influence ED, including spinal cord injuries, psychological distress, diabetes, and medications such as beta-blockers. There are several medications that can treat ED. The corpus cavernosa is a region of erectile tissue that fills with blood during an erection. Medications that dilate the corpora cavernosa are used to treat ED. These medications are known as PDE5 inhibitors. A common PDE5 inhibitor is sildenafil (Viagra). Viagra relaxes the blood vessel walls and increases blood flow to specific areas of the body. Due to blood vessel relaxation, Viagra can cause a sudden decrease in blood pressure. Common side effects include flushing of the skin and headache. Other PDE5 inhibitors used for the treatment of ED include vardenafil (Levitra) and tadalafil (Cialis).

Hypospadias/Epispadias

Hypospadias and epispadias are both birth defects where the urethra does not develop in the proper position. In normal development, the opening to the urethra is located at the tip of the penis in males or below the clitoris in females. In males, **hypospadias** occurs when the urethral opening is on the underside of the penis. **Epispadias** occurs when the urethral opening is on the top side of the penis, anywhere from the top of the glans, along the shaft, or near the pubic bone. In females, it is located close to the clitoris or up to the lower abdomen. While the cause is largely unknown, there are a few risk factors including genetics, advanced maternal age, and exposure to high levels of progesterone. It is difficult to identify on an ultrasound, so is typically diagnosed at birth through a physical examination. If present, a referral to pediatric urology will be placed for surgical treatment.

Paraphimosis/Phimosis

Paraphimosis and phimosis are conditions of the foreskin in uncircumcised males. In **paraphimosis**, the foreskin cannot be brought forward over the glans penis due to tightness of the foreskin. This is considered a medical emergency, as it can cut off circulation to the penis. **Phimosis** occurs when the foreskin cannot be retracted from the glans penis due to tightness of the foreskin. It is common in boys younger than four years of age. Though phimosis is typically painless, symptoms can include pain, swelling of the foreskin, and purple discoloration of the head of the penis. It may impact sexual function and normal urination. Poor hygiene and penile piercings can increase the risk of both conditions. Diagnosis is completed by a physical examination. Paraphimosis may be treated in the office by manual replacement of the foreskin. However, if the foreskin is unable to be replaced, surgery may be required, and circumcision may be recommended. For phimosis, treatment recommendations include application of a topical steroid cream to the penis as well as stretching exercises to improve the elasticity of the foreskin.

Priapism

Priapism is a urological emergency manifested by the enlargement of the penis that is unrelated to sexual stimulation and is unrelieved by ejaculation. Low-flow priapism is the most common form and is not associated with evidence of trauma but is due to dysfunction of the detumescence mechanism that is responsible for the relaxation of the erect penis. High-flow priapism results from abnormal arterial blood to the penis as a result of trauma to the GU system. The cause of low-flow priapism is most often idiopathic; however, the most common cause of the condition in children is sickle cell disease. Additional conditions that may cause this form of priapism include dialysis, vasculitis, spinal cord stenosis, bladder and renal cancer, and some medications, including heparin, cocaine, and omeprazole. High-flow priapism is due to straddle injuries or, most commonly, injury to the arteries of the penis by the injection of medications into the vasculature of the penis.

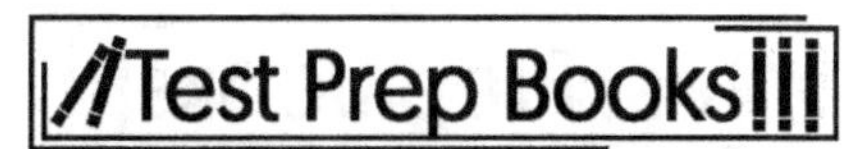

Prompt treatment of low-flow priapism within twelve hours of the onset of symptoms is necessary to prevent long-term alterations in erectile function. The primary cause is identified and treated, if possible, followed by aspiration of fluid from the corpora cavernosa at the base of the penis, with or without saline irrigation, which is an effective treatment in thirty percent of cases. If aspiration and irrigation are unsuccessful, a vasoconstrictive agent such as phenylephrine can be instilled at 5-minute intervals until the erection is entirely resolved. If these interventions fail to eradicate the priapism, temporary or permanent surgical placement of a shunt between the corpus cavernosum and the glans penis or corpus spongiosum is necessary to restore venous drainage. Treatment of high-flow priapism involves cauterization and/or evacuation of areas of bleeding. Care is focused on identification of the specific condition and prompt resolution of the erection.

Testicular Disorders

Hydrocele/Varicocele

Hydrocele is the collection of fluid within the tunica vaginalis of the scrotum. The primary symptom is swelling of the scrotum, which may be accompanied by discomfort or pain. The primary risk factor is age, with hydroceles being most common in infants and rarely occurring in adults. Diagnosis is completed with a physical exam, although an ultrasound may be completed to confirm the diagnosis. Most hydroceles will resolve on their own. If it does not, a hydrocelectomy performed by a urologist may be necessary.

Varicocele is the enlargement of the veins of the scrotum, and it can be more common in the left testicle than the right. There are typically few symptoms, but these may include dull pain or a bump in the scrotum. Contributing factors include lack of physical activity and age between fifteen and twenty-five. Diagnosis will start with a physical exam and may require a pelvic ultrasound. Treatment may not be required; however, supportive measures can be used, such as ice, supportive underwear or jock strap, and NSAIDs for pain or discomfort.

Testicular Torsion

Torsion refers to the abnormal twisting of the structures of the spermatic cord, which results in ischemia in the ipsilateral testicle that causes irreversible damage to fertility if not relieved within six hours. The condition is most common in infants, due to the mobility of the undescended testicles, and in adolescents, due to the abnormal attachment of fascia and muscles to the spermatic cord.

The **Testicular Workup for Ischemia and Suspected Torsion** (**TWIST**) is the scoring system used to quantify the risk associated with the condition. The TWIST is used by emergency providers and then validated by the physician, most commonly a urologist, and the score is based on swelling of the testicle, hardened texture of the testicle, absence of the cremasteric reflex, nausea and vomiting, and placement of the testicles at a higher-than-normal position in the scrotum. The resulting risk factor may be low, intermediate, or high. A low TWIST score may indicate an alternative cause for the patient's manifestations. An intermediate risk requires the use of ultrasound to confirm the diagnosis, while the patient with a high-risk TWIST score requires immediate surgical intervention to prevent long-term dysfunction.

Nonoperative treatments include manual manipulation of the testicle guided by Doppler imaging. If the procedure is successful, surgical stabilization of the spermatic cord structures is required. Immediate surgical repair is required if the procedure is unsuccessful. If the affected testicle is nonviable and is removed, a testicular prosthesis will be inserted after wound healing is complete. Analgesics and antianxiety medications will be included in the treatment plan. Caregivers must be aware that the condition can reoccur. Emergency care of the patient requires immediate intervention based on the calculation of the TWIST score to prevent necrosis of the affected testicle.

Sexuality

Sexuality remains a complex and evolving subject that affects the life of every patient in one way or another. The **LGBTQ+ community**, in particular, is subjected to stigma, prejudice, and even hate and violence around the world that threatens their mental and cardiovascular health. Sexuality encompasses a variety of terms that shape a person's identity and experiences. Key terms include gay or lesbian, meaning a male or female, respectively, who identifies as such and is attracted to others of the same sex; bisexual, meaning attracted to both males and females; cisgender, or those whose gender identity aligns with their sex assigned at birth; transgender, meaning gender identity aligning with the opposite sex of that assigned at birth; and queer/questioning, or those who are unsure of their sexuality or gender identity. Gender itself refers to social, emotional, or other traits that portray masculinity or femininity. Patients who confide about such issues or their personal experiences place an incredible degree of trust in their provider. This is a monumental responsibility and must not be taken lightly. Clinicians who listen and display open-mindedness and compassion can cultivate strong and long-lasting patient-provider relationships for the betterment of their patients' mental and physical health.

Contraception

Contraception refers to mechanical or pharmacologic measures to prevent pregnancy and, in the case of male or female condoms, STIs. Each carries its own benefits and drawbacks. Barrier contraceptives include condoms, diaphragms, cervical caps, sponges, and spermicides. These either prevent the entry of sperm into the uterus and fallopian tube or cause their demise before ascending that far. Importantly, the efficacy of these options relies on proper use; thus, they are more prone to failure than some long-acting contraceptive options. Pharmacologic measures include hormonal contraceptives, which may be administered orally on a daily basis, injected intramuscularly on a monthly basis, placed transdermally via a patch, inserted vaginally via a ring, or implanted via a hormone-secreting rod or intrauterine device (IUD). Longer-acting options such as injections, rods, and IUDs have become more popular in recent years and carry the lowest failure rates, as they do not rely on the patient remembering to administer them daily. Patients should be counseled on each option and how it would be discontinued; they must also be informed that only condoms help prevent STIs and that they should use condoms for this purpose regardless of other contraceptive use.

Infertility

Infertility is diagnosed in patients after 12 months of correctly timed sexual intercourse in patients under age 35 or after 6 months if over age 35. Evaluation begins with comprehensive histories and physical exams for both the male and female partner. Semen analysis should also occur early in the process, as the male factor contributes to up to half of infertility cases. If this analysis reveals normal sperm count and motility, then workup proceeds to evaluation of ovulatory function, which accounts for another 25 percent of cases of infertility. Ask female patients about their menstrual history, including the length and regularity of cycles. Consider obtaining a day-21 progesterone and measuring levels of FSH, LH, TSH, and prolactin. If all are normal, imaging such as ultrasound will be required to assess for tubal patency and anatomical abnormalities. Treatment depends on the underlying cause. In vitro fertilization (IVF) has become a popular and effective treatment for many cases of infertility. Patients diagnosed with infertility and others who desire IVF should be given referral to a reproductive endocrinology and infertility (REI) specialist for further evaluation and counseling.

Sexually Transmitted Infections

Sexually transmitted infections (STIs) include a great variety of bacterial, viral, and protozoal organisms. HPV is by far the most common STI in the world and is not curable. However, its most serious consequence of

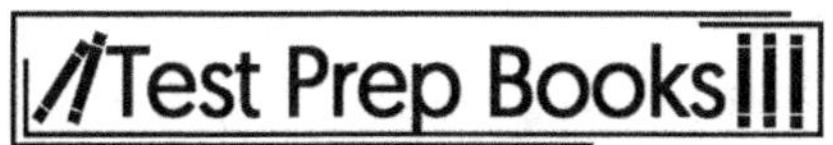

cervical cancer is highly preventable with the Gardasil® vaccine. The most common curable STIs are chlamydia and gonorrhea, both bacterial infections treated with antibiotics. Certain variants of *Chlamydia trachomatis* can also cause a longer-term infection known as lymphogranuloma venereum. Syphilis is caused by a spirochete bacterium that is highly treatable with penicillin but causes long-term, life-threatening complications if untreated. HIV, the virus that causes AIDS, affects those in poverty, those who engage in high-risk sexual behavior, and men who have sex with men (MSM) at disproportionate rates; however, significant advancements have been made in treatment and prevention of progression to AIDS. *Trichomonas vaginalis* is a protozoal organism that causes trichomoniasis, an STI characterized by vaginal discharge, erythema, and pruritus; it is curable with metronidazole. Many other STIs exist with greater prevalence in the developing world than the US, but these above are the most important with which every clinician must be familiar.

LGBTQ+ and Gender Non-conforming Individuals

Gender equity aims to provide all people with equal access to healthcare, regardless of gender or sexual orientation. Women report that they find health services less accessible, and studies indicate that women pay more for health services and health insurance premiums than men. However, men tend to have poorer health outcomes due to behaviors that may be influenced by social and cultural norms. For example, some studies indicate that men are more likely to feel stigmatized for seeking out mental health services and therefore have worse mental health outcomes than women. They also are less likely to practice hygienic behaviors that prevent disease transmission, such as handwashing.

People in the lesbian, gay, bisexual, trans, queer, intersex, asexual, and other sexual identities (LGBTQIA+) face significant health disparities that lead to poor health outcomes such as depression, suicidal ideation, and participation in risky behaviors. This appears to be due to a lack of education and understanding about these groups' health preferences and goals by healthcare providers. Additionally, many healthcare providers may harbor internal biases against these groups. People in the LGBTQIA+ community are also less likely to have access to health insurance through a spouse, as most employers do not recognize same-sex partnerships for insurance benefits. People who undergo gender transition undergo numerous health procedures in their lifetime that must be handled with sensitivity.

In order to achieve gender equity, healthcare providers must educate themselves on specific diseases faced by vulnerable populations, as well as specific health outcomes desired by these populations. For example, some healthcare providers may assume a young woman who does not want children may change her mind later in life and deny her a tubal litigation without acknowledging the patient's true health wants. Healthcare providers should consider any subconscious internal beliefs or stereotypes they may hold about patient populations, work to address them, and recognize culturally sensitive ways of delivering care.

Practice Quiz

1. The WHNP is caring for a 26-year-old female patient with abnormal uterine bleeding. Which of the following tests does the WHNP order first?
   a. Pap smear
   b. Uterine biopsy
   c. Pelvic ultrasonography
   d. Pregnancy test

2. Billie is a 20-year-old college student who faints in the campus recreation center weight room while exercising. She is rushed to health services where she regains consciousness, but the medical personnel order blood and urine tests. Billie's blood tests show iron levels of about 10 grams of hemoglobin per deciliter. Her urine is darker and a bit bloody. Billie shares that she has had very heavy and long menstrual cycles lately. Billie is suffering from which of the following?
   a. Iron-deficiency anemia
   b. Anabolic steroid use
   c. Polycystic ovary syndrome
   d. An eating disorder

3. The WHNP is assessing a 38-year-old male who presents with marked left-sided scrotal swelling and distention of the abdomen. The WHNP understands that which of the following is NOT an expected finding in this patient?
   a. Diarrhea
   b. Tachycardia
   c. Rebound tenderness
   d. BUN 27

4. Resnick's criteria address which of the following conditions?
   a. Urinary incontinence
   b. Benign prostatic hyperplasia
   c. Peripheral vascular disorders
   d. Intraductal papilloma

5. Which screening test is useful in decreasing the incidence and mortality of cancer and is generally recommended once every three years for women aged 21 to 65?
   a. HPV
   b. PAP
   c. Colonoscopy
   d. Mammogram

See answers on the next page

Answer Explanations

1. D: A pregnancy test is performed first to determine if the patient is pregnant. A Pap smear, uterine biopsy, and pelvic ultrasound may be performed, based on the patient's history and physical findings, but they would not be the first test performed, making *A*, *B*, and *C* incorrect answers.

2. A: Iron deficiency anemia is characterized by iron levels lower than 12 g/dL in women, and Billie's tests showed she was below this level. She also shared that she has heavy, long menstrual periods, and it appears she is currently in her cycle. This heavy blood loss can deplete iron levels. Her fainting episode is also a symptom of anemia.

3. A: The patient's manifestations are consistent with an incarcerated or strangulated hernia that is progressing to a small-bowel obstruction as evidenced by the abdominal distention. This complication is associated with decreased peristalsis and eventual absence of bowel activity, which means that diarrhea would be an uncommon manifestation. Tachycardia and a BUN of 27 are related to fluid volume losses resulting from the accumulation of fluid proximal to the obstruction in the small bowel; therefore, choices *B* and *D* are incorrect. Rebound tenderness is also an expected finding in a bowel obstruction due to the trapped gas and fluid proximal to the obstruction; therefore, Choice *C* is incorrect.

4. A: Resnick's criteria (DIAPPERS) address multiple risk factors for urinary incontinence. The list includes delirium, symptomatic urinary infection, atrophic vaginitis, pharmaceuticals, psychological disorders (especially depression), excessive urine output, restricted mobility, and stool impaction. The remaining conditions are not addressed by Resnick's criteria; therefore, Choices *B, C,* and *D* are incorrect.

5. B: The Papanicolaou (PAP) test is useful for reducing the incidence and mortality of cervical cancer, and providers generally recommend that women between the ages of 21 and 65 get the test performed once every three years. Choice *A* is incorrect because the human papillomavirus (HPV) test, which is performed to detect a virus that may lead to cervical cancer or genital warts, is generally recommended for women over age 30, though it is also given to some men to detect the virus on the penis or scrotum. Choice *C* is incorrect because a colonoscopy is generally recommended for women and men once every ten years to screen for colon cancer or polyps. Choice *D* is incorrect because a mammogram is generally recommended once a year for women over age 40 to screen for breast cancer.

Obstetrics

Anatomy and Physiology of Pregnancy

The Process of Conception and Gestation

Conception describes the process whereby a sperm cell from a fertile man travels into a woman's uterus and merges with her egg cell while it goes down a fallopian tube from the ovary to the uterus. The order of the three stages of prenatal development includes germinal, embryonic, and fetal. The **germinal stage** takes place between conception and the first two weeks, which is when the **zygote** (a single cell formed from the fusion of a man's sperm and a woman's egg) begins to undergo rapid division. The **embryonic stage** occurs between the second and eighth week of pregnancy, which is when organs start to develop (**organogenesis**), and it's during this process that the fetus is most prone to birth defects caused by various types of external factors, including drugs, toxins, and extreme environments. The **fetal stage** transpires between week nine up to the fetus's birth. The brain continues to grow and develop during this stage.

Normal Fetal-Placental Development

Placental and fetal growth go hand in hand; without the function of the placenta, there would be no sustainable fetal life. The **placenta** performs multiple processes for the fetus, including metabolic functions as well as physiological functions like the exchange of nutrients, waste, gases, and electrolytes. The placenta forms after fertilization of the ovum, which then develops into a morula before becoming a blastocyst that will implant into the uterus after around 6 days. This will initiate the production of human chorionic gonadotropin (hCG) and grow to form the chorion, which will develop into the fetal placenta. During the first trimester of pregnancy, the placental growth is slow but will correlate to the size of the uterus and fetus by the start of the second trimester. The amnio-chorionic membrane is developed due to the growth of the amniotic sac, which is quicker than that of the chorionic sac and leads to their fusion. The fetomaternal junction acts as support for the chorion and involves the development of endometrial blood vessels, which assist in the exchange of maternal and fetal blood. Typically, maternal and fetal red blood cells will not be mixed during this process. The placental membrane facilitates the exchange of substances such as nutrients, gases, and waste from the mother to the fetus. This membrane consists of cytotrophoblast, embryonic connective tissue (Wharton's jelly), fetal blood vessels, and syncytiotrophoblast. Two umbilical arteries carry deoxygenated blood from the fetus to the chorionic arteries in the placenta, which perform the exchange of substances at the capillary beds and then return the oxygenated blood via one umbilical vein back to the fetus.

Alterations in Maternal Anatomy/Physiology

Many maternal anatomic and physical changes occur throughout pregnancy, including alterations to the respiratory, endocrine, cardiovascular, urinary, and gastrointestinal systems. Many of these changes are related to fluctuating hormone levels, particularly due to the production of hCG and, more precisely, beta-hCG by the syncytiotrophoblastic cells of the placenta. Beta-hCG is essential in the production of progesterone and estrogen as well as the halting of ovulation through the activation of the corpus luteum. The production of the hormone **relaxin** from both the corpus luteum and the placenta is also increased in pregnant individuals. Relaxin works to soften connective tissues, as well as the birth canal, to prepare for fetal development and the physiological requirements of pregnancy.

The respiratory system is altered by hormone fluctuations as well as anatomy changes. Increased levels of progesterone result in increased ventilation and minor respiratory acidosis, which is compensated for

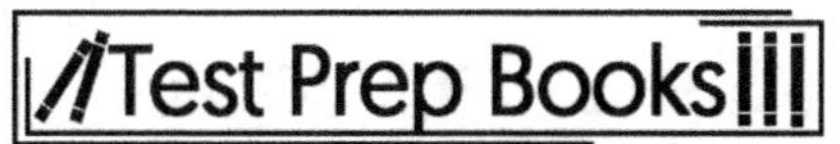

metabolically by increased bicarbonate production via the kidneys. Anatomically, the position of the diaphragm is pushed upward 5 centimeters to adjust for the growing fetus, which results in decreased expiratory reserves, increased work of breathing, and shortness of breath.

The cardiovascular system of a pregnant patient undergoes numerous changes, including increased stroke volume and heart rate resulting in greater cardiac output. Heart contractility and cardiac compliance are also increased. Renal blood flow rises by as much as 80 percent due to the improved cardiac output, which results in a 50 percent higher glomerular filtration rate (GFR). Overall, this leads to a total fluid volume increase of 1.5 liters of water to the body.

Finally, the gastrointestinal system is affected by a relaxed esophageal sphincter and slowed gastric emptying due to increased progesterone. These changes increase the risk of gastroesophageal reflux disease (GERD) during pregnancy.

Prenatal Care

Excellent nursing care prior to, during, and immediately following childbirth is essential. Pregnancy as a medical state comprises several distinct stages: antepartum, intrapartum, postpartum, and newborn care. **Antepartum** care can be defined as care during pregnancy. During this period, the pregnant patient must be assessed periodically for appropriate fetal growth, responsiveness in-utero, and the mother's overall health status. Any fluctuations in these areas signal the potential for maternal or fetal distress. It is necessary to obtain a complete medical, gynecological, and obstetrical history. The provider must be aware of any sexually transmitted diseases, previous abortions or full-term pregnancies (gravida), any complications, and the number of vaginal and cesarean births (para), as well as estimated date of delivery (EDD) and current birth plan.

Gestational Age Determination

Determining **gestational age** is vital to ensure proper assessments and screenings are completed in a timely manner to improve the health outcomes of the mother and fetus. Gestational age can be determined through many different assessment techniques, including history of last menstrual period, physical measurement of fundal height, and transvaginal or transabdominal ultrasounds.

Ultrasound is the gold standard of gestational age determination and has increased accuracy in the first trimester of pregnancy with the transvaginal probe. Ultrasound allows for visualization of the uterus along with the surrounding area, including the bladder, rectum, and uterine wall, which can assist in determining the position and size of the fetus. The uterus grows by approximately 1 centimeter each week after 4 weeks of gestation, with the most accurate gestational age being measured prior to week 14 of pregnancy.

Naegele's Rule is often used when calculating gestational age based on last menstrual period. To utilize this method, add 1 year and 7 days to the date of the last menstrual period, and then subtract 3 months to determine the patient's estimated due date.

Fundal height can also be palpated and measured to determine gestational age. At 12 weeks of gestation, the uterus will be palpable right above the pubic symphysis. By 16 weeks, the fundus will be between the pubic symphysis and umbilicus. At 20 weeks, the fundus will be palpable by the umbilicus. After 20 weeks, the fundal height can be measured in centimeters from the pubic symphysis, which should equal the number of weeks in gestation.

Risk Assessment

Risk assessment is vital to ensure the health and safety of both the mother and fetus during pregnancy. Risk assessments allow for early detection and intervention of potential health complications while also helping low-risk patients avoid unnecessary interventions and costs. Low-risk pregnancies are typically defined as singleton (one fetus), vertex presentation, normal fetal development, and no significant obstetric or medical history, typically delivering when the baby is term (37–40 weeks of gestation). Low-risk pregnancies typically require less testing and fewer interventions and are a good indication of fewer maternal and fetal complications. **High-risk pregnancies** are characterized by any diagnosis that may pose an increased risk of complications for the mother and fetus. Patients with medical conditions such as diabetes, hypertension, obesity, heart disease, autoimmune disorders, and kidney disease are at a higher risk of experiencing further complications during pregnancy. Obstetric factors, such as multiple gestation pregnancies (e.g., twins or triplets), placental issues (e.g., placenta previa), preeclampsia or eclampsia, gestational diabetes, and previous preterm birth or birth complications all increase the maternal and fetal risks.

Nutrition

Both before and during pregnancy, nutrition and weight management each have a significant impact on infant development. **Prenatal nutrition** relates to nutrient contents that affect a fetus's growth and development. Sustaining a healthy weight while carrying an embryo (**gestation**) decreases the prospect of negative risks associated with congenital birth defects. Prenatal development is a crucial time for healthy infant development, and nutrients are a prime component in ensuring the infants' optimal health and general wellness. Some examples of nutritious foods for infants during prenatal development include lean meats, fruits, low-fat dairy products, vegetables, and whole grains.

Immunizations

Immunizations play an important role in ensuring the health and safety of the mother and fetus during pregnancy. Certain vaccinations are important to have prior to becoming pregnant, such as the measles, mumps, and rubella (**MMR**) vaccine to prevent rubella, which can lead to serious pregnancy complications, miscarriage, and birth defects. During pregnancy, patients are advised to obtain the pertussis (**TDAP**) immunization to pass antibodies on to the fetus that will protect them after birth. Seventy percent of deaths from pertussis occur in newborns to 2-month-old babies who have not yet had the immunization. Therefore, it is vital for the pregnant patient to receive this immunization between the 27th and 36th week of gestation to allow for the greatest effect. It is also recommended to get a flu shot before October to lower the risk of illness in the mother or baby. The respiratory syncytial virus (**RSV**) vaccination can be either received by the pregnant patient during the 32nd to 36th week of gestation or given to the newborn baby during their first RSV season. The **COVID-19** vaccine is now also recommended by the American College of Obstetricians and Gynecologists (ACOG) for pregnant patients.

Medication Reconciliation

Medication reconciliation is an important part of prenatal care to ensure the patient is only taking pregnancy-safe medications when necessary. Studies have shown that 70 percent of women in the US take one or more medications during the first 3 months of pregnancy. This is important due to the lack of information available on the effects of many medications during pregnancy. Medication reconciliation involves interviewing the patient to compile a complete list of current medications. This list can then be examined by the health care team to determine if each medication is safe to continue taking during pregnancy or needs to be switched to an alternative, pregnancy-safe option. Many medications have teratogenic effects and can cause serious birth defects when taken during pregnancy.

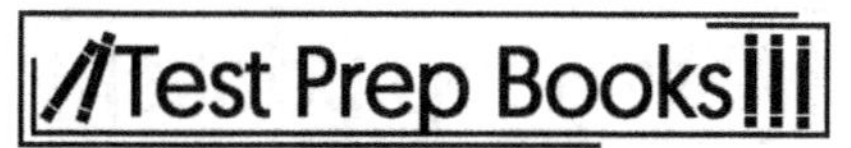

Health Guidance

Prenatal health guidance is very important to promote healthy maternal and fetal outcomes. Prenatal guidelines include categories such as nutrition, exercise, stress, sleep, and vaccination recommendations. Patients should take at least 400 micrograms of **folic acid** or methylated folate, preferably starting prior to pregnancy, to assist in the prevention of congenital defects. No more than 200 milligrams of **caffeine** should be consumed due to an increased risk of low birth weight and miscarriage. **Non-steroidal anti-inflammatory drugs (NSAIDs)** should be avoided due to increased risks to the fetus, such as kidney issues and premature ductus arteriosus closure. Instead, low doses of Tylenol should be used as the pregnancy-safe alternative for pain.

Screening Tests

After conception, pregnancy normally lasts forty weeks divided into three trimesters. The first and second trimesters last 14 weeks each, while the third trimester lasts from week 28 until delivery. Initial prenatal visits should include lab work: CBC, quantitative hCG, blood type and Rh antibody screening, and hepatitis and STI panels.

Throughout **prenatal care**, fetal ultrasound can be utilized to assess gestational age and growth, and patients are screened for pre-eclampsia with vital signs and urinalysis. Between 18–20 weeks' gestation, blood work and full anatomical ultrasound evaluates for chromosomal and anatomic abnormalities. Additionally, screening for gestational diabetes occurs at 24 to 28 weeks.

Glucose tolerance tests challenge the body to regulate glucose upon ingestion. After fasting, a drink containing liquid glucose will be administered to patients. After 1 to 3 hours, blood sugar levels are measured. Normal findings are 140 mg/dL or less. Blood sugar levels of 200 mg/dL are characteristic of diabetes.

Common Discomforts of Pregnancy

Pregnancy brings many common discomforts for patients, which can be brought on by hormone fluctuations, physical challenges, and emotional changes. Back pain is a common issue, with around 50 percent of patients reporting some form of backache during their pregnancy. Postural changes such as lordosis, ligament and intravertebral joint relaxation (due to the hormone relaxin), and abdominal muscle strain can contribute to back pain; these should be assessed to determine the correct plan for management. Leg muscle cramps are also a common complaint, particularly in the third trimester. Sudden muscle contractions can cause severe, sharp pain in the legs, which may be related to decreased serum calcium and increased phosphate levels. Assessment should be completed to rule out thrombophlebitis, which would present with redness, edema, pallor, and Homan's sign. Hormonal fluctuations are also known to cause increased headaches, breast tenderness, and fatigue, as well as nausea and vomiting.

Prenatal Exam

From conception until 28 weeks' gestation, **prenatal visits** can be scheduled monthly. From then until 36 weeks' gestation, visits should be biweekly, followed by weekly visits until delivery.

The provider performs the prenatal pelvic exam to assess the development of the fetus and the status of the maternal reproductive system. The pelvic exam is done at the first visit but is not repeated with every visit. In a normal pregnancy, it may not be repeated until the third trimester. The provider performs the postpartum exam to assess the return of the maternal reproductive organs to the nonpregnant state.

Assessment of Fetal Well Being

Amniotic Fluid Index (AFI)

A normal amount of amniotic fluid is vital to healthy fetal outcomes. Amniotic fluid is the substance that surrounds the fetus, providing protection, cushion for the umbilical cord, fluid, nutrition, and antibacterial properties. High or low levels of amniotic fluid are both associated with an increased risk of poor fetal health outcomes. The **amniotic fluid index** (**AFI**) is a measurement calculated during ultrasound examination that allows the provider to estimate the amount of amniotic fluid surrounding the fetus. This test is part of the biophysical and modified biophysical profile (BPP). **Polyhydramnios**, or increased amniotic fluid, is characterized by an AFI of 24 centimeters or more. Polyhydramnios can be related to congenital disorders, gastrointestinal obstructions, or musculoskeletal conditions. **Oligohydramnios**, or low amniotic fluid, is characterized by an AFI of less than 5 centimeters. Oligohydramnios can be related to intrauterine growth restriction (IUGR), renal issues, or genitourinary infections. Invasive testing of amniotic fluid, or amniocentesis, may be required to diagnose certain conditions (e.g., trisomy 21).

Biophysical and Modified Biophysical Profile (BPP)

Biophysical and modified biophysical profile (**BPP**) testing is vital in evaluating fetal health outcomes. BPP testing includes a reactive nonstress test (NST) and fetal ultrasound to assess fetal breathing, movement, tone, and amniotic fluid level. These five indicators are scored on a scale of 0–2, with 2 being sufficient and 0 being nonexistent. Sufficient fetal breathing should involve one or more episodes of breathing that last for 30 or more seconds within a 30-minute time frame. Sufficient movement is classified as three or more movements within a 30-minute time frame. Fetal tone is sufficient if one or more flexions or extensions are observed. Amniotic fluid volume is sufficient if one pocket of amniotic fluid can be measured at 2 centimeters or more without any presence of umbilical cord or fetus. A modified BPP includes an NST as well as an amniotic fluid measurement and is typically used during the second or third trimester. The modified BBP is used to determine placental perfusion or insufficiency, which can cause decreased amniotic fluid volume and inadequate perfusion of the fetal kidneys.

Genetic Screening and Diagnostic Tests

Genetic screening and diagnostic testing are available for all patients throughout pregnancy, although they should be discussed with the patient early in the first trimester. Assessing the patient for risk factors, such as family history of genetic conditions, is also important to determine whether further testing is necessary.

During the first trimester, maternal blood work should be performed to measure biomarkers such as free beta-human chorionic gonadotropin (β-hCG), estriol, pregnancy-associated plasma protein A (PAPP-A), and maternal serum alpha-fetoprotein (MSAFP). A sonogram is also commonly performed between 11 and 14 weeks of gestation to determine **nuchal translucency**, which is an indication of chromosomal abnormalities. **Cell-free DNA** (**cfDNA**) testing is also completed in the first trimester to screen for chromosomal abnormalities.

During the second trimester, triple, quadruple, and penta screenings can be performed via maternal blood work. The triple screen is characterized by testing for serum levels of unconjugated estriol, MSAFP, and β-hCG. The quadruple screen involves the same testing as the triple screen panel with the addition of the inhibin A test. The penta screening involves testing for hyperglycosylated hCG in addition to the tests in the quadruple screening. These screenings assess for the presence of trisomies 13, 18, and 21, as well as disorders relating to the sex chromosomes.

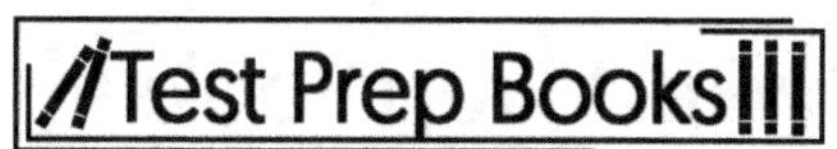

Nonstress Testing (NST)

Nonstress testing (**NST**) during the antenatal period is a vital part of fetal surveillance. NSTs monitor fetal heart rate (FHR) and movement to ensure that the fetus is healthy and sufficiently oxygenated. NSTs assist in preventing stillbirth by allowing the health care team to noninvasively assess fetal well-being and determine any indications for early induction or delivery. Indications for an NST include history of previous pregnancy complications, reduced fetal movement, fetal anomalies, fetal growth restriction (FGR), or maternal conditions such as hypertension, diabetes, preeclampsia, obesity, and advanced maternal age. NSTs are typically performed with the patient positioned in semi-Fowler's or left lateral to ensure there is no compression on the vena cava. Most patients can begin receiving NSTs at 37 weeks of gestation when the fetus is able to show reactivity. The FHR is typically assessed for a minimum of 20 minutes via external monitors. An NST would be considered reactive if the fetus has a heart rate acceleration of at least 15 beats per minute higher than baseline that lasts at least 15 seconds in response to their movement. A reactive NST is a good indicator of fetal health and oxygenation. On the other hand, a nonreactive NST is characterized by an absence of heart rate accelerations associated with movement or no movement, indicating that additional testing is necessary.

Ultrasound

Ultrasonography is an important tool that enables practitioners to assess the fetus prior to delivery. Typically, ultrasounds are performed in the first, second, and third trimesters of pregnancy to ensure fetal well-being prior to delivery. In the first trimester, patients typically receive an ultrasound between 7 and 12 weeks of gestation. This ultrasound is commonly transvaginal and assists in determining FHR, gestational age, fetal size, and number of fetuses. First-trimester ultrasounds are also commonly used to test for nuchal translucency or when concerns (e.g., vaginal bleeding) arise. The **fetal anatomy scan** should be performed in the second trimester between 18 and 22 weeks of gestation. This ultrasound studies the fetus in detail to survey fetal size and anatomy, confirm gender, rule out birth defects and congenital conditions, and determine the location of the placenta. Early diagnosis of fetal anomalies is essential to ensure prompt care after delivery to increase the chances of positive outcomes for both the mother and fetus. If any anomaly or placental issue is present during the second-trimester scan, this would warrant additional scans in the third trimester (and possible referral to maternal-fetal medicine) to determine the best course of action for delivery and newborn care. Additional reasons for ultrasound use in the third trimester include growth scans (e.g., IUGR or macrosomia) as well as confirmation of fetal presentation and positioning.

Medical and Obstetrical Complications of Pregnancy

Maternal Medical Disorders

Diabetes

Diabetes that develops during pregnancy is known as **gestational diabetes mellitus** (**GDM**). GDM is a type of hyperglycemia that, if left untreated, could negatively affect the mother and fetus. There are two types of GDM: diet-controlled (A1GDM) and pharmacologically controlled (A2GDM). Risk factors for developing GDM include history of GDM, body mass index (BMI) over 25, hypertension, polycystic ovarian syndrome (PCOS), family history, decreased activity level, and previous newborn weight over 4000 grams at birth. Insulin resistance is a common issue in pregnancy due to the release of progesterone, prolactin, estrogen, growth hormone, and human placental lactogen from the placenta. Maternal β-cell dysfunction, due to the increase in hormones, also results in less insulin being secreted. Screening for GDM should be performed between 24 and 28 weeks of gestation. There are two types of initial tests for GDM: the 1 hour 50-gram glucose test and the 2 hour 75-gram glucose test. Most patients will choose to undergo the 1-hour non-fasting test, in which

80 percent of patients will pass and around 20 percent of patients will require additional testing with a secondary 3 hour 100-gram fasting glucose test to confirm a GDM diagnosis. The criteria required to pass the 3-hour glucose test include the following: fasting glucose under 95 mg/dL, 1 hour glucose under 185 mg/dL, 2-hour glucose under 155 mg/dL, and 3-hour glucose under 140 mg/dL. To be positive for GDM, two or more of the above criteria must exceed the listed glucose level. Treatment involves lifestyle changes such as increase in activity level and diet modification. Patients will typically need to monitor their glucose levels four times a day. Pharmacological treatment or insulin therapy may be required if lifestyle modification does not work to lower glucose levels.

STI/HIV

Sexually transmitted infection (STI) and human immunodeficiency virus (HIV) testing is imperative to a healthy pregnancy and fetus. STIs during pregnancy can cause serious birth defects, miscarriage, and still birth. If a newborn is exposed in the birth canal during delivery, they are at high risk of developing eye or lung infections. If the mother is infected with syphilis, the newborn is likely to have issues with their brain, eyes, skin, bones, and teeth. HIV, when left untreated, can be life threatening for the mother as well as the newborn. Screening for STIs and HIV must be completed as soon as possible to ensure prompt treatment and increase the chances of positive health outcomes for the fetus. During the first trimester, all pregnant patients should be screened for hepatitis B, hepatitis C, syphilis, HIV, chlamydia, and gonorrhea. During the third trimester, all patients should be rescreened for syphilis and HIV, with chlamydia and gonorrhea rescreening added for those at an increased risk.

Hypertension

Hypertension in pregnancy can pose significant risks for both the mother and fetus. There are several different kinds of hypertension in pregnancy, including chronic hypertension, preeclampsia with or without severe features, eclampsia, and gestational hypertension, as well as hemolysis, elevated liver enzymes, and low platelet count (HELLP) syndrome. Early detection and intervention are vital to mitigate adverse effects of these conditions along with lowering the risk of maternal and fetal morbidity. Risk factors for these conditions include preexisting hypertension, history of preeclampsia in a previous pregnancy, family history of hypertension or preeclampsia, BMI >30, renal conditions, diabetes mellitus, twin or multiple fetuses, and autoimmune disorders. Hypertension is classified as systolic blood pressure over 140 mmHg and diastolic pressure over 90 mmHg. Severe-range blood pressure is defined as a systolic blood pressure over 160 mmHg and diastolic pressure over 110 mmHg. Preeclampsia is typically diagnosed with elevated blood pressures and common symptoms, including increased edema in the face and extremities, vision changes, headache or change in mental status, hepatic issues, pulmonary edema, and proteinuria. Treatment involves 81 mg of aspirin started at time of diagnosis and continued until delivery, along with antihypertensive therapies if the patient's blood pressure is over 140/90 mmHg. Common antihypertensive medications used in pregnancy include labetalol, nifedipine for acute treatment, and hydralazine.

Epilepsy

Uncontrolled electrical impulses in the brain that appear suddenly and excessively can cause a **seizure**. There are two types of seizures. **Primary seizures** are not associated with a specific disease process or lesion in the brain. **Secondary seizures** have an underlying cause. Duration and a description of the seizure will help guide treatment. Family members who were present during the seizure can provide important details about the event. The provider must assess for several risk factors when a patient voices seizure activity. Comorbidities, such as heart disease, stroke, and cerebral palsy, can contribute to seizures.

Acute alcohol intoxication or drug withdrawal can alter the electrical impulses in the brain. Electrolyte irregularities, such as a deficiency in serum glucose or an excess in serum potassium, may cause disturbances. Providers should ask about head injuries or diagnosis of brain tumors. There are various classifications of seizures. The most common is the **tonic-clonic seizure**. It lasts between two and five minutes and is

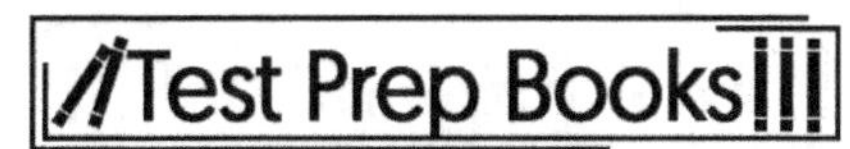

characterized by two phases. Stiffening of the muscles in the extremities and loss of consciousness is the first, **tonic phase**. During the second phase, known as the **clonic phase**, involuntary jerky movements happen throughout the body. Incontinence may be present.

Patients will be confused and fatigued after seizure activity. Diagnostic tests will include an electroencephalogram (EEG), CT scan, and MRI. The most important part of treatment is to prevent injury during a seizure. Two or more seizures that are unprovoked is known as epilepsy.

Anticonvulsants are also called antiepileptic or anti-seizure medications. They are used in the treatment of epileptic seizures. They suppress excessive firing of neurons and therefore prevent the initiation and spread of seizures. The common side effects are dizziness, sedation, weight gain, hepatotoxicity, hair loss, blood disorders, etc. Anticonvulsants are teratogenic and can cause significant harm to a fetus and result in birth defects. Therefore, female patients on anticonvulsant therapy should consult with their physicians before planning pregnancy.

Focal Seizures

In partial seizures, the excess neuronal discharge occurs in one cerebral cortex, and most often results from structural abnormalities. **Partial (focal) seizures** may evolve into a generalized seizure (called secondary generalization), which causes loss of consciousness. Secondary generalization occurs when a partial seizure spreads and activates the entire cerebrum bilaterally. Activation may occur so rapidly that the initial partial seizure is not clinically apparent or is very brief.

Generalized Seizures

In **generalized seizures**, the aberrant electrical discharge diffusely involves the entire cortex of both hemispheres from the onset, and consciousness is usually lost. Generalized seizures result most often from metabolic disorders and sometimes from genetic disorders.

Status Epilepticus

Prolonged seizure activity is defined as **status epilepticus**, which is the occurrence of multiple seizures, each lasting more than five minutes over a thirty-minute period. This condition is life-threatening, as the brain does not have sufficient recovery time to reoxygenate. Causes of this condition include epilepsy, metabolic imbalances, stroke, uncontrolled infections, and acute drug/alcohol withdrawal. Care of this condition includes the immediate administration of the first-line pharmacological therapy, benzodiazepines. The second-line therapy is any compatible antiseizure medication, with the third-line therapy typically being general anesthesia and endotracheal intubation.

Eclampsia

Eclampsia is the life-threatening complication of severe preeclampsia that is manifested by the onset of seizure activity and/or the development of coma and is associated with hypertension, proteinuria, intrauterine fetal growth delay, and diminished amniotic fluid. There are no specific diagnostic tests, and while the specific etiology is unknown, there are indications that the condition results from the interchange of maternal and fetal tissue or allografts. **Magnesium sulfate** is recommended for short-term use for 24 to 48 hours to stabilize the patient for delivery, which is the only curative measure.

Substance Use

Research has demonstrated that pregnant women using drugs such as alcohol, tobacco, marijuana, opioids, and other illicit substances, as well as misusing prescription drugs, can significantly affect the health of a fetus, and even increase the risk of a stillbirth. Many of these substances can easily pass through the woman's placenta, so when a pregnant woman engages in substance use, these substances can also reach the fetus. Another potential result of drug use during pregnancy is **neonatal abstinence syndrome**, which involves the fetus experiencing withdrawal symptoms soon after being born. Drugs that increase this risk during pregnancy include opioids, alcohol, benzodiazepines, barbiturates, and even caffeine. The full extent of a fetus's withdrawal symptoms is contingent on which drugs were used, how frequently the pregnant mother used these drugs, the manner in which her body metabolized the drugs, and whether the infant was born prematurely or underwent a full term before birth.

Tobacco use while pregnant can result in birth defects or an increased risk of **sudden infant death syndrome**, which is the unexplained death of an infant before they reach their first year of life. Using illegal drugs such as cocaine and methamphetamine, or misusing prescription drugs such as opioids, can also possibly result in birth defects, withdrawal symptoms, underweight babies, or even the loss of the baby.

Alcohol Exposed Pregnancy (FASD)

Fetal alcohol spectrum disorders (**FASD**) are associated with exposure to alcohol during pregnancy and pose significant risks to fetal physical and neurological well-being. There are five categories that comprise FASD: partial fetal alcohol syndrome (pFAS), neurobehavioral disorder associated with prenatal alcohol exposure (ND-PAE), alcohol-related neurodevelopmental disorder (ARND), fetal alcohol syndrome (FAS), and alcohol-related birth defects (ARBD). Alcohol is highly teratogenic, and exposure in pregnancy is the leading contributor to preventable congenital disabilities. No amount of alcohol should be consumed at any point during pregnancy. Alcohol exposure in the first trimester has been linked to brain damage and facial asymmetry characterized by short palpebral fissures, thin upper lips, smooth philtrum, and low-set ears. Alcohol consumption in the second trimester increases the risk of miscarriage as well as decreased brain volume, height, and weight during the third trimester. While there is no cure for FASD, there are resources available to help lessen the neurological effects, such as educational aids.

Thrombocytopenia

Idiopathic Thrombocytopenia Purpura (ITP)

Thrombocytes are cells in the blood that help with the clotting process that achieves hemostasis. A normal count of thrombocytes or platelets is 140,000 to 440,000, though that number can vary in the case of pregnant women or persons with inflammatory conditions. A significant drop below that number is considered thrombocytopenia. **Idiopathic thrombocytopenia purpura** (**ITP**) is a type of thrombocytopenia that occurs in the absence of systemic disease, marked by bleeding, and often has no known cause, hence the idiopathy.

ITP is a chronic condition in adults, but usually resolves spontaneously in children. Typically, the patient will present with petechiae, purpura, and mucosal bleeding. **Petechiae** are small red or purple spots that appear on the skin and mark small points of bleeding in the capillary beds. **Purpura** is a slightly larger point of collected blood under the skin that indicate uncontrolled bleeding in the capillary beds. Ecchymosis, or bruising, which is the largest of the bleeding lesions, may also be present in ITP.

Diagnosis of ITP is made via blood tests, with other causes of thrombocytopenia excluded to confirm diagnosis. Corticosteroids will be used to try and stop bleeding. In very severe cases of ITP, a splenectomy, in which the spleen is removed, is considered to resolve ITP. In the case of severe, uncontrolled bleeding, the patient may be given a platelet transfusion.

Disseminated Intravascular Coagulation (DIC)

Disseminated intravascular coagulation (**DIC**) is a medical emergency in which the coagulation cascade has been activated by exposure to a tissue factor. The fibrinolytic pathway is also activated. Usually onset of DIC is rapid, with bleeding and occlusion of the small blood vessels present. The result of a sudden onset of DIC is thrombocytopenia, a prolonged PT and PTT time, high d-Dimer, and lowered plasma fibrinogen.

Causes of DIC can include obstetric complications such as abruptio placentae, retained dead fetus, or amniotic fluid embolism. Infections with gram-negative organs that release an endotoxin that causes tissue factor release may cause DIC. Cancers usually produce a slow-onset DIC in which more clotting activities are part of the clinical presentation.

Treatment of DIC will include replacement therapy of platelets, cryoprecipitate, and fresh frozen plasma. In patients with a slower onset of DIC, heparin may be used to treat the condition.

Heparin-induced Thrombocytopenia (HIT)

Heparin-induced thrombocytopenia (**HIT**) occurs when the anticoagulation caused by the administration of heparin leads to thrombosis and thus, thrombocytopenia. This condition results when the patient's body has an abnormal antibody response to the heparin that activates platelets.

Two forms of heparin-induced thrombocytopenia have been identified: HIT type I and HIT type II. HIT type I, also called heparin-associated thrombocytopenia, occurs at the beginning of therapy, is most often a benign condition that does not result in thrombotic events, is not the end-product of an immune response, and quickly resolves spontaneously. HIT I results in a transient decrease in the platelet count, which recovers rapidly when heparin is discontinued and rarely results in a thrombotic event.

HIT type II is defined as an immune-mediated reaction resulting in platelet activation and hypercoagulability that is caused by the presence of heparin. HIT type II can result in increased risk of a thrombotic event or life-threatening gangrene. Since it is an immune-mediated response, the onset is typically five to fourteen days after receiving any type or amount of heparin product. The immediate medical intervention is to discontinue any heparin products and initiate a non-heparinized anticoagulant.

Gestational Thrombocytopenia

Gestational thrombocytopenia is the most common cause of low platelet counts in pregnancy, accounting for 70–80 percent of pregnancy-related thrombocytopenia. While the exact cause of gestational thrombocytopenia is unknown, there are many theories, including increased placental use of platelets, the creation of platelet-targeting autoantibodies, changes in von Willebrand factor, increased plasma volume leading to decreased platelet dilution, and difficulties associated with thrombopoietin. Gestational thrombocytopenia will typically resolve after the delivery of the newborn, which excludes typical autoimmune etiologies. Diagnosis is made via the following criteria: asymptomatic mother with no platelet count issues in the fetus, patient in the second or third trimester, absence of bleeding, full recovery within 1 to 2 months following delivery of the fetus, and occurrence in prior or future pregnancies. Typically, gestational thrombocytopenia is diagnosed when all etiologies have been ruled out and requires no further treatment, as it spontaneously resolves 1 to 2 months after delivery. If the patient's platelet counts falls below 70×10^9 per liter, additional testing will be necessary, as this is unlikely with gestational thrombocytopenia alone.

Anemia

Anemia is a nonhereditary blood disorder in which an individual's blood has a low number of red blood cells. Mild forms of anemia may have no symptoms or manageable symptoms such as tiredness. Severe forms of anemia can result in extreme fatigue, shortness of breath, or unconsciousness. Anemia can be caused by low iron levels as a result of poor diet, heavy menstrual cycles in women, or stomach and intestinal cancers. In these instances, low iron levels can typically be remedied with iron supplementation or dietary changes. Sometimes, iron-deficiency anemia will need to be treated with blood transfusions; however, this is quite rare. A type of anemia called pernicious anemia is caused by vitamin B-12 deficiencies. Other forms of anemia are caused by chronic diseases, especially diseases related to the kidney, disorders within the bone marrow (aplastic anemia), or autoimmune disorders (autoimmune hemolytic anemia). These situations usually require stronger medication, synthetic hormones, blood transfusions, and sometimes transplants to rectify the low red blood cell count.

Infection

Congenital Varicella

Congenital varicella is a condition caused by transmission of the varicella virus, also known as chicken pox, to the fetus during pregnancy. The infection causes low birth weight, skin abnormalities (consisting of hypertrophic scar tissue on areas of the body), malformed extremities, and damage to the nervous system (causing developmental delays and vision issues). Infection is uncommon due to high rates of vaccinations in the population; however, women who are unvaccinated are at a higher risk of contracting varicella and passing it to the fetus. If the mother has a confirmed varicella infection through history, physical exam, and culture of the lesions, the amniotic fluid should be analyzed by PCR assay, and fetal ultrasound can be used to determine if there are abnormalities of the limbs, head, or soft tissue. While the best treatment is prevention, varicella-zoster immune globulin (VZIG) and acyclovir can be used to treat the infection and reduce the severity of disease.

Cytomegalovirus (CMV)

Cytomegalovirus (CMV) is a commonly occurring herpes virus (HHV-5) that can lay dormant in the body for many years before reactivating and causing symptoms later in life. CMV can be passed from a pregnant woman to the fetus, resulting in congenital CMV. In healthy patients, symptoms are non-existent to mild and include fever, sore throat, fatigue, and swollen lymph nodes. Infected infants may be born with hearing loss, vision issues, seizures, microcephaly, and developmental delays. Immunocompromised individuals may exhibit more severe symptoms, such as pneumonia, hepatitis, and seizures. Risk factors for infection include working with children under five years of age, living in close contact with others, and being in an immunocompromised state. Blood, urine, and saliva tests can be used to confirm diagnosis. Antiviral medications, such as ganciclovir or valganciclovir, can be used to treat the infection. These will typically be used for immunocompromised individuals and infants to lessen the risk of future health problems.

Group B Streptococcus

Group B streptococcus (GBS) is a commonly found bacteria in the normal flora of the genitals and intestinal tracts. For pregnant women, the bacteria can cause serious infection of the newborn due to transmission during birth. Although the mother may not exhibit any symptoms, a urinary tract infection is associated with infection. Infants may show symptoms such as fever, seizures, meningitis, and skin, joint, and bone infections, which may lead to sepsis. Pregnant women should be screened between thirty-five and thirty-seven weeks through a vaginal swab. If GBS is present, the mother should receive treatment with antibiotics, such as penicillin, amoxicillin, or cephalexin, to prevent transmission.

Hepatitis

Hepatitis is an inflammatory condition of the liver, which is further categorized as infectious or noninfectious. Causative infectious agents for hepatitis may be viral, fungal, or bacterial, while noninfectious causes include autoimmune disease, prescription and recreational drugs, alcohol abuse, and metabolic disorders. More than 50 percent of the cases of acute hepatitis in the United States are caused by a virus. Transmission routes include fecal-oral, parenteral, sexual contact, and perinatal transmission. There are four phases of the course of viral hepatitis. During phase 1, which is asymptomatic, the host is infected and the virus replicates; the onset of mild symptoms occurs in phase 2; progressive symptoms of liver dysfunction appear in phase 3; and recovery from the infection occurs in phase 4. These phases are specific to the causative agent and the individual.

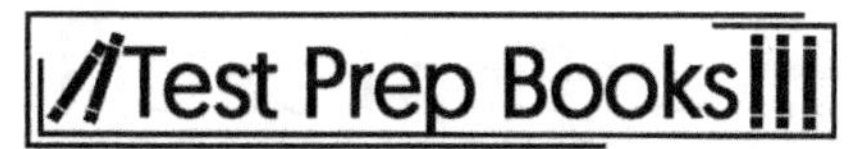

The most common viral agents are hepatitis A (HAV), hepatitis B (HBV), and hepatitis C (HCV). Less commonly, hepatitis D (HDV), hepatitis E (HEV), CMV, Epstein-Barr virus, and adenovirus may cause hepatitis. HAV and HBV often present with nausea, jaundice, anorexia, right upper quadrant pain, fatigue, and malaise. HCV may be asymptomatic or, alternatively, may present with similar symptoms. Approximately 20 percent of acute infections with HBV and HCV result in chronic hepatitis, which is a risk factor for the development of cirrhosis and liver failure. The care of the patient with acute hepatitis due to HAV and HCV is focused on symptom relief, while the antiviral treatment for HBV is effective in decreasing the incidence of adenocarcinoma.

Chronic hepatitis is a complication of acute hepatitis and frequently progresses to hepatic failure, which is associated with deteriorating coagulation status and the onset of hepatic encephalopathy due to alterations in the blood-brain barrier that result in brain cell edema. Care of the patient with hepatic failure is focused on fluid volume, homeostasis, and reduction of encephalopathy.

Herpes Simplex Virus

Herpes simplex virus, either **HSV-1** or **HSV-2**, can be passed from the mother to the child either in utero, during birth, or after birth. Infection of the infant with HSV often results in permanent disability or death. HSV causes painful blisters or ulcers in adults. HSV-1 is spread by oral contact and typically presents around the oral cavity. HSV-2 is spread through sexual contact and results in genital sores. Women who have an outbreak of HSV during the third trimester are more likely to transmit the virus to their infant. Infected infants will show symptoms of fever, failure to thrive, and irritability. Early diagnosis can be difficult but is achieved through testing of blood or cerebrospinal fluid. Prevention through the identification of high-risk mothers, subsequent administration of antiviral therapies, and completion of birth through C-section is ideal. However, antiviral drugs such as acyclovir, famciclovir, and valacyclovir can be given to newborns.

Human Papillomavirus

Human papillomavirus (HPV) is a sexually transmitted virus that can be passed from mother to baby during birth, though this type of transmission is uncommon. Infected infants may show symptoms such as warts on the skin, warts in the respiratory system leading to benign tumors, or no symptoms at all. To diagnose HPV in infants, nasal swabs should be collected and tested for HPV DNA shortly after birth. There is no treatment, as many infants will clear the infection on their own.

Rubella

Rubella is a viral infection often known as German measles or three-day measles. It commonly affects infants and children who have not received MMR vaccinations. Symptoms are mild and include fever, headache, arthralgias, swollen lymph nodes, and rash that begins on the face, spreads to the trunk, and then to the arms and legs. Symptoms typically last one to five days, although a person can be infectious the week prior to symptoms appearing and a week after resolution of symptoms. While the infection is mild, it can be dangerous for pregnant women, as it can pass to the fetus, resulting in growth delays, deafness, congenital heart defects, miscarriage, and stillborn birth. Rubella presents as similar to other illnesses; therefore, antibody tests should be run on blood samples and a viral culture should be completed to confirm diagnosis. The infection will typically resolve on its own, and supportive care measures such as rest, fluids, antipyretics, and pain relievers should be encouraged.

Zika Virus

Zika virus, which is transmitted through mosquito bites and sexual exposure, is especially dangerous to pregnant women and the fetus. Women who are pregnant should be advised to not travel to areas where Zika is active. Symptoms of infection are mild and include fever, rash, arthralgias, headache, and conjunctivitis. The virus is diagnosed through a PCR test of the blood. The infection will typically clear on its own and does not require treatment. When acquired during pregnancy, complications such as miscarriage, stillbirth, and preterm birth can occur. Additionally, the infant may be born with birth defects such as microcephaly, abnormal brain development, eye abnormalities, and hearing loss.

Pregnancy-Specific Conditions

Gestational Trophoblastic Disease

Gestational trophoblastic disease (GTD) involves abnormal and rapid growth of trophoblastic tissue that can become cancerous. The primary risk factor is advanced maternal age. The most common GTD is known as a hydatidiform mole (HM, or "molar pregnancy"). GTD is never a viable pregnancy, though some HMs include partial fetal tissue. Examples of malignant GTD include choriocarcinomas and invasive moles. Clinical features of GTD include a uterus larger than expected for gestational age. This typically coincides with quantitative hCG levels that are extremely high, such that it is considered a tumor marker. Patients may also experience hyperemesis gravidarum and hypertension at earlier stages than usual. The most common presenting symptom, though, is vaginal bleeding. Ultrasound is first-line imaging; classically, a "snowstorm" or "cluster of grapes" appearance suggests GTD, though their absence does not negate the condition. Treatment involves tumor evacuation via suction curettage. Patients must also undergo six months of hCG surveillance to ensure eradication, during which time they must take a contraceptive as pregnancy would falsely elevate hCG.

Placenta Previa

Placenta previa is defined as the abnormal placement of the placenta with either complete coverage of the internal cervical os (complete) by the placenta, or location of the placenta within two centimeters of the internal cervical os (marginal). The condition generally presents with painless vaginal bleeding during the third trimester of pregnancy and is associated with the possibility of hemorrhage at the onset of labor, due to cervical dilation and the relative inability of the lower uterine segment to effectively contract the vessels of the exposed maternal implantation site. Risk factors for this condition include maternal age greater than thirty-five years, infertility treatments, increased number of previous pregnancies, multiple births, previous C-sections, previous abortions, previous placenta previa, and smoking or cocaine use.

Once the condition is identified, the patient can be safely observed as long as the maternal and fetal monitoring parameters remain stable. Betamethasone therapy is indicated for the maturation of the fetal lungs if the pregnancy duration is less than thirty-four weeks. At the first sign of bleeding, immediate surgery is necessary. The care of the patient who presents with hemorrhage without prior identification of the placenta previa will trigger the agency protocol for obstetrical emergencies, which will include the transvaginal ultrasound confirmation of the condition and preparations for emergency surgery, including coagulation studies and type and cross match for six units of blood. Depending on the cause of the placenta previa, surgical removal of the uterus may be the only alternative surgical approach.

Abruptio Placenta

Abruptio placenta refers to the premature separation of the placenta from the uterine wall and is the most significant cause of hemorrhage in the third trimester. Descriptive terms for the condition include the identification of the degree of separation (either partial or complete), or the location of the separation (either marginal or central). Clinically, Class 0 indicates only the identification of a blood clot in the expelled placenta, while the manifestations in Classes 1, 2, and 3 progress from mild vaginal bleeding to hemorrhage, from mild uterine pain to tetanic or continuous contractions, from normal vital signs to maternal shock, from absent fetal distress to fetal demise, and from normal clotting to fibrinogen deficiency and hemorrhage. The exact cause is not known. However, there are several common risk factors, including maternal hypertension, which occurs in 40 percent of the cases of abruptio placenta; smoking; trauma in the form of car accidents, falls, or assaults; cocaine or alcohol abuse; maternal age greater than thirty-five or less than twenty years old; and previous history of abruptio placenta.

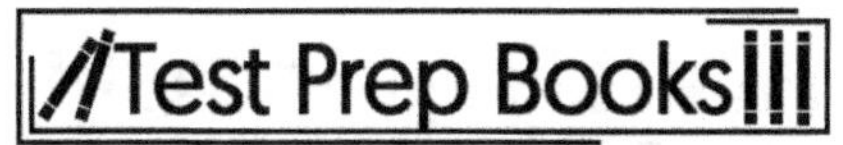

Depending on the patient's presenting manifestations, diagnostic studies include CBC, coagulation tests, type and screen, Kleihauer-Betke test in Rh-negative mothers to identify fetal-to-maternal transfer of blood, a nonstress test, fetal monitoring, and the possible use of ultrasonography; however, ultrasounds have a low sensitivity for identifying the separation of the placenta. The emergency care of the patient starts with fetal monitoring, initiation of IV access for fluid resuscitation with crystalloids and colloids, assessment and correction of any coagulopathy, administration of RhoGAM as needed, consideration of steroids for fetal lung maturity in preterm newborns, and preparation for delivery of the newborn.

Placenta Accreta

Placenta accreta occurs when the placental tissue grows beyond its normal barrier of the endometrium and starts to invade the uterine myometrium. There are several categories of placenta accreta based on the severity of the tissue growth into the myometrium, including placental increta, accreta, and percreta. Risk factors for the development of placenta accreta include history of cesarean section or other uterine surgery, multiparity, and advanced maternal age. Diagnosis typically follows an ultrasound, color Doppler, and possibly magnetic resonance imaging. Placenta accreta commonly presents along with a placenta previa, which would also be shown with ultrasonography. Management of placenta accreta involves the early delivery of the neonate between 34 and 36 weeks of gestation to prioritize fetal development while minimizing maternal risks. Delivery should be performed via C-section, which may involve prophylactic hysterectomy to lower the chances of maternal hemorrhage. Patients should be treated at a high acuity level facility to sufficiently monitor blood loss, hemoglobin and hematocrit, blood gases, and electrolyte levels. Massive transfusion protocols may be required if maternal hemorrhage occurs.

Vasa Previa

Vasa previa is characterized by fetal vessels that are present near or over the cervical os and are unprotected by the umbilical cord or placental tissue. This is very dangerous for the mother and fetus and could lead to vessel rupture during delivery. Vasa previa can occur in bilobate or succenturiate placentas, in which the vessels stretch between the lobes, leaving them exposed, as well as with velamentous insertions. Other conditions may occur alongside the vasa previa, including lower-lying placentas, multiparity, and placenta previa. Typically, diagnosis can be made following a color Doppler, in which the arterial and venous blood flows can be observed to determine their location in relation to the cervical os. However, diagnosis through color abdominal ultrasound can be difficult in obese patients, fetuses in difficult positions, and those with scar tissue from prior abdominal surgeries. Diagnosis is critical for a positive prognosis, as 56 percent of neonates with undiagnosed vasa previa will not make it through delivery due to ruptured vessels.

Bleeding in Pregnancy

Bleeding in pregnancy can be a benign occurrence or point to a more serious pregnancy complication, depending on when it presents and the amount of blood present. In the first trimester, bleeding is often a common occurrence and can be related to many different potential causes. These may include implantation bleeding at 1–2 weeks postfertilization, post-Pap exam, and sexual intercourse. Infection, ectopic pregnancy, and early miscarriage are more serious causes of first-trimester bleeding, which would require further evaluation. Light bleeding in the second or third trimester of pregnancy can be due to inflammation or growths and nodules formed on the cervix. Heavier bleeding later in pregnancy is more concerning and may be due to a placental issue, such as placenta previa, placenta accreta, or placental abruption. Each of these conditions can cause increased morbidity for the mother and fetus and therefore should be diagnosed as soon as possible.

Cervical Insufficiency

Cervical insufficiency involves cervical weakness such that, despite the absence of uterine contractions, pregnancy cannot be sustained into the third trimester. Risk factors include prior cervical insufficiency, abnormal anatomy, connective tissue diseases, and past procedures such as dilation or cervical biopsy. The typical presentation entails asymptomatic cervical shortening and/or dilation; bleeding, fluid discharge, or contractions likely represent a different diagnosis. It is usually identified on cervical exam during routine prenatal visits; ultrasound may be necessary for proper assessment of cervical length. If identified, cervical insufficiency merits hospitalization with fetal monitoring to rule out active labor and monitor fetal vital signs. Testing for STIs, UTIs, and amniotic membrane rupture may also be considered. For treatment, vaginal or intramuscular progesterone may help to improve cervical strength. More commonly, **cervical cerclage** is placed in the second trimester and often remains until the onset of labor. Providers should counsel all patients with cervical insufficiency to avoid sexual intercourse to maintain cervical integrity.

Intrauterine Fetal Demise (IUFD)

Intrauterine fetal demise (**IUFD**), also known as **stillbirth**, is defined as the death of a fetus weighing at least 350 grams or at least 20 weeks of gestation in which no signs of life are apparent once the fetus has been separated from its mother. There are a variety of maternal, placental, and fetal complications that can ultimately lead to stillbirth. Maternal complications include hypertension, diabetes, substance use, advanced maternal age, multiple gestations, and obesity. Placental factors include FGR, placental abnormalities, and placental abruption, which can all greatly increase the chances of stillbirth. Umbilical cord torsions, knots, or strictures along with vasa previa, umbilical cord prolapse, and umbilical cord anomalies also contribute to an increased risk of stillbirth. Fetal contributing factors include polyhydramnios, oligohydramnios, fetal infection, and genetic abnormalities. Each of these potential etiologies leads to a decrease in blood flow to the fetus, which results in fetal hypoxia and ultimately fetal death. Diagnosis typically follows fetal ultrasound, in which an absence of cardiac activity is observed along with Apgar scores of 0 at 1 and 5 minutes. Laboratory testing, imaging, genetic testing, and autopsy can all be completed to help determine the cause of death of the fetus.

Multiple Gestation

Multiple gestation typically involves fraternal twins; identical twins, triplets, and further multiples occur far less frequently. Advanced maternal age, high BMI, and family history of multiple gestation raises the likelihood of its occurrence in any pregnancy. Multiple gestation is commonly identified early and incidentally on routine prenatal ultrasound, and fetal heart tone auscultation may reveal multiple heartbeats. Additional features include a uterus that is large for gestational age, severe morning sickness, and increased weight gain. β-hCG and α-fetoprotein may also be elevated, though these are not specific to multiple gestation. Once multiple gestation is diagnosed, assessment should be completed via ultrasound for the number of amniotic sacs and placental chorions. Sharing of either structure by the fetuses raises the risk of complications, such as twin-twin transfusion syndrome in monochorionic fetuses. Patients must be counseled regarding increasing intake of folic acid and calories to accommodate the additional gestation(s). Though multiple gestation increases the risk of premature delivery, delivery should still be scheduled prior to forty weeks. This helps mitigate increased risks of pre-eclampsia, gestational diabetes, and complicated delivery.

Gestational Diabetes

Gestational diabetes is a form of diabetes that some women develop during the second to third trimester of pregnancy, when their systems temporarily become resistant to insulin—typically due to hormonal shifts and potential weight gain. High blood sugar in a pregnant woman can affect fetal growth and influence the baby's risk of becoming obese. Pregnant women with gestational diabetes are encouraged to exercise daily, avoid excessive weight gain, and carefully monitor their diet. Gestational diabetes is similar to type 2 diabetes in the way symptoms present and in treatment options.

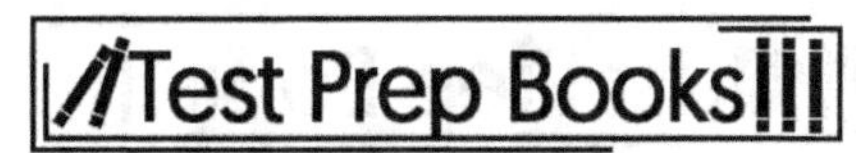

Postdates Pregnancy

Post-dates or post-term pregnancies are defined as pregnancies that go past 42 weeks of gestation. This condition has been shown to occur at a higher rate in patients with hormonal disorders, obesity, or inaccurate gestational dating. **Post-dates pregnancies** lead to an increased risk of complications and increased morbidity rates for both the mother and the fetus. The incidence of stillbirth at 42 weeks of gestation is almost twice the rate at term (40 weeks) and quadruple the term rate by 43 weeks of gestation. Higher risk of meconium aspiration syndrome as well as fetal macrosomia are seen in neonates who are delivered after 40 weeks of gestation. Fetal macrosomia can increase the risk of shoulder dystocia during delivery and may require cesarean section. It is vital to ensure that the gestational age has accurately been dated with routine ultrasounds prior to discussing interventions for postdates, such as induction of labor. If the gestational age is accurate, it is recommended to induce labor at term to reduce the risk of maternal and fetal morbidity.

Ectopic Pregnancy

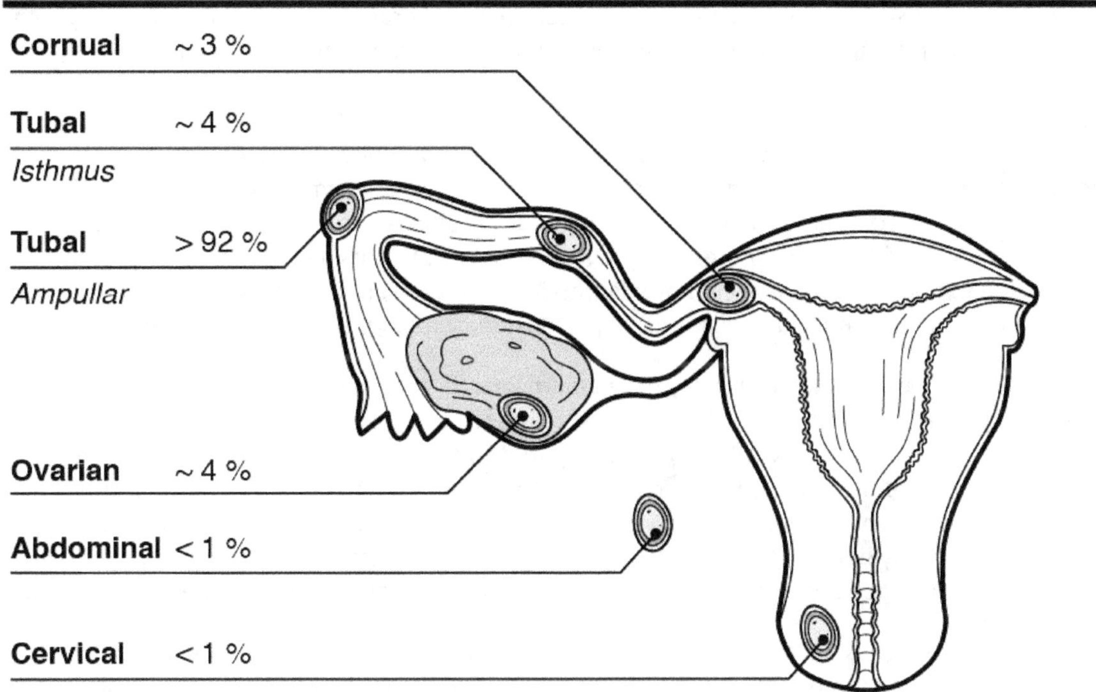

An **ectopic pregnancy** results from the abnormal implantation of the fertilized ovum at an alternative anatomical site—most commonly the fallopian tube—that is physiologically incapable of sustaining the pregnancy. An undetected or untreated ectopic pregnancy is a life-threatening emergency. The majority of patients do not have any identifiable risk factors; however, the most common defect is an alteration in the structure of the fallopian tubes that impedes the movement of the fertilized ovum to the appropriate site in the uterus.

Common causes of damage to the fallopian tubes include PID, a history of previous ectopic pregnancies, smoking (because it decreases the motility of the fallopian tube), the use of intrauterine devices (IUDs), and assisted reproduction, which doubles the risk for this disorder. Although the three classic symptoms are pain, amenorrhea, and vaginal bleeding, only 40 to 50 percent of patients with an ectopic pregnancy present with all three manifestations. Additional manifestations will be dependent on the implantation site, most commonly the fallopian tube, or rarely, the abdomen, and the "age" of the pregnancy, and may include signs of early pregnancy or abnormal signs such as dizziness, weakness, flu symptoms, and in the extreme, cardiac arrest.

To decrease the morbidity associated with undiagnosed ectopic pregnancies, all women of childbearing age who present with pain, vaginal bleeding, and amenorrhea must be screened for pregnancy. Testing of the urine and serum for beta human chorionic gonadotropin (βhCG) will be positive before the first missed menstrual period, and transvaginal ultrasonography is the recommended imaging modality. Laparoscopy is the treatment of choice for patients who are experiencing pain or hemodynamic instability. Intramuscular methotrexate, which impedes DNA synthesis and prevents cellular replication, is the recommended expectant treatment for ectopic pregnancy. The protocol requires an initial assessment of βhCG, liver and kidney function, blood type, Rh status, and bone marrow function. Methotrexate is administered in a single dose, and its effectiveness is measured by evidence of decreasing βhCG levels. Emergency treatment of an ectopic pregnancy is focused on identification of the location and characteristics of the abnormal pregnancy and the patient's systemic manifestations, which may include hemorrhage and cardiac arrest.

Preterm Labor

Most neonatal deaths in the United States are due to **preterm labor**, which is defined as the onset of uterine contractions that are of adequate strength and frequency to result in effacement and dilation of the cervix between 20–37 weeks' gestation. Although the exact etiology is unclear, the most significant predictor for preterm labor is a positive history for preterm labor. Additional risk factors include abruptio placenta, cervical incompetence due to prior surgery, uterine fibroids, cervical infections, fetal distress, and placental defects due to systemic conditions that include diabetes, hypertension, smoking, and alcohol and drug abuse.

The routine testing for a patient with a history of second-trimester pregnancy loss includes coagulation studies, cultures for chlamydia and gonorrhea, glucose tolerance assessment, and immune antibody studies. Two additional parameters—the cervical length as measured by transvaginal ultrasonography and the fetal fibronectin level (fFN)—are used to assess the risk for preterm labor in a patient with inconclusive manifestations. Preterm labor is treated with tocolytic agents and progesterone. The primary purpose of tocolytic therapy is to delay delivery for up to 48 hours to optimize the effect of betamethasone therapy on fetal lung maturation, thereby decreasing the incidence of respiratory distress syndrome in the newborn.

Tocolytic therapy with magnesium sulfate is recommended for preterm labor from twenty-four to thirty-three weeks of gestation. Common side effects of magnesium sulfate are headache, lethargy, blurred vision, and facial flushing. Toxic manifestations include respiratory depression and cardiac arrest. Progesterone is believed to prevent preterm labor by direct effect on the uterus after the placenta is fully formed, and it may also be used to delay delivery. The care of the patient with preterm labor is focused on confirming the presence of true labor, assessing fetal health, and administering tocolytic agents and progesterone, which help inhibit the labor process.

Hyperemesis Gravidarum

Hyperemesis gravidarum is an acute form of nausea and vomiting that is associated with fluid volume depletion, resulting in ketosis and up to a 5 percent weight loss. This extreme form of "morning sickness" may also be manifested by fatigue, weakness, dizziness, sleep disturbance, and mood changes. Diagnostic studies include urinalysis to assess acid-base balance and to rule out UTI, liver function studies to rule out

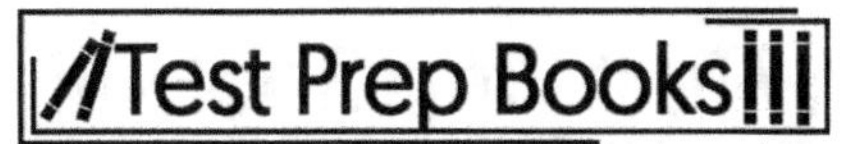

hepatitis, CBC, and thyroid function studies. Obstetrical ultrasonography is done to assess the condition of the pregnancy and to confirm the number of fetuses.

The condition typically begins before eight weeks of gestation and rarely persists beyond twenty to twenty-two weeks of gestation. The symptomatic treatment includes close assessment of the fluid volume status and vital signs, antiemetics, and IV fluid replacement. In the event of severe nutritional deficits, acid-base dysfunction, or electrolyte imbalance, hospitalization may be required. The care of the patient with hyperemesis gravidarum is focused on correction of fluid volume deficit, resolution of ketosis and electrolyte imbalances, and relief from nausea and vomiting.

Hypertensive Disorders of Pregnancy

Preeclampsia

Preeclampsia is characterized by the onset of hypertension and proteinuria after twenty weeks of gestation and may persist for four to six weeks postpartum. The cause is unknown; however, there is evidence of alterations in the endothelium of the vasculature accompanied by vasospasm. Risk factors include nulliparity, maternal age over forty years old, family history, chronic renal disease, obesity, hypertension, and diabetes. Early manifestations include visual disturbances, altered mental state, dyspnea, facial edema, and possible upper right quadrant pain. Severe manifestations include hypertension on bedrest, increasing liver enzymes with increased pain, progressive renal dysfunction, pulmonary edema, and thrombocytopenia. Routine labs, fetal nonstress testing, and corticosteroids for lung maturation are done prior to delivery, which is the only known cure.

Eclampsia

Eclampsia is the life-threatening complication of severe preeclampsia that is manifested by the onset of seizure activity and/or the development of coma and is associated with hypertension, proteinuria, intrauterine fetal growth delay, and diminished amniotic fluid. There are no specific diagnostic tests, and while the specific etiology is unknown, there are indications that the condition results from the interchange of maternal and fetal tissue or allografts. Magnesium sulfate is recommended for short-term use for 24 to 48 hours to stabilize the patient for delivery, which is the only curative measure.

HELLP Syndrome

HELLP syndrome is also associated with significant maternal and fetal mortality, resulting from liver rupture and strokes due to cerebral edema or hemorrhage. The syndrome is characterized by hemolysis of RBCs, elevated liver enzymes, and low platelet levels (HELLP). Some authorities consider HELLP syndrome to be a severe form of preeclampsia, while others view it as a separate entity. The coagulation defects and liver dysfunction are the result of microvascular changes in the endothelium in the presence of hypertension; however, the cause is unknown. Risk factors are similar to risk factors for preeclampsia. Manifestations include elevated liver enzymes, coagulation defects including thrombocytopenia and hemolytic anemia, and right upper quadrant pain, and there are classification systems that assess the condition according to the extent of hepatic dysfunction. The treatment involves stabilization of the patient and prompt delivery with attention to correction of the coagulation defects and liver dysfunction. The emergency care of all of these life-threatening conditions is focused on treating hypertension, safe delivery of the fetus, and prevention of associated complications.

Malpresentations

Breech Presentation

Breech presentation is an umbrella term for any of three abnormal fetal positions wherein the presenting body part is the feet or buttocks. It occurs more often in premature births; usually, the fetus naturally turns to the proper head-first presentation during the third trimester. If this does not occur, breech presentation may manifest as frank, incomplete, or complete breech. **Frank breech** refers to hip flexion and knee extension, with the feet near the head. **Incomplete breech** involves extension of one or both hips and of one or both knees. With **complete breech**, both hips and knees are flexed. Breech presentation is identified by Leopold maneuvers, which will demonstrate a hard, round structure at the fundus; this is the fetus' head. Ultrasound can confirm diagnosis. Before the onset of labor, a mechanical maneuver called external cephalic version can shift the fetus into proper position. However, if labor is progressing, cesarean delivery is typically indicated as breech deliveries are frequently complicated.

Compound Presentation

Compound presentation occurs when a fetal hand presents alongside the fetal head in the birth canal. This increases the risk of injury to the fetal hand and arm and can lead to obstructed labor. Obstructed labor may occur due to the increased circumference of fetal parts required to pass through the birth canal. If there is insufficient space, the fetus can become stuck, and a cesarean section may be necessary. The fetal arm is at risk of mechanical and nerve injury due to the possible use of traction and maneuvers needed to safely deliver the fetus.

Cord Presentation

Cord presentation or funic presentation is characterized by the umbilical cord lying between the fetal head or fetal presenting part and the cervical os. This is a very rare condition that poses significant fetal and maternal risks. This condition is typically diagnosed via abdominal or vaginal ultrasound but can also be assessed during a cervical dilation check. Cord presentation precedes the event of a cord prolapse, which greatly increases the risk of fetal morbidity. Cord prolapse can occur during labor with the rupture of membranes, and a cervical exam should be performed to ensure the practitioner feels the fetal head rather than the umbilical cord. Cord presentation can resolve on its own during the third trimester and should be confirmed with an ultrasound examination prior to delivery. Quick resolution of this issue is necessary, with a stat cesarean section typically advised.

Umbilical Cord Prolapse

Umbilical cord prolapse (UCP) constitutes an obstetric emergency. It involves protrusion of the cord through the cervix and subsequent compression by the fetus, leading to fetal hypoxia and bradycardia. Fetal malpresentation, prematurity, multiple gestation, and polyhydramnios raise the risk of UCP. It may be either overt, in which the cord prolapses before the presenting fetal part, or occult, wherein the cord and fetal part present alongside each other. UCP should be suspected in any case of fetal bradycardia as well as late or severe variable decelerations. Palpation of a pulsatile structure confirms UCP; however, this is not always present, such as in occult UCP. This is a clinical diagnosis; imaging is both unnecessary and costs valuable time. Once recognized, the presenting fetal part must be manually elevated off of the cord. This is a temporizing measure to allow for preparation for emergency C-section, which is the definitive treatment. If delivery is delayed and decelerations persist, tocolytic drugs like terbutaline may reduce pressure on the umbilical vessels.

Face Presentation

Face presentation is a rare type of cephalic presentation in which the fetal head leads with the chin (mentum) rather than typical cephalic presentation, in which the fetal chin flexes down towards the neck. This is dangerous, as it increases the circumference of the fetal presenting part and may lead to obstruction at birth. The fetal neck is typically hyperextended toward the fetal back and can usually be assessed with ultrasonography or digital exam during labor to confirm diagnosis. Cesarean section is recommended in patients with face presentation and a fetal mentum positioned posteriorly or transversely, which increases the circumference of the fetal presenting part to be larger than the birth canal. Vaginal delivery is possible in some cases of face presentation if the patient is aware of the associated risks.

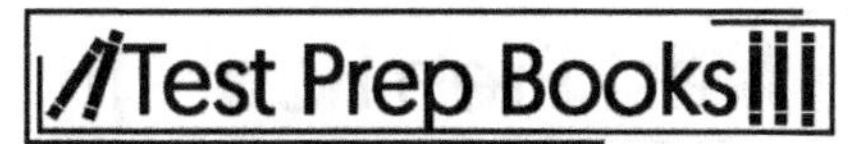

Oblique/Transverse Lie

Oblique or **transverse fetal lie** occurs when the fetus is positioned with their head at an angle, which often leads to shoulder presentation at the cervical os. This condition can occur due to a short umbilical cord or placenta previa and commonly requires a cesarean section in the event of shoulder presentation. An **external cephalic version** (**ECV**) can be performed to attempt to move the fetus into a cephalic position by manually pressing on the mother's abdomen. However, this intervention comes with many risks, including compressing the umbilical cord, which would require a stat cesarean section.

Unstable Lie

Unstable lie is characterized by the frequent movement and position change of a fetus after 37 weeks of gestation. Frequent position change late in pregnancy creates an increased risk of malpresentation at the time of labor, cord prolapse, and cesarean delivery. Unstable lie may be due to fetal anomalies, placenta previa, uterine anomalies, or polyhydramnios, in which there is an excess of amniotic fluid, which keeps the fetus from being able to engage in the pelvis. Unstable lie will typically resolve prior to the onset of labor; however, if the fetus is still unstable or in transverse lie, an ECV or cesarean section may be indicated.

Rh Alloimmunization

The Rh ("Rhesus") factor is expressed after a patient's A, B, AB, or O blood type and refers to the presence or absence of the Rh antigen on red blood cells. Rh(D) is the most common such antigen. **Rh incompatibility** involves exposure of a woman with Rh-negative blood to an Rh-positive fetus. This exposure causes **alloimmunization**, characterized by anti-Rh antibody formation, such that subsequent exposure in future pregnancies produces an immune attack on fetal RBCs. This causes the catastrophic complications of fetal hydrops and erythroblastosis fetalis.

Rh incompatibility is asymptomatic and must be screened for at the initial prenatal visit for every pregnancy. Patients who are Rh-negative should be tested for the presence of anti-Rh antibodies at their twenty-eight-week visit. If the fetus is Rh-positive and the mother is Rh-negative with a negative antibody screen, anti-D immunoglobulin (**RhoGAM**) is administered at that time and again within seventy-two hours postpartum. Those with a positive anti-Rh antibody screen should be referred to a high-risk pregnancy specialist, and delivery should be considered at thirty-four weeks.

Coping with Pregnancy Loss

Abortion is defined as any form of early pregnancy loss; however, the term **miscarriage** appears more commonly in lay literature. Up to 80 percent of spontaneous abortions occur in the first trimester and may be categorized as threatened, inevitable, incomplete, complete, or missed. In addition, abortions are labeled as sporadic or recurrent. Chromosomal anomalies of the fetus are generally accepted as the most common cause of early abortions. In addition, several maternal risk factors have been identified that may be associated with first- or second-trimester pregnancy losses. Advanced maternal age and a history of type 1 diabetes, renal disease, severe hypertension, thyroid dysfunction, anatomical defects of the uterus, illicit drug use, smoking, alcohol abuse, and non-ASA NSAID use have all been associated with an increased risk of an initial or recurrent early pregnancy loss.

The diagnosis of a threatened **spontaneous abortion** will be based on the patient's history and physical, lab studies, and ultrasonography. The first priority is to confirm the presence of the pregnancy; therefore, lab studies will include the assessment of βhCG (human chorionic gonadotropin) in addition to CBC with differential, blood and Rh typing, hemoglobin and hematocrit, and coagulation studies. Transabdominal and transvaginal ultrasonography are the recommended imaging modalities. Treatment is dependent on the stage of the pregnancy, the presenting manifestations, and in some cases, the patient's preference for the treatment approach. A threatened abortion of a first-trimester pregnancy will be treated with expectant management, which includes close observation of maternal hemodynamic status and blood loss. If the abortion continues to an incomplete abortion, surgical or pharmacologically induced evacuation of the products of conception will be considered. Treatment is focused on the prevention and/or treatment of hemorrhage and the prevention of infection.

Fetal Growth Aberrations

Fetal Growth Restriction

Fetal growth restriction (**FGR**) is defined as an estimated fetal weight (EFW) that falls below the 10th percentile for their gestational age. This is calculated with an ultrasound examination or maternal fundal height to measure the EFW or abdominal circumference of the fetus. Some fetuses may just be small for their age, while others are pathogenically growth-restricted due to placental insufficiencies, small intrauterine space, and fetal genetic abnormalities. Although the 10th percentile is typically used for FGR diagnosis, fetal morbidity is significantly increased when the fetus measures at or below the 3rd percentile. There are two types of FGR: early-onset (prior to 32 weeks of gestation) and late-onset (at 32 weeks or longer gestation). Some fetuses may require early delivery as soon as the benefits outweigh the risks of premature delivery. Every scenario will be slightly different, and EFW should be serially assessed after FGR diagnosis to ensure the appropriate delivery timing is attained.

Macrosomia

Macrosomia refers to a fetal birth weight between 4000 and 4500 grams and is associated with both maternal and fetal risks. Macrosomia is formally diagnosed by birth weight, but it can be estimated antenatally with ultrasound examinations and maternal fundal height measurements, although these methods are not always very accurate. Both maternal and fetal etiologies can lead to macrosomia, including maternal obesity, diabetes, post-dates pregnancy, male fetal gender, or fetal genetic anomalies. Excessive fetal growth can potentially be mitigated with blood sugar control, increased exercise, and maternal weight management. Cesarean section is typically recommended for a fetus exceeding 5000 grams in non-diabetic patients or 4500 grams in diabetic patients to reduce the risk of birth complications such as shoulder dystocia, fetal distress, perineal laceration, and postpartum hemorrhage (PPH). However, this recommendation is controversial considering the varying accuracy of fetal weight estimations.

Shoulder Dystocia

Shoulder dystocia is an obstetric emergency wherein delivery of a fetus' shoulder is obstructed, usually by the mother's pubic symphysis. It typically involves the anterior shoulder. Key risk factors include gestational diabetes, fetal macrosomia, and gestational age over forty weeks; however, it frequently occurs without any risk factors. Signs include delayed presentation (over sixty seconds) of the fetal body; inability to manually guide the fetal head downward to promote shoulder expulsion; and the "turtle sign," which describes presentation followed by retraction of the head. Emergent treatment is imperative and begins with attempts to relieve the obstruction via hyperflexion of the mother's hips (**McRoberts maneuver**) and/or suprapubic pressure. If unsuccessful, rotation of the shoulders or traction on the posterior shoulder may be attempted. Last-resort measures include intentional clavicular fracture to increase shoulder flexibility; manual pushing of the head back into the uterus (**Zavanelli maneuver**) followed by emergent C-section; or symphysiotomy, which is an incision of the cartilage at the pubic symphysis.

Thromboembolic Disorders

Amniotic Fluid Embolism (AFE)

Amniotic fluid embolisms are a risk in pregnant and postpartum individuals. They can occur when amniotic fluid or other fetal cells enter the parent's bloodstream; this results in an inflammatory immune response that causes the parent to experience extreme blood clotting and internal bleeding. Symptoms are sudden and rapid; they are primarily seen in the parent. Symptoms include difficulty breathing, a drop in blood

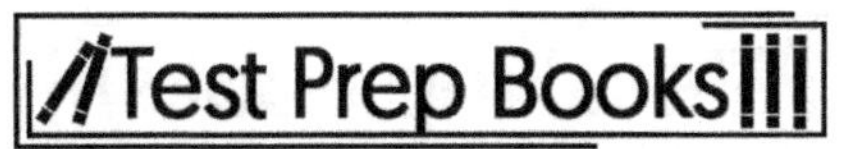

pressure, bleeding (usually from the uterus or incision sites), significant mood shifts, and seizures. More severe complications include heart failure and a positive feedback loop of blood clotting and clot breakdown, which leads to internal hemorrhage. In some cases, the fetus or newborn may also show signs of distress.

Deep Vein Thrombosis (DVT) and Pulmonary Embolism (PE)

A **pulmonary embolism** (**PE**) is the abnormal presence of a blood clot, or thrombus, causing a blockage in one of the lungs' pulmonary arteries. It is not a specific disease, but rather a complication due to thrombus formation in the venous system of one of the lower extremities, which is termed **deep venous thrombosis** (**DVT**). Other rarer causes of PEs are thrombi arising in the veins of the kidneys, pelvis, upper extremities, or the right atrium of the heart. Occasionally, other matter besides blood clots can cause pulmonary emboli, such as fat, air, and septic (infected with bacteria) emboli. PE is a common and potentially fatal condition.

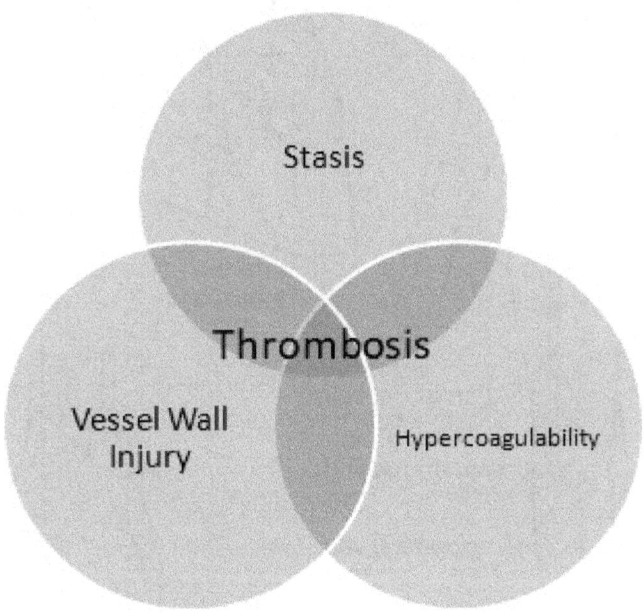

The primary influences on the development of DVT and PE are shown in **Virchow's triad**: blood hypercoagulability, endothelial injury/dysfunction, and stasis of blood.

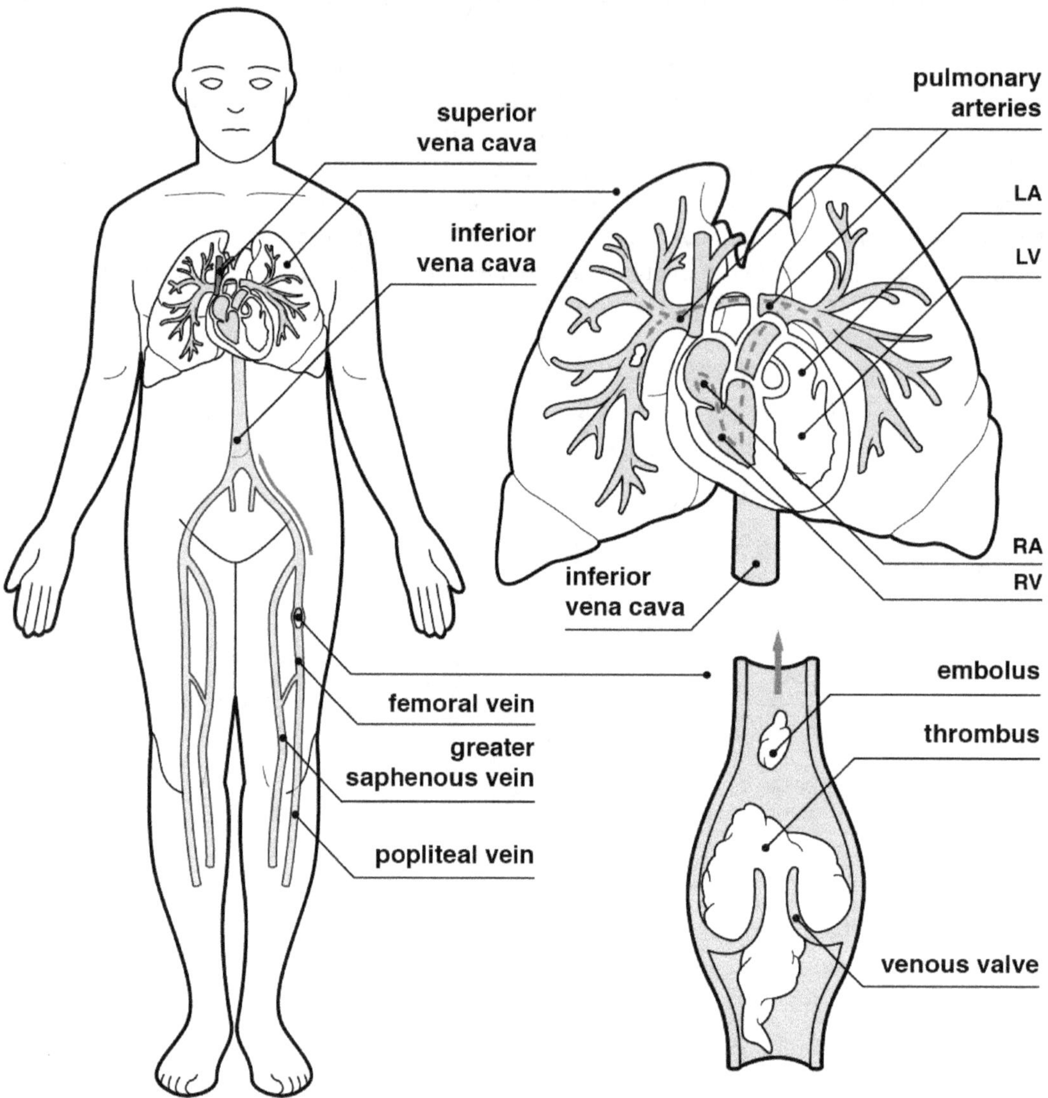

Risk factors for DVT and PE include:

- Cancer
- Heart disease, especially congestive heart failure (CHF)
- Prolonged immobility (such as prolonged bedrest or lengthy trips in planes or cars)
- Surgery (one of the leading risk factors, accounting for up to 15 percent of all postoperative deaths)
- Overweight/obesity
- Smoking
- Pregnancy
- Supplemental estrogen from birth control pills or estrogen replacement therapy (ERT)

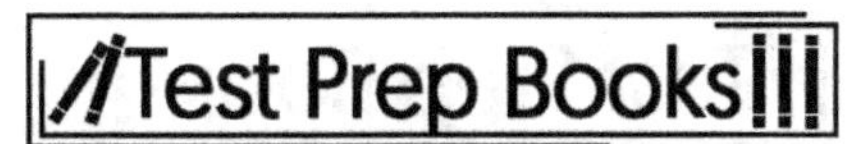

The signs and symptoms of PE are nonspecific, which often presents a diagnostic dilemma and a delay in diagnosis. Nearly half of all individuals with PE are asymptomatic. The signs and symptoms of PE can vary greatly depending on the size of the blood clots, how much lung tissue is involved, and an individual's overall health. Signs and symptoms of PE can include:

- Pleuritic chest pain
- Dyspnea
- Cough
- Tachypnea
- Hypoxia
- Fever
- Diaphoresis
- Rales
- Cyanosis
- Unilateral lower extremity edema (symptom of DVT)

The diagnosis of PE can be a difficult task. Many clinicians support determining the clinical probability of PE before proceeding with diagnostic testing. This process involves assessing the presence or absence of the following manifestations:

- Pulmonary Signs: Tachypnea, rales, and cyanosis
- Cardiac Signs: Tachycardia, S3 or S4 gallop, attenuated second heart sound, and cardiac murmur
- Constitutional Signs: Fever, diaphoresis, signs and symptoms of thrombophlebitis, and lower extremity edema

Once the clinical probability of PE has been determined, diagnostic testing ensues. Duplex ultrasonography is the standard for diagnosing a DVT. A spiral computed tomography (CT) scan with or without contrast has replaced pulmonary angiography as the standard for diagnosing a PE. If spiral CT scanning is unavailable or if individuals have a contraindication to the administration of intravenous contrast material, ventilation-perfusion (V/Q) scanning is often selected. Magnetic resonance imaging (MRI) is usually reserved for pregnant women and individuals with a contraindication to the administration of intravenous contrast material. A D-dimer blood test is most useful for individuals with a low or moderate pretest probability of PE, since levels are typically elevated with PE. Arterial blood gas (ABG) analysis usually reveals hypoxemia, hypocapnia, and respiratory alkalosis.

A chest x-ray, though not diagnostic for PE since its findings are typically nonspecific, can exclude diseases that mimic PE, as can an echocardiogram. Electrocardiography is also useful because it can assess right ventricular heart function and serve as a prognostic indicator, since there is a 10 percent death rate from PE with right ventricular dysfunction. Lastly, transesophageal echocardiography (TEE) can reveal central PE.

Treatment of PE should begin immediately to prevent complications or death. PE treatment is focused on preventing an increase in size of the current blood clots and the formation of new blood clots. Supportive care treatment of PE can include:

- Supplemental oxygen to ease hypoxia/hypoxemia
- Dopamine (Inotropin®) or dobutamine (Dobutrex®) administered via IV for related hypotension
- Cardiac monitoring in the case of associated arrhythmias or right ventricular dysfunction
- Intubation and mechanical ventilation

Medications involved in treatment can include: thrombolytics or clot dissolvers (such as tissue plasminogen activator (tPA), alteplase, urokinase, streptokinase, or reteplase). These medications are reserved for individuals with a diagnosis of acute PE and associated hypotension (systolic BP < 90 mmHg). They are not given concurrently with anticoagulants. Anticoagulants or blood thinners may also be used. The historical standard for the initial treatment of PE was unfractionated heparin (UFH) administered via IV or subcutaneous (SC) injection, which requires frequent blood monitoring. Current treatment guidelines recommend low-molecular weight heparin (LMWH) administered via SC injection over UFH IV or SC as it has greater bioavailability than UFH and blood monitoring is not necessary. Fondaparinux (Arixtra®) administered via SC injection is also recommended over UFH IV or SC; blood monitoring is not necessary.

Warfarin (Coumadin®), an oral anticoagulant was the historical standard for the outpatient prevention and treatment of PE. It is initiated the same day as treatment with UFH, LMWH, or fondaparinux. It is recommended INR of 2-3 with frequent blood monitoring, at which time IV or SC anticoagulant is discontinued. Alternatives to Warfarin include oral factor Xa inhibitor anticoagulants such as apixaban (Eliquis®), rivaroxaban (Xarelto®), and edoxaban (Savaysa®), or dabigatran (Pradaxa®), an oral direct thrombin inhibitor anticoagulant. Blood monitoring is not necessary with these medications. The most significant adverse effect of both thrombolytics and anticoagulants is bleeding.

An embolectomy (removal of emboli via catheter or surgery) is reserved for individuals with a massive PE and contraindications to thrombolytics or anticoagulants. Vena cava filters (also called inferior vena cava (IVC) filters or Greenfield filters) are only indicated in individuals with an absolute contraindication to anticoagulants, a massive PE who have survived and for whom recurrent PE will be fatal, or documented recurrent PE.

Postpartum Care and Complications

Postpartum Care

The **postpartum** phase is considered to begin immediately after childbirth and ends after six weeks. Once the infant is delivered, it becomes a second patient and must be cared for separately from the mother. The nurse must assess both patients every 15 minutes for 2 hours to confirm that both mother and infant are adjusting well. Continued hospitalization is generally no longer than one day for a vaginal birth and two to three days for a cesarean section. Upon discharge—with infant care manual, feeding plan, and patient education completed—the couplet and other caregivers return to the home environment. Within weeks, the couplet will visit the physician, for well checks. This nursing assessment includes a depression inventory and discussions of progress with infant feeding.

Infants born prior to thirty-seven weeks gestation are considered to be preterm and at a high risk for complications at birth and throughout infancy. Specialized care of preterm infants and those born with twice-repeated Apgar scores below 7 must occur in the neonatal intensive care unit. Well infants are roomed in with their mothers, as a couplet. The postpartum nurse must be prepared to teach the parent(s) on feeding, changing, and general care of the infant. Umbilical cord care, as well as proper cleaning of a circumcised penis, is also vital in preparation for the discharge home. Within the first 24-to-48 hours after birth, careful assessment must be performed to ascertain if the infant is not adjusting to their new environment.

Uterine Involution

Uterine involution occurs during the first 6 weeks following delivery and involves the uterus shrinking back down to roughly the size it was prior to pregnancy. After delivering the fetus and placenta, a large wound is left where the placenta was attached to the uterus. Uterine involution begins following the passing of the placenta and assists in preventing postpartum hemorrhage by contracting the uterus to decrease its blood flow. This uterine contraction is accompanied by postpartum bleeding and cramping, with the highest amount in the first 12 hours postdelivery; however, cramping may continue for several days and bleeding for

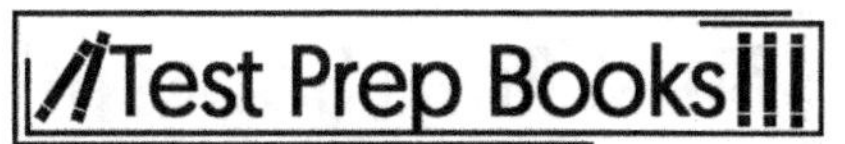

several weeks. Breastfeeding mothers may notice increased cramping during feeds, as breastfeeding induces the release of oxytocin, which causes uterine contraction. **Fundal massage** is vital during the first few hours after the delivery of the placenta to ensure the uterus is firm and contracted to prevent excess bleeding. If the uterus is soft during the fundal exam, additional pressure should be applied to expel any clots and assist the uterus in contracting.

Perineal Care

Perineal care is a vital part of the postpartum process, whether there are tears, episiotomies, or intact skin. A tear is characterized by a rip in the tissue or muscle from the vaginal opening to the anus or labia. An **episiotomy** is an incision made in the perineal tissue from the vaginal wall to provide additional space to aid in the delivery of the fetus. There are different levels of tears: first-degree (involves only superficial tissue), second-degree (involves superficial tissue of the perineum along with perineal muscles), third-degree (a tear in the tissue and perineal muscle that extends to the anal sphincter), and fourth-degree (a tear in the tissue and perineal muscle through the anal sphincter and around or beneath it). Tears or episiotomies can both require stitches along with extra care to prevent infection or additional pain. It is important to keep the perineum clean by spraying warm water with a perineal bottle after urination. Ice packs can be helpful to decrease pain and swelling, while increased fluid consumption dilutes urine to reduce irritation. Pain medication can be prescribed, and position changes are encouraged to reduce prolonged sitting or standing.

Breast Care

In the first few days after delivery, the mother will produce **colostrum**, a thick, nutrient-dense substance for the neonate. After 2–3 days, the mother's milk will start to come in, which may cause painful engorgement. Pain may be relieved by acetaminophen or ibuprofen, while engorgement can be aided by ice packs and gentle hand expression to help the neonate achieve a correct latch. Mastitis can develop from a blocked milk duct, which can be caused by prolonged engorgement or incomplete emptying during feedings. Redness, pain, fever, and swelling are all indications of inflammation and possible infection of the breast tissue. Antibiotics may be necessary in the case of infection, and complete emptying of each breast during feedings along with ensuring a correct latch is essential to preventing recurrence. If the patient is planning to feed with a bottle, breast binding or wearing a tight-fitting bra along with avoiding any nipple stimulation will help stop milk production.

Fatigue and Sleep Disturbances

Fatigue and sleep disturbances are a large part of the postpartum process and greatly affect maternal patients. Between infant night wakings for feedings, diaper changes, or comfort, these patients suffer from large amounts of mental and physical exhaustion. Typically, sleep will be the most interrupted in the weeks following delivery and slowly improve, although some patients may not see improvement for several months. Lack of sleep has been shown to contribute to early weaning from breast milk, depression, and decrease in overall functionality. Studies have shown that populations in a lower socioeconomic status are at a higher risk for increased length of sleep disturbances in the postpartum period. Practitioners should monitor the fatigue and sleep disturbances of patients to recommend different interventions, such as sleep training.

Lochia

Lochia is characterized by the discharge following the delivery of the fetus and placenta, which is composed of blood, endometrial tissue, amniotic fluid, and mucus. There are three phases of lochia: lochia rubra, lochia serosa, and lochia alba. **Lochia rubra** occurs directly following delivery for 3 or 4 days and is typically the heaviest flow of dark red discharge with possible small clots. **Lochia serosa** is the second phase, which lasts for the following 4 to 12 days and is characterized by a moderate amount of pink or brown discharge with few to no clots. **Lochia alba** is the third phase, which consists of light amounts of yellowish discharge with little or no blood and can last until 6 weeks postpartum. Patients will still have lochia following a cesarean delivery to expel the endometrial tissue, blood, amniotic fluid, and mucus from pregnancy, although it may be lighter than is typical for a vaginal delivery.

Breastfeeding

Breastfeeding should be initiated within the first hour of the newborn's life to begin to develop a proper latch, support the maternal-infant bond, and ensure the neonate is getting adequate nutrition. If possible, skin-to-skin contact should be implemented directly following delivery to support oxytocin production, temperature management, and bonding. Signs that the newborn is ready to start breastfeeding include the infant "rooting" or looking around while opening their mouth to find the nipple. If the mother is able, the newborn should be fed following these cues on demand to ensure they are receiving adequate nutrition. In the first 1–3 days postpartum, the mother will only produce colostrum, which is a small quantity of an incredibly nutrient-dense milk. Colostrum ensures that the newborn is receiving the proper nutrients and immunity factors in the right amount of substance that will fit in their small abdomen. After 2–3 days, the patient will start to produce breast milk, which comes in larger quantities and may lead to breast engorgement.

Contraception

Contraception during the postpartum period is often recommended early on for patients who want to prevent an unplanned pregnancy. Ovulation can begin as soon as 3 weeks postpartum and can occur before the normal menstrual cycle resumes. Some methods of contraception can be initiated directly following delivery, such as a hormonal or copper intrauterine device (IUD), contraceptive implants, and progesterone-only pills. These methods are all safe for breastfeeding and help delay or prevent future pregnancy. Sterilization surgery can also be performed at the time of cesarean section if the patient has decided prior to delivery that their family is complete.

Nutrition

Postpartum patients who are breastfeeding require 340–400 additional kilocalories a day to support their milk production. This will amount to a calorie goal of around 2,000 to 2,800 kilocalories a day for breastfeeding mothers. In addition, breastfeeding patients should increase both their choline and iodine intake to support lactation, which can be done through consuming a proper diet. Choline-dense foods include eggs, meats, dairy, beans, lentils, and some seafood. Iodine-rich foods include eggs, dairy, iodized salt, and seafood. Continued use of prenatal multivitamins is often recommended, although this may lead to excessive amounts of folic acid and iron that are beyond the needs of a postpartum patient.

Emotional Changes

Emotional changes occur with every postpartum patient, as this is a very emotionally charged experience that comes with rapidly changing hormones. **Oxytocin** is known to be very high in the postpartum period, which helps form the maternal-newborn bond. However, progesterone drops during this time and is typically at a very low level until the first menstrual cycle. This low level of progesterone is speculated to be the cause of postpartum "baby blues" and postpartum depression or anxiety. It is vital to screen postpartum patients after delivery and again at their 6 week checkup to ensure they are coping well with their emotional needs. Support groups are available, along with medication when necessary.

Postpartum Complications

Bladder Distention and Urinary Retention

Postpartum bladder distension and **urinary retention** can lead to severe complications, including renal failure and bladder rupture. Urinary retention should be monitored in the postpartum patient by tracking intake and output via number of trips to the bathroom or by measuring the urine output. There are several risk factors

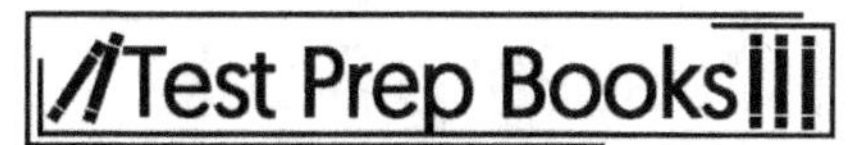

for urinary retention, including prolonged labor, epidural anesthesia, episiotomy, and fetal macrosomia. Symptoms involve a feeling of bladder fullness, pain, or distention along with urinary frequency, dysuria, or incomplete emptying. Assessment involves feeling for a displaced fundus, palpating for a distended bladder, increased bleeding, or decreased urine output. There are three types of urinary retention in the postpartum period: covert, overt, and persistent/ chronic. Covert bladder distention occurs when the patient reports a feeling of fullness after voiding and has a postvoid residual volume of 150 mL or more when assessed via ultrasound. Overt bladder distention occurs when a patient is unable to void for 6 or more hours following catheter removal. Persistent or chronic bladder distention is characterized by urinary retention that lasts for more than 3 days and may require self-catheterization.

Hematoma

There are several types of **hematomas** that can occur during the postnatal period, including vulvar, puerperal, and retroperitoneal. Vulvar hematomas often occur due to injury to the pudendal artery and cause pooling of blood near the urogenital areas. These will typically resolve on their own, although surgical excision may be necessary depending on the size. Puerperal hematomas are very severe and can result in maternal morbidity. Puerperal hematomas are caused by injury to the pelvic vessels, typically from episiotomy, vaginal tear, or assisted delivery. Retroperitoneal hematomas are rare but can be very severe when they do occur. The retroperitoneal space can contain a large amount of blood before being diagnosed, which greatly increases the maternal risk of morbidity. It is vital to assess and diagnose these hematomas as soon as possible to increase the chances of a positive health outcome.

Postpartum Hemorrhage

Postpartum hemorrhage is commonly defined as the loss of more than 500 milliliters following a vaginal delivery or 1000 milliliters after a Cesarean section (C-section) in a pregnancy that has progressed for at least twenty weeks. Less substantial losses can result in alterations in fluid volume status in patients with comorbidities such as anemia, cardiac disease, dehydration, or preeclampsia, which means that postpartum hemorrhage is the loss of any amount of blood that results in altered hemodynamic status. There are multiple contributing factors; however, the most common precipitating pathophysiology for hemorrhage is **uterine atony**. These factors are related to tone, tissue, trauma, or thrombosis. Alterations in tone may be due to uterine atony resulting from distention of the uterine muscles in prolonged labor or with a large-for-gestational-age (LGA) newborn. Tissue alterations include retained placental tissue or placenta accreta. Trauma may result from manipulation of the fetus during delivery, history of previous C-section, prolonged labor, and internal version and extraction of a second twin. Alterations in coagulation may be due to preexisting coagulopathies.

The diagnosis depends on the presenting manifestations of postpartum vaginal bleeding and deteriorating hemodynamic status. Commonly, the emergency care of postpartum hemorrhage includes notification of obstetrical, anesthesia, and surgical suite providers; type and cross match for six units of packed red blood cells (PRBCs); assignment of data recording to one provider; aggressive fluid management, including appropriate blood products; assessment of the placenta for missing fragments of tissue; baseline lab studies, including CBC, coagulation studies, renal function tests, and electrolytes; and oxygen by mask. The goal of treatment is to reverse the coagulopathy, resolve the underlying defect, and maintain close surveillance of the contractility of the uterus, or surgical intervention in the event of massive hemorrhage.

Transfusion Reaction

Transfusion reactions occur when a patient has an adverse response to receiving a blood transfusion. Blood transfusions are routinely administered to patients who have experienced significant blood loss. Generally, donated blood is matched to a patient based on blood type. If a patient does not receive blood that matches their own blood type, they will experience an adverse reaction due to the mismatch in protein markers that denote each blood type. Patients will experience a strong immune response that will cause their immune cells to attack the transfused blood. Additionally, they may have an allergic response to an entity in the donated blood. Transfusion reactions typically occur within twenty-four hours. Patients may experience symptoms such as physical pain, dark urine, fever, dizziness, shortness of breath, widespread itching, organ failure, lung injury, or death. Based on the intensity of the reaction, treatment can range from administering an antihistamine to performing emergency surgery.

Hemorrhoids

Hemorrhoids or piles are a common ailment during the postpartum period and are the result of increased intra-abdominal pressure during pregnancy. This increase in pressure leads to enlarged vessels around the anus, which can swell and lead to discomfort and bleeding. Constipation due to pregnancy is also a common cause of hemorrhoids due to the increased pressure when bearing down for bowel movements. Typically, a vein uses valves to push blood back up to the heart. However, when intra-abdominal pressure is increased, it becomes difficult for the valves to push the blood back against the pressure. This results in a pooling of blood and the creation of hemorrhoids. There are several factors that can help alleviate hemorrhoids, including adequate fiber and water intake as well as exercise, stool softeners, ice, avoiding sitting for long periods of time, and using a cushion when sitting. This condition is typically self-limiting and will resolve on its own within days or a few weeks. Witch hazel pads and prescription steroid creams can be used to lessen symptoms and promote healing.

Postpartum Mood Disorders

Postpartum psychiatric disorders include postpartum blues, perinatal depression, and postpartum psychosis. Risk factors include history of psychiatric disorders, poor social support, high-risk pregnancy, sleep deprivation, and unhealthy lifestyle. **Postpartum blues** are common, occurring in up to one-third of new mothers; they typically resolve within two weeks. However, the condition can devolve into **postpartum depression**, which carries a high risk of maternal suicide. Features include persistent depressed mood, feelings of guilt or worthlessness, impaired sleep or concentration, weight fluctuations, or suicidal ideation.

Multifaceted treatment may entail antidepressant medications, cognitive-behavioral therapy, and various lifestyle modifications. Conversely, **postpartum psychosis** is rare but extremely high risk. It shares the same risk factors and may feature paranoia, confusion, delusions, mania, and/or hallucinations. Fortunately, it responds well to treatment, such as lithium, atypical antipsychotics, or antiseizure medications. Providers should maintain a low threshold for specialty referral as this is a psychiatric emergency. Patients prescribed lithium should refrain from breastfeeding while taking it. Patients should be routinely screened for psychiatric disorders at postpartum visits using the Edinburgh Postnatal Depression Scale and Mood Disorder Questionnaire.

Postpartum Infection

There are several infectious conditions that may occur after a vaginal or Caesarean birth or during breastfeeding. There is rarely sufficient postpartum observation of the new mother to identify the onset of infection, usually from the second to the tenth postpartum day, which is manifested by a temperature greater than 38 °C (100.4 °F). Common infectious conditions include endometritis, postsurgical wound infections, perineal cellulitis, urinary tract infections, mastitis, and inflammation of the pelvic veins. The manifestations are specific to the anatomical site of the infection, while the causative agents are most often commonly occurring pathogens in the vagina and abdomen. Research indicates that the occurrence of severe sepsis is associated with preexisting conditions, including chronic liver disease, chronic kidney disease, congestive heart failure, and lupus.

Routine diagnostic studies include CBC; electrolytes; coagulation studies; blood, cervical, and wound cultures; and urinalysis. Ultrasonography is used to identify abscess formation, while CT and MRI scans are used to identify septic pelvic thrombosis or other systemic infection such as appendicitis. Antimicrobial treatment is

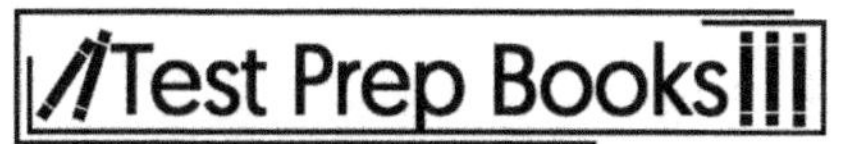

specific to site of the infection. Emergency care of the patient with a postpartum infection is focused on aggressive fluid replacement to support hydration and hemodynamic status, identification of the source of the infection, and administration of the appropriate antimicrobial agent. Patients who present with thrombosed pelvic veins may also require anticoagulant therapy that will necessitate in-hospital care. All patients with systemic manifestations will be considered for admission, and all patients who present with infection will require follow-up care with an obstetrician.

Thromboembolic Disorders

Postpartum patients are at a high risk of developing a thromboembolic disorder for the first 6 weeks after delivery. Injury to the vasculature during delivery leads to an increased risk of developing a blood clot, deep vein thrombosis (DVT), or pulmonary embolism (PE). Cesarean section patients are at an even higher risk due to the trauma of the vasculature. There are several types of thromboembolic disorders, including DVT, PE, and septic pelvic thrombophlebitis. DVTs typically present with leg pain, redness, edema, and erythema. A Doppler ultrasound should be used to diagnose a DVT, and computed tomography (CT) with contrast may be used if further imaging is necessary. A PE can present with chest pain, shortness of breath, and a cough, which can be diagnosed following a helical CT, with a possible need for pulmonary angiography. Septic pelvic thrombophlebitis occurs when a blood clot carries a bacterial infection and typically presents as a fever for 3–5 days that is unresponsive to treatments. Low molecular weight heparin should be initiated for treatment, as warfarin should be avoided for the first 6 weeks postpartum due to bleeding risk.

Endometritis

Endometritis is a condition in which the uterus becomes infected by bacteria from the vaginal canal after birth. Only 1–3 percent of patients who delivered vaginally and 10–30 percent of patients who delivered via cesarean section may be diagnosed with endometritis. This condition typically presents with pain or tenderness to the lower abdomen and uterus, fatigue, vaginal discharge, and fever. Patients who experienced a prolonged labor and delivery process, cesarean section, chorioamnionitis, prolonged rupture of membranes, retained placenta, or diabetes are at an increased risk of developing endometritis. Prior to diagnosis, other causes of symptoms should be ruled out via urinalysis and urine cultures. A broad-spectrum antibiotic is typically used for treatment, including clindamycin and gentamicin.

Mastitis

Mastitis refers to inflammation of the breast tissue and most commonly occurs in breastfeeding women. Inflammation results from mechanical trauma from lactation, duct blockage, or introduction of bacteria through broken skin. When infection does occur, *Staphylococcus aureus* is the most common causative organism. Patients with mastitis present with unilateral findings typical of inflammation: pain, warmth, and swelling of the affected breast. Physical exam reveals asymmetric size, erythema, and tenderness to palpation. Diagnosis is made based on history and physical exam with no need for labs or imaging. Treatment involves supportive measures, such as warm compresses and acetaminophen for pain relief as well as antibiotics with coverage against *S. aureus* to reduce the risk of abscess. Patients who are lactating should be advised to continue doing so to prevent duct blockage, which can prolong or worsen mastitis. However, it is important to note that patients who are not currently lactating should be assessed for inflammatory breast cancer as this malignancy can resemble mastitis.

Practice Quiz

1. What amount of total body blood loss is considered life-threatening and will throw a patient into hypovolemic shock?
    a. 1/8
    b. 1/7
    c. 1/5
    d. 1/10

2. When assessing a pregnant woman at 24 weeks gestation, which early manifestation would alert the nurse to a possible diagnosis of preeclampsia?
    a. Hypertension on bedrest
    b. Facial edema
    c. Increasing liver enzymes
    d. Thrombocytopenia

3. The WHNP is caring for a 19-year-old woman who presents in the emergency department with manifestations of acute hepatitis. She tells the WHNP that she thinks she might be pregnant and asks how this disease could affect her baby. The WHNP understands that which of the following genotypes is associated with the most significant risk for perinatal transmission of the hepatitis virus?
    a. HAeAb negative
    b. HBeAg positive
    c. HCeAg negative
    d. HDeAb positive

4. The WHNP is preparing a discharge plan for a patient who has chronic urinary retention and will be performing self-catheterization at home. Which of the following statements indicates the need for additional teaching?
    a. "My doctor told me that I can use my catheters more than once."
    b. "If I have chills and fever, it may mean that I am not emptying my bladder."
    c. "The acid in coffee will help to maintain the acidity of my urine, which decreases infection."
    d. "I should have about 700 milliliters to 1000 milliliters of urine output every day."

5. Which of the following is true about testing for herpes zoster?
    a. Viral cultures are the gold standard for identifying the herpes zoster virus.
    b. The Tzanck smear does not differentiate between varicella zoster virus and herpes simplex virus.
    c. The direct fluorescent antibody test is readily available in primary care facilities.
    d. The polymerase chain reaction analysis is less sensitive than the Tzanck smear.

See answers on the next page

Answer Explanations

1. C: Losing 1/5 (or 20 percent) of one's blood volume will throw a person into hypovolemic shock and is considered life threatening. Organ failure with profound hypotension will likely follow; fluid resuscitation and blood transfusions will be needed as soon as possible. Choices *A*, *B*, and *D* represent values less than 15–20 percent, or the amount of blood volume loss required to cause hypovolemic shock.

2. B: Early manifestations of preeclampsia include hypertension, facial edema, visual disturbances, altered mental state, dyspnea, and possible right upper quadrant pain. Severe manifestations include seizure activity, increasing liver enzymes with increased pain, thrombocytopenia, progressive renal dysfunction, and pulmonary edema, making Choices *A*, *C*, and *D* incorrect answers.

3. B: The greatest risk for perinatal virus transmission occurs with the antigen-positive hepatitis B virus. Hepatitis A virus spreads most commonly by the fecal-oral route, and perinatal transmission has not been established; therefore, Choice *A* is incorrect. Hepatitis C is rarely transmitted to the fetus, and the antigen-negative genotype would be less likely than the antigen-positive genotype to affect the fetus; therefore, Choice *C* is incorrect. Perinatal transmission of the hepatitis D virus is rare, and release of the hepatitis D virions requires coinfection with the hepatitis B virus; therefore, Choice *D* is incorrect.

4. C: While it is recommended that patients maintain an acidic pH in the urine to limit the growth of *E. coli*, coffee is to be avoided because caffeine intake is associated with increased feelings of the need to void and urgency. Therefore, Choice *C* indicates the need for additional instruction and is the correct answer. The correct catheter will be prescribed for the individual patient, and usually clean technique and the reuse of the catheter is appropriate. The providers must be convinced that the patient and/or caregiver understand the procedure and the identification of complications that require medical intervention; therefore, Choice *A* is incorrect. The onset of chills and fever may indicate an infection of the bladder or kidney due to incomplete emptying of the bladder and should be immediately reported to the healthcare provider. Therefore, Choice *B* is incorrect. Urine output will depend on the patient's intake and diet; however, an average output of 30 mL/h is acceptable in most instances; therefore, Choice *D* is incorrect.

5. B: The Tzanck test can identify herpes viruses, but it is not able to differentiate the individual viruses. Choice *A* is incorrect because the viral culture takes the longest of all of the tests to complete and the results are also less useful. The direct fluorescent antibody test is relatively new and is not widely available; therefore, Choice *C* is incorrect. The polymerase chain reaction analysis is more sensitive than the Tzanck smear, but it is not as widely available. Many researchers recommend the Tzanck smear because it is seventy-nine percent sensitive and one hundred percent specific to the herpes viruses.

Pharmacology

Pharmacokinetics and Pharmacodynamics

Pharmacokinetics

Pharmacokinetics traces the progress of a drug from the point of administration to the final intended effect of the drug on the target tissue or organ, followed by excretion of the drug. Kinetics means movement, and pharmacokinetics studies the movement or progress of a drug through human tissue in four phases: absorption, distribution, metabolism, and excretion.

The process and timeline for absorption depend on the route of administration, the membrane solubility of the drug, blood flow at the point of administration (with consideration of the first-pass action by the liver), and gastric emptying rates for drugs administered by mouth.

Distribution occurs through the circulatory system, which means that the vascularity of three defined body compartments determines the rate of distribution for any single drug. The three compartments are the highly vascular central compartment, which consists of the heart, brain, kidney, and liver; the peripheral compartment, which consists of adipose tissue and muscle; and the special tissues, which include the cerebral spinal fluid (CSF) and the blood-brain barrier of the central nervous system. Metabolism is a two-part process that prepares lipid-soluble drugs to assume a water-soluble form in order to facilitate excretion. Excretion is a process that occurs most often in the liver and gastrointestinal (GI) tract. Excretion of the drug metabolites is largely through the urine and bile, but, depending on molecular size, waste may be excreted through the feces and through expired air.

Pharmacodynamics

Pharmacodynamics is the study of the body's response to a drug, including the identification of all possible adverse effects. More specifically, pharmacodynamics studies a drug's dynamic properties in terms of affinity, efficacy, and potency. Every drug is either an agonist or antagonist. The reaction between the cell and the drug occurs most often between specific cell receptor sites, either on the cell surface or in the intracellular fluid. Affinity refers to the original attraction between cell-specific drug receptors and cell receptor sites. A drug's **potency** concerns the amount that is necessary to trigger the therapeutic response.

Efficacy refers to the scale of the reaction produced by a drug at the same receptor site. Continuous stimulation of the receptor site by a drug can decrease the response, which is called desensitization. Patient conditions such as aging, genetic alterations, thyroid disorders, Parkinson's disease, and some forms of type 1 diabetes can alter reactions at the binding sites. The resulting reaction may be an increase or a decrease in the therapeutic effect. Thus, for example, the analgesic effect of opioid medications is enhanced in the elderly, while the therapeutic effect of some bronchodilators is decreased. Elderly patients who are cognitively impaired are at significant risk for increased deficits when treated with anticholinergic agents, some anti-Parkinson's drugs, and CNS-altering drugs that cause sedation.

Pharmacogenetics

Pharmacogenetics, which is one part of pharmacogenomics, is the identification of a patient's inherited pattern of response to a drug. The genetically-determined response to a drug can vary as much as one-

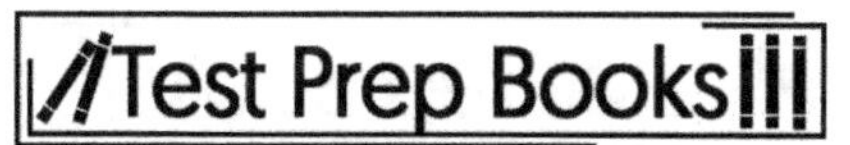

thousand-fold from one individual to another under similar circumstances. There are four kinds of pharmacogenetic alterations:

- Change in the plasma concentration of the drug due to changes in the metabolic process
- Alteration in the pharmacodynamic process that results in reduced binding of the drug at the receptor site
- Idiosyncratic alterations that increase the possibility for a hypersensitivity reaction to the drug
- Systemic pathogenesis, such as tumor formation

If these differences can be better understood, there is potential for developing individual drug therapies that improve outcomes while saving money. Genetic tests for many of these genetic patterns either do not exist, are prohibitively expensive, or require large populations of subjects for test development. One variation that has been identified with currently available genetic testing is an alteration in the enzymes involved in the reaction with the anti-platelet drug clopidogrel. This alteration is linked to life-threatening cardiac events. Genetic testing for this alteration identifies at-risk patients that should be treated with alternative anti-platelet drugs. This form of individual drug therapy is supported by the database maintained by the Clinical Pharmacogenetics Implementation Consortium of the National Institutes of Health's Pharmacogenomics Research Network, which is a clearinghouse for research data related to all possible genetic alterations that affect individual responses to drug therapy.

Pharmacotherapeutics

Pharmacotherapeutics is the study of the therapeutic uses and effects of drugs. Pharmacotherapeutics may also include the identification of a drug's adverse effects as well as possible interactions with other prescription drugs. The women's health care nurse practitioner (WHNP) understands that the original efficacy and safety of all medications is established by the United States Food and Drug Administration (FDA). Pharmacotherapeutics may also focus on the stated outcome for the therapy, which may be prevention, cure, or control of illness.

Comprehensive databases that include all drug categories have been developed and maintained by government-associated agencies such as the United States Pharmacopeia, interested professional groups such as the American Society of Health-System Pharmacists, and commercial groups that categorize the drugs for marketing purposes. Through these groups' websites, the WHNP has access to current prescribing resources, including patient education materials. As a cost-saving measure, care institutions use the databases to establish agency-specific formularies that define and limit the drugs in each pharmacotherapeutic category that are available for use in that agency. Additional cost savings include the use of generic drugs whenever possible. Generic drugs are identical to name brand drugs but may be available at a fraction of the cost.

Pharmacotherapeutic Selection

Pharmacotherapeutic intervention selection is a form of clinical judgment that is based on the findings of the WHNP's comprehensive assessment. The selection of pharmacotherapeutic interventions is based on: indications for the therapy; contraindications; cost and compliance; efficacy; adverse effects; dose; duration; and patient directions. As previously noted, the patient's pharmacokinetic response to any drug is related to the patient's inherited metabolic pathways, comorbidities, and the drug characteristics for all prescribed and over the counter (OTC) drugs. The potential for altered drug metabolism can also be the result of the binding of one or more prescribed drugs to liver enzymes, which can decrease (inhibition) or increase (induction) excretion of the drugs through that same enzyme pathway. Inhibition is more common than induction, which potentially results in an adverse drug reaction (ADR) due to increases in the plasma concentration of the drugs. The risk for ADRs also exists when two drugs compete for the same enzyme pathway. These potential sources for ADRs are not always predictable. This means that the WHNP will be aware of common ADRs while maintaining close monitoring for patient-specific reactions.

Another issue that is associated with the selection of pharmacotherapeutic agents is the use of **off-label use of drugs**, which means that the drug is being used for a treatment that has not been approved by the FDA. This practice is common in the treatment of cancer when a drug that has been evaluated for the treatment of one form of cancer is used to treat a different form of cancer without being evaluated by the FDA for that specific use. These new therapies can be related to adverse reactions that may be unpredictable. This practice is common in pediatric populations, especially in children with rare diseases because there is insufficient research data to support the providers' clinical decisions.

Pharmacotherapeutic Monitoring

Ongoing assessment and documentation of the effectiveness of the plan of care is an essential function of the WHNP's professional practice. The initial assessment by the WHNP is the foundation for all future assessments and evaluations. With respect to the pharmacotherapeutic plan, patient safety requires a full accounting of all agents that the patient consumes, including OTC and prescription drugs, herbs, and all other supplements.

Ongoing monitoring of the effectiveness of the pharmacotherapeutic plan also requires an accurate assessment of the patient's adherence to the plan. **Adherence** may also be identified as compliance, but however it is defined, there is evidence that up to 50 percent of all patients who take five or more drugs rarely demonstrate 100 percent adherence to the prescribed regimen. The result is the sub-optimal treatment of a chronic disease that can progress to a more acute form of the condition. WHNPs should understand that there are several contributing factors for this finding, including the cost of the drug, the complexity of the pharmacotherapeutic plan, and the adverse effects associated with the prescribed drugs. Factors that enhance adherence include comprehensive patient education, a cooperative relationship with the WHNP, and provider attempts to limit drug costs. The WHNP is aware that in addition to the use of generic drugs, many national pharmaceutical providers have a lower cost formulary that can provide an alternative to the newer but more costly drugs.

Cardiovascular System Medications

Antihypertensive Medications

Antihypertensive medications are used to treat high blood pressure. Although hypertensive individuals generally do not have symptoms, some people experience headaches, blurred vision, and dizziness. When high blood pressure is left untreated, it can lead to different clinical conditions including coronary artery disease, heart failure, kidney failure, or stroke. There are two values that comprise a blood pressure measure. The top number is the systolic pressure (the pressure on the arterial walls when the heart muscle contracts) and the bottom number is the diastolic pressure (the pressure on the arterial walls when the heart muscle

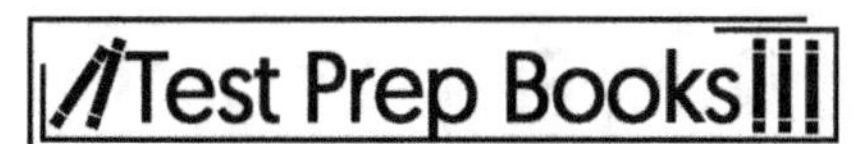

relaxes). Normal, healthy blood pressure in adults should be a systolic reading less than 120 mmHg and a diastolic reading less than 80 mmHg.

There are three stages of high blood pressure, as outlined below:

- **Prehypertension** is characterized by systolic pressure between 120-139 mmHg and diastolic pressure between 80-89 mmHg.
- **Stage 1 hypertensive** is characterized by systolic pressure between 140-159 mmHg and diastolic pressure between 90-99 mmHg.
- **Stage 2 hypertensive** is characterized by systolic pressure of 160 mmHg and higher and diastolic pressure of 100 mmHg and higher.

ACE Inhibitors (ACEIs)

"**ACE inhibitors**," or angiotensin-converting enzyme inhibitors, are used to treat hypertension and cardiovascular diseases. The most common side effect of ACE inhibitors is a chronic dry cough, which, in many cases, is so annoying for a patient that it results in switching the medication to a different class. Other frequent side effects are low blood pressure (hypotension), dizziness, fatigue, headache, and hyperkalemia (increased blood potassium levels).

Examples of some ACE Inhibitors include the following:

- Ramipril
- Enalapril
- Lisinopril
- Captopril
- Quinapril
- Perindopril

ARBs

Angiotensin Receptor Blockers (ARBs) have similar therapeutic effects as ACE Inhibitors; however, they tend to have better compliance due to their lower incidence of persistent cough. They block the effect of angiotensin at the receptor site and are widely used for hypertension and cardiovascular disease. The common side effects are hypotension, fatigue, dizziness, headache, and hyperkalemia.

Examples of ARBs include the following:

- Losartan
- Irbesartan
- Valsartan
- Candesartan
- Telmisartan
- Olmesartan

CCBs

Calcium Channel Blockers (CCBs) work by decreasing calcium entry through calcium channels. By regulating the movement of calcium, contraction of vascular smooth muscle is controlled, which causes blood vessels to dilate. This reduces blood pressure and workload on the heart, so this type of medication is used to treat hypertension and angina and to control heart rate. Common side effects of CCBs include dizziness, flushing of the face, headache, edema (swelling), tachycardia (fast heart rate), bradycardia (slow heart rate), and constipation. In combination with other medications that treat hypertension, calcium channel blocker toxicity is possible. Combinations, like verapamil with beta-blockers, can lead to severe bradycardia.

The following are examples of common calcium channel blockers:

- Amlodipine
- Nifedipine
- Felodipine
- Verapamil
- Diltiazem

Beta Blockers

Beta blockers are an important class of antihypertensive medications and are widely used to treat hypertension and cardiovascular disease. Some of them are also used to treat migraines, agitation, and anxiety. The side effects of beta blockers include hypotension, dizziness, bradycardia, headache, bronchoconstriction (trouble breathing), and fatigue.

Commonly prescribed beta blockers include the following:

- Atenolol
- Metoprolol
- Propranolol
- Sotalol
- Nadolol
- Carvedilol
- Labetalol

Vasodilators

Vasodilators cause blood vessels to dilate, lowering resistance to flow and reducing the workload on the heart. Vasodilators are used to treat hypertension, angina, and heart failure. The common side effects associated with their use include lightheadedness, dizziness, low blood pressure, flushing, reflex tachycardia, and headache. Vasodilators should not be combined with medications for erectile dysfunction, as this interaction can cause a fatal drop in blood pressure.

Examples of common vasodilators include the following:

- Nitroglycerin (available as sublingual tablets, sprays, patches, and extended-release capsules)
- Isosorbide mononitrate
- Isosorbide dinitrate
- Hydralazine
- Minoxidil (limited use)

Alpha-1 Receptor Blockers

Alpha-blockers decrease the norepinephrine-induced vascular contraction, causing relaxation of blood vessels and a resultant reduction in blood pressure. This type of medication is used to treat high blood pressure and benign prostatic hyperplasia (BPH). The common side effects of this class of medications include hypotension, dizziness, headache, tachycardia, weakness, and nausea.

Examples of alpha blockers include the following:

- Prazosin
- Doxazosin
- Terazosin
- Tamsulosin (primarily used to treat BPH)
- Alfuzosin (primarily used to treat BPH)

Diuretics

Diuretics are used alone and in combination with other medications to treat hypertension. They are often used to eliminate excess body fluid to treat swelling/edema. Diuretics inhibit the absorption of sodium in renal tubules, resulting in increased elimination of salt and water. This action increases urine output, decreases blood volume, and lowers blood pressure. Side effects of diuretics include hypotension, dizziness, hypokalemia, dehydration, hyperglycemia, polyuria (frequent or excessive urination), fatigue, syncope (fainting), and tinnitus (ringing in ears).

Examples of commonly prescribed diuretics include the following:

- Furosemide
- Bumetanide
- Hydrochlorothiazide
- Spironolactone
- Amiloride
- Triamterene

Endocrine System Medications

Anti-Diabetic Medications

Anti-diabetic medications are used to treat diabetes, which is a chronic metabolic disease in which the body cannot properly regulate blood sugar levels. This dysregulation is caused by either inadequate or absent insulin production from the pancreas (Type 1 diabetes) or inadequate action of insulin in peripheral tissues (insulin resistance in Type 2 diabetes). Type 1 diabetes usually occurs in early childhood and is typically treated with insulin injections or medications. Type 2 diabetes generally develops later in adolescence or adulthood and is related to poor diet, lack of physical activity, and obesity. Diabetes often does not cause daily symptoms, but symptoms do arise when blood sugar is either too high (from inadequate control) or too low (from inappropriate dosing of hypoglycemic [antidiabetic] agents, including insulin). A few of the symptoms of diabetes include increased thirst and hunger, fatigue, blurred vision, a tingling sensation in the feet, and frequent urination.

Examples of some antidiabetic medications include the following:

- Insulin
- Metformin
- Acarbose
- Gliclazide, glyburide, glimepiride
- Rosiglitazone and pioglitazone
- Sitagliptin and saxagliptin

The most effective way of treating Type 2 diabetes is to combine both drug and non-drug therapies. As a part of the treatment, drug therapy can stimulate the pancreas to produce more insulin or help the body better use the insulin produced by the pancreas.

Gastrointestinal System Medications

Gastric Acid Neutralizers/Suppressants

Gastric acid neutralizers/suppressants either neutralize stomach acid or decrease acid production and, therefore, provide relief of symptoms associated with **hyperacidity**. They are also used to treat gastroesophageal reflux disease, or GERD. In GERD, the lower esophageal sphincter does not close properly, which causes the contents of the stomach to back up into the esophagus. This leads to irritation, which is why the common symptoms of GERD include heartburn, coughing, nausea, difficulty swallowing, and a strained voice. There are many factors that can cause or exacerbate GERD including obesity, pregnancy, eating a large meal, acidic foods, a hiatal hernia, and smoking. Lifestyle modifications such as avoiding trigger foods, losing weight (if obesity is a component), decreasing meal size, and trying not to lie down immediately after eating, can reduce symptoms.

The medications used to treat hyperacidity in the stomach include the following:

- Antacids (e.g., calcium carbonate)
- Ranitidine
- Famotidine
- Omeprazole
- Esomeprazole
- Lansoprazole
- Rabeprazole
- Pantoprazole

Genitourinary System Medications

UTIs occur within the urethra, kidney ureters, or bladder. UTIs that travel can extend into the kidneys and cause pyelonephritis. UTIs are caused by bacteria. Pharmacological treatment includes antibiotics. A **culture and sensitivity test** should be performed to determine the type of bacteria for proper antibiotic selection. Trimethoprim-sulfamethoxazole (Bactrim DS®) may be prescribed to non-pregnant females with no comorbidities over a period of 3 days. Patients should be informed that the most common side effects of Bactrim include GI disturbances such as nausea and vomiting. Another antibiotic commonly used in treating UTIs is nitrofurantoin (Macrobid®). Common side effects include nausea, vomiting, and headache. UTIs may cause a burning sensation when urinating.

Phenazopyridine HCL (Pyridium®) is a pain reliever that targets the lower urinary tract. Pyridium helps relieve bladder spasms. Patients should be alerted that Pyridium causes orange discoloration of the urine and may stain surfaces and clothing. BPH is the age-related enlargement of the prostate gland in males. BPH can constrict the urethra and alter the flow of urine. Patients with BPH can have urinary retention, urethral obstruction, and bladder distention. Pharmacological treatment includes decreasing the volume of the prostate and lowering the resistance of the bladder outlet. Medications that decrease the resistance of the bladder outlet include alpha-adrenergic blockers. A common medication is tamsulosin (Flomax®). Headache and dizziness are very common side effects, and patients should be instructed to change positions slowly. Other common symptoms include stuffy nose and abnormal ejaculation. Medications such as finasteride (Proscar®) reduce dihydrotestosterone serum levels that decrease the volume of the prostate. Proscar may cause impotence and is a reason for discontinuation by patients. Medications that decrease the volume of the prostate may take 6 to 12 months for a full response.

Hematologic Pharmacology

Anemia is a general term for the reduction of RBCs circulating within the body or the decrease in hemoglobin that helps transport oxygen to the tissues. The goal of anemia treatment is to increase the number of RBCs and raise the hemoglobin levels. There are different types of anemias, and supplemental medications are necessary to correct the deficiencies. Iron-deficiency anemia is the lack of sufficient amounts of iron used for hemoglobin synthesis. The most cost-effective medication to treat iron-deficiency anemia is ferrous sulfate (iron). Practitioners should expect to see blood levels return to normalcy after approximately 2 months of use. Patients should be instructed to take ferrous sulfate on an empty stomach and informed that milk products and antacid medications interfere with the absorption of iron. **Pernicious anemia** is the insufficient production of hydrochloric acid in the stomach.

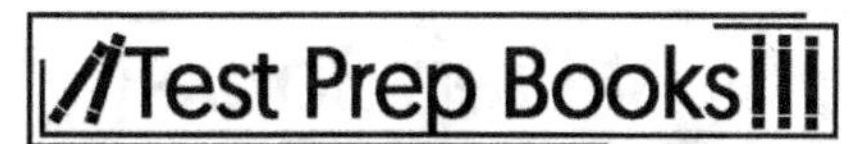

The intrinsic factor found in the gastric mucosa that is necessary for the absorption of vitamin B12 in the small intestine is decreased in pernicious anemia. Replacement of vitamin B12 in parenteral form is preferred and will increase the regeneration of RBCs. Patients should be encouraged to eat vitamin B12–rich foods such as animal proteins and eggs. Folic acid deficiency anemia is due to a decrease in folic acid levels that interferes with the DNA synthesis and maturation of RBCs. Pharmacological treatment is aimed at increasing folic acid levels. Oral folate is recommended. Serum folic acid levels should increase within a period of 3 to 4 months. **Aplastic anemia** results from bone marrow dysfunction. RBCs, WBCs, and platelets are produced in the bone marrow. Decreased levels of erythrocytes, leukocytes, and platelets is termed pancytopenia. Autoimmune disorders are a prevalent cause of aplastic anemia. Pharmacological treatment is aimed at reducing the immune response. Immunosuppressants such as cyclosporine can help prevent further damage to the bone marrow. Hematopoietic growth factors stimulate the production of WBCs and RBCs. Filgrastim (Neupogen®) is a colony-stimulating medication. Common side effects involve the musculoskeletal system and can cause muscle and bone pain.

Immune System Medications

Antivirals

Antivirals are used to fight viruses in the body by either stopping replication or blocking the function of a viral protein. They are used to treat HIV, herpes, hepatitis B and C, and influenza, among other viruses. Vaccines are also available to prevent some viral infections. Side effects of antivirals include headache, nausea, blood abnormalities including anemia and neutropenia (low neutrophil count), dizziness, cough, runny or stuff nose, etc.

Some examples of disease-specific antivirals include the following:

- Acyclovir, valaciclovir (Valtrex®): Herpes simplex, herpes zoster, and herpes B
- Ritonavir, indinavir, darunavir: Protease inhibitor for HIV
- Tenofovir (Viread®): Hepatitis B and HIV infection
- Interferon: Hepatitis C
- Oseltamivir (Tamiflu): Influenza

Antibiotics

Antibiotics are antimicrobial agents that are used for treatment and prevention of bacterial infections. The mechanism of action of an antibiotic involves either killing bacteria or inhibiting their growth. Antibiotics are not effective against viruses, and therefore, they should not be used to treat viral infections. Antibiotics are often prescribed based on the result of a bacterial culture to ascertain which class of antibiotic(s) the respective strain will respond to. The common side effects of antibiotics include allergies, hypersensitivity reactions or anaphylaxis, stomach upset, diarrhea, candida (fungal) infections, and bacterial resistance (superinfection, in which a strain of bacteria develops resistance to broad classes of antibiotics).

Commonly prescribed antibiotics include the following:

- Penicillin V
- Amoxicillin (with or without clavulanic acid)
- Ampicillin
- Cloxacillin
- Cephalexin
- Cefuroxime
- Cefixime
- Tetracycline
- Doxycycline

- Minocycline
- Gentamicin
- Tobramycin
- Ciprofloxacin
- Levofloxacin
- Erythromycin
- Azithromycin
- Clarithromycin
- Clindamycin

Antimetabolites

Antimetabolites are used to treat diseases including severe psoriasis, rheumatoid arthritis, and several types of cancer (breast, lung, lymphoma, and leukemia). The most commonly used medication of this class is methotrexate, which suppresses the growth of abnormal cells and the action of the immune system. Methotrexate is widely used to treat rheumatoid arthritis. This medication is typically prescribed as a once per week dose, and it should not be prescribed for daily dosing because overdosing can be lethal. Pharmacists should be alerted to any prescriptions for daily methotrexate, as the doctor must be contacted to confirm and correct the dosing.

The following are the potential side effects of methotrexate:

- Dizziness
- Drowsiness
- Headache
- Swollen gums
- Increased susceptibility to infections
- Hair loss
- Confusion
- Weakness

Steroids

Steroids are used to treat allergies, asthma, rashes, swelling, and inflammation. These medications are available in different forms, such as oral tablets, nasal sprays, eye drops, topical creams and ointments, inhalants, and injections. The common side effects of steroids include insulin resistance and diabetes, osteoporosis, depression, hypertension, edema, glaucoma, etc.

The following are examples of commonly prescribed corticosteroids:

- Prednisone
- Hydrocortisone
- Fluticasone
- Triamcinolone
- Mometasone
- Budesonide
- Fluocinolone
- Betamethasone
- Dexamethasone

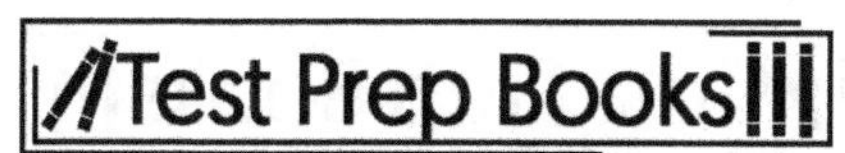

Nervous System Medications

Antidepressants and Anxiolytics

Antidepressants are used to treat different mood disorders including depression, anxiety, phobias, and obsessive-compulsive disorder (OCD). Treatment for depression includes various medications, in addition to cognitive behavioral therapy (e.g., counseling).

Antidepressants exert their therapeutic effects by modulating the release or action of various neurotransmitters in the brain. **Neurotransmitters** are chemical messengers that transmit signals from one neuron to another. The common side effects of antidepressants are serotonin syndrome (headache, agitation, tremor, hallucination, tachycardia, hyperthermia, shivering and sweating), sexual dysfunction, weight changes, gastric acidity, diarrhea, sleep disturbances, and suicidal ideation.

Commonly prescribed antidepressant medications include the following:

- Sertraline
- Fluoxetine
- Paroxetine
- Citalopram
- Escitalopram
- Venlafaxine
- Desvenlafaxine
- Duloxetine
- Trazodone
- Bupropion
- Amitriptyline
- Nortriptyline

Benzodiazepines are a class of medications used for the short-term treatment of anxiety. They are often combined with antidepressants during initial treatment to increase treatment compliance. Benzodiazepines have the potential for significant physical dependence and withdrawal symptoms. These drugs can be used as sedatives and hypnotics and are also utilized as an add-on therapy with anti-convulsant medications. Benzodiazepines are often used to treat symptoms from alcohol withdrawal. The majority of benzodiazepines are labeled as Class IV controlled substances. The common side effects of these medications include physical dependence, sedation, drowsiness, dizziness, and lack of coordination.

The following are commonly prescribed benzodiazepines:

- Diazepam
- Lorazepam
- Clonazepam
- Alprazolam
- Midazolam
- Temazepam

Antipsychotics

Antipsychotics are used to treat psychosis, including schizophrenia and bipolar disorder. Psychosis is often characterized by a cluster of symptoms including delusions (false beliefs), paranoia (fear or anxiety), hallucinations, and disordered thoughts. The most common side effects of antipsychotics are dyskinesia (movement disorder), loss of libido or sex drive, gynecomastia (breast enlargement) in males, weight gain, heart diseases (QT prolongation), and metabolic disorders including type 2 diabetes.

The following are examples of commonly prescribed antipsychotics:

- Chlorpromazine
- Fluphenazine
- Haloperidol
- Aripiprazole
- Olanzapine
- Risperidone
- Ziprasidone
- Clozapine

Stimulant Medications

Stimulant medications are also called sympathomimetic agents, as they work by augmenting the sympathetic neurotransmitter activity (e.g., epinephrine and norepinephrine). These drugs are often used during emergencies to treat cardiac arrest and shock. Stimulant medications are also commonly used to treat attention-deficit hyperactivity disorder (ADHD). The common side effects of such medications include irritability, weight loss, insomnia, dizziness, agitation, headache, abdominal pain, tachycardia, growth retardation, hypertension, cardiovascular disturbances, and death.

The following are examples of sympathomimetic drugs that are used in the treatment of ADHD:

- Methylphenidate
- Dextroamphetamine
- Lisdexamfetamine
- Mixed salts of amphetamine
- Atomoxetine

Anticonvulsant Medications

Anticonvulsants are also called antiepileptic or anti-seizure medications. They are used in the treatment of epileptic seizures. They suppress excessive firing of neurons and therefore prevent the initiation and spread of seizures. This class of medications is often used to stabilize mood in bipolar disorder or for the treatment of neuropathic pain. The common side effects are dizziness, sedation, weight gain, hepatotoxicity, hair loss, blood disorders, etc. Anticonvulsants are teratogenic and can cause significant harm to a fetus and result in birth defects. Therefore, female patients on anticonvulsant therapy should consult with their physicians before planning pregnancy.

The common medications in this class include the following:

- Carbamazepine
- Oxcarbazepine
- Phenytoin
- Valproic acid
- Divalproex
- Levetiracetam
- Lamotrigine
- Topiramate
- Clobazam

Pain Management

Pain is a subjective symptom. Every person will experience pain in different proportions. It is estimated that more than 60 percent of people who experience acute pain will not receive adequate pain management. Up to 75 percent of people who have chronic pain throughout their life span will suffer from partial or total disability that can become permanent. A person's perception of pain varies. The pain threshold is influenced by social and environmental factors. Pain tolerance is a person's ability to endure pain. Tolerance can be influenced by gender, sociocultural background, and age. **Acute pain** is characterized by a sudden onset that is localized and usually temporary. Acute pain will last 6 months or less and has an identified cause, such as surgery, infectious process, or trauma. Physical symptoms include elevated heart rate, dilated pupils, pale skin, diaphoresis, and increased blood pressure and respirations.

Chronic pain is present for more than three months and is not always linked to a direct cause. Medical treatment is difficult and may not provide relief to the patient. Chronic pain is usually dull and aching. Conditions that can cause chronic pain include back pain, cancer, and postoperative pain. It is important for practitioners to educate patients on pain intensity rating scales. One of the most common pain assessment tools is the numeric rating scale. This scale measures pain from 0 to 10 and is commonly used in clinical settings. Pediatric patients and patients who are cognitively impaired may use the face, legs, activity, cry, consolability (FLACC) and FACES scales. The FLACC scale is based on observation of activity and body movement, and the FACES scale provides a pictorial perception of pain. Practitioners should attempt to determine the etiology of the pain and treat the disease process. When a cause cannot be found, treatment is aimed at controlling pain. Pharmacological treatment includes nonsteroidal anti-inflammatory drugs (NSAIDs), opioid analgesics, topical anesthetics, and nerve block injections. Complementary therapies can enhance the patient's quality of life. Alternative therapies include herbal medications, meditation, imagery, music, and aromatherapy.

Pain Assessment

Pain is a subjective topic that varies by patient; therefore, healthcare professionals have a responsibility to combine clinical knowledge, personal expertise, and patient involvement in developing a safe and effective pain management plan. Unmanaged pain can lead to reduced quality of life and the inability to complete basic tasks like eating, can affect mood, and often leads to prolonged depression. In complex surgical cases, unmanaged pain can lead to poor recovery outcomes, including increased rates of infection and hormonal disruption. Pain management plans can employ a number of different techniques depending on the severity of the case.

Pain can be assessed in a number of ways, including visual and physical assessments, obtaining reports from the patient, and administering formal pain measurement scales. Visual and physical pain assessments may include noticing any conditions or injuries a patient has (for example, patients with a noticeable degree of kyphosis in their backs are expected to report a significant degree of muscular pain and tension along the spine) or noticing the intensity of pain that occurs with certain movements.

Patient self-reports of pain should be noted and taken seriously; however, patients who have previous prescriptions for narcotics or appear to desperately want them should be treated with extreme caution.

Finally, formal pain measurement instruments include numeric rating scales and verbal rating scales that patients work through with their healthcare providers to determine pain intensity. For preoperative patients, medical teams may choose a specific instrument with the patient prior to the procedure. During the preoperative period, medical teams may choose to review the instrument in detail with patients to ensure that they know how to properly report their pain levels. The selected instrument should then be utilized to continuously assess pain during the recovery period.

Medications for Pain Management

Pain is the most commonly seen symptom. However, since cases often vary widely in scope and every patient will have a different personal threshold for pain tolerance, best practices are difficult to develop when it comes to pain management. It is often done on a case-by-case basis. However, when a patient's pain is not managed in a way that seems appropriate to that individual, it can cause patient and family dissatisfaction in the healthcare organization. As a result, medical staff must try to provide effective and safe pain management options that can make the patient comfortable at the present time, but that also do not cause harm over time. In some cases, like a sprained muscle, ice therapy and time can provide adequate pain management. More serious cases, defined as pain that does not subside after an objectively reasonable period of time for the injury, may require topical, intramuscular, or oral pain medication. These can include stronger doses of common over-the-counter pain medications, or prescription pain medications.

Prescription pain medications, especially opioids and muscle relaxers, are known for causing debilitating addiction; therefore, when prescribing them to a patient, the lowest dose and dosing frequency necessary should be utilized. Additionally, patients should be closely monitored for their reactions to their pain medications. Finally, some individuals who are addicted to prescription pain killers and muscle relaxers may feign injuries in order to receive another prescription. Therefore, all patients' medical histories should be thoroughly evaluated to note their history of pain medication usage. Patients should also be assessed for showing any signs of drug abuse history and withdrawal symptoms (such as damaged teeth, shaking, and agitation).

Procedural sedation allows patients to remain somewhat alert during medical procedures that may be uncomfortable but not unbearably painful, such as resetting bones. Unlike general anesthesia, where patients are completely sedated and do not feel any sensations, procedural sedation allows patients to be somewhat conscious and aware of bodily functions. It can be utilized with or without pain-relieving medications. Practitioner awareness is crucial when administering procedural sedation, especially when pain relief is also utilized. Recently, overuse and improper use of common procedural sedation agents, such as propofol, and common pain relief medications that are often used in conjunction, such as fentanyl, have caused high profile deaths.

Analgesia, Narcotics, NSAIDS, and Opioids

Analgesics is an umbrella term for a variety of pain-relieving pharmaceuticals that can include mild over-the-counter medications as well as prescription-strength medications that require close monitoring by a medical professional. Different categories of analgesics work by targeting different pathways to pain.

Nonsteroidal anti-inflammatory drugs (**NSAIDS**) include commonly recognized medications such as ibuprofen; prescription strength doses are simply much more concentrated than versions that can be bought over the counter. NSAIDS work by targeting areas of inflammation in the body that result in pain; consequently, they are most effective for pain situations involving muscles or soft tissues.

Opioids, a type of narcotic, are prescription-only medications that work by targeting nociceptors in the brain to reduce pathway signaling that result in the physical perception of pain. While these medications are often able to eliminate pain quickly, they can also cause extremely uncomfortable side effects, like severe nausea and dizziness, in some patients. Additionally, most narcotics are highly addictive, and an opioid epidemic is well-documented in the United States. These types of prescriptions should be carefully prescribed and monitored if they are required in patient treatment plans. As patients near the end of their prescription, they may need tailored treatment to avoid withdrawal symptoms.

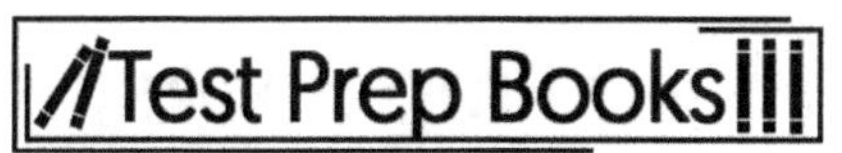

Multimodal Chronic and/or Acute Pain Management

Multimodal pain management refers to using pharmacological, non-pharmacological, and alternative medicine to treat pain. Pharmacological management includes everything from over-the-counter (OTC) pain medication to anesthetics. **Non-pharmacological pain management** refers to modalities such as heat, ice, compression, and physical therapy. Alternative medicine, or **complementary and alternative medicine** (**CAM**), is often viewed as a more natural or non-westernized type of medicine. This includes treatments such as meditation, yoga, supplements, massage, and chiropractic therapy. These pain management types can each be used separately or in combination. CAM is becoming more and more popular in the United States, and patients often ask about non-pharmacologic or alternative treatments. Nurses are in an excellent position to educate patients on all their choices.

Acute mild pain is generally treated with OTC pain medications and non-pharmacologic modalities such as the RICE (rest, ice, compression, and elevation) technique for musculoskeletal injuries. Acute, moderate-to-severe pain is often treated with a short course of powerful, pharmacologic pain medications such as opioids. If pain lasts for longer than three months, it is considered chronic pain. Chronic pain is multi-factorial and often requires a combination of the three different types of treatment.

Patient Pain Management Expectations

Patients often expect to be pain-free after receiving pain treatment. Managing this expectation can have a considerable impact on the patient's outcome. Asking the patient what a positive outcome would be for them can give the nurse insight into their expectations. If a patient expects to be pain-free, the nurse can educate on how the goal is to make the patient comfortable, not necessarily free of pain. Educating the patient that some pain is normal and means the body is healing can help manage expectations as well. Understanding a patient's thoughts, perceptions, and goals around pain can help the nurse form an individualized plan to best meet that patient's needs.

The opposite is also true. If a patient is terrified of a procedure due to fear of the pain, the nurse can set realistic expectations on the level of pain they may experience. It is important to be truthful when describing the level of pain that a patient might face during a procedure. The nurse should not underplay the pain and let the patient be caught off guard during the procedure. Be truthful and the patient will enter the procedure with the right mindset regarding pain.

Respiratory System Medications

Antiasthmatics

Antiasthmatics are used to prevent and treat the acute symptoms of asthma, which is a disease characterized by wheezing, cough, chest tightness, and shortness of breath. Acute asthma can be life-threatening and needs to be treated promptly. Asthma is caused by inflammation and constriction of the airways, which results in difficulty breathing. Acute asthma may be exacerbated by certain triggering factors including environmental allergens, certain medications (e.g., aspirin), stress or exercise, smoke, and lung infections. It is important to avoid the triggering factors to prevent acute symptoms. The common side effects of antiasthmatics are cough, hoarseness, decreased bone mineral density, growth retardation in children, mouth thrush, agitation, tachycardia, and a transient increase in blood pressure.

There are two categories to asthma medications that can be used alone or in combination:

- Bronchodilators (dilate the airway to ease breathing):
    - Salbutamol
    - Formoterol (generally used in combination with inhaled corticosteroids)
    - Salmeterol (generally used in combination with inhaled corticosteroids)

- Anti-inflammatory agents:
    - Fluticasone (inhaled corticosteroid)
    - Budesonide (inhaled corticosteroid)
    - Beclometasone (inhaled corticosteroid)
    - Montelukast
    - Zafirlukast

Pharmacological Agents Used for Acute Asthma

Various classes of pharmacological agents are used for the treatment and control of status asthmaticus. The following discussion concentrates on pharmacological agents to treat and control acute asthma rather than chronic asthma. Urgent care of asthma can include the following:

Beta-2 Adrenergic Agonists (Beta-2 Agonists)

Short-acting preparations of **Beta-2 agonists** relax the muscles in the airways, resulting in bronchodilation (expanding of the bronchial air passages) and increased airflow to the lungs. It is important to remember that one of the underlying factors in asthma is bronchoconstriction. Albuterol is the most commonly used short-acting Beta-2 agonist. Adverse effects of albuterol include tachycardia, tremors, and anxiety. Another short-acting Beta-2 agonist used to treat acute asthma is levalbuterol (Xopenex). This medication is related to albuterol and has the same result, but without the adverse effects. However, it must be noted that the frequent use of adrenergic agents prior to receiving emergency care can decrease a patient's response to these medications in a hospital setting.

Anticholinergics

Anticholinergics block the action of the neurotransmitter acetylcholine which, in turn, causes bronchodilation. Anticholinergics can also increase the bronchodilation effect of short-acting Beta-2 agonists. The most commonly used anticholinergic is ipratropium, which is used in combination with short-acting Beta-2 agonists for the treatment of status asthmaticus. Adverse effects can include dry mouth, blurred vision, and constipation.

Corticosteroids

Corticosteroids are potent anti-inflammatory medications that fight the inflammation accompanying asthma. Corticosteroids commonly used in the treatment of status asthmaticus include prednisone, prednisolone, and methylprednisolone. Methylprednisolone is typically administered once intravenously (IV) in cases of status asthmaticus and then followed by a taper of oral prednisone over seven to ten days. The intravenous administration of corticosteroids is equal in effectiveness to oral corticosteroid administration. Corticosteroids have numerous adverse effects, and they should not be used for more than two weeks. Adverse effects of long-term corticosteroid use can include weight gain, osteoporosis, thinning of skin, cataracts, easy bruising, and diabetes. Therefore, it is necessary to monitor blood glucose routinely and use regular insulin on a sliding scale. Electrolytes (particularly potassium) must also be monitored.

Methylxanthines

Methylxanthines are used as bronchodilators and as adjuncts to Beta-2 agonists and corticosteroids in treating status asthmaticus. The primary methylxanthines are theophylline and aminophylline. At therapeutic doses, methylxanthines are much weaker bronchodilators than Beta-2 agonists. The adverse effects of methylxanthines can include nausea, vomiting, tachycardia, headaches, and seizures. As a result, therapeutic monitoring is mandatory. Therapeutic levels of theophylline range from 10 mcg/mL to 20 mcg/mL. Methylxanthines aren't frequently used to treat status asthmaticus because of their possible adverse effects and the need for close monitoring of drug blood levels.

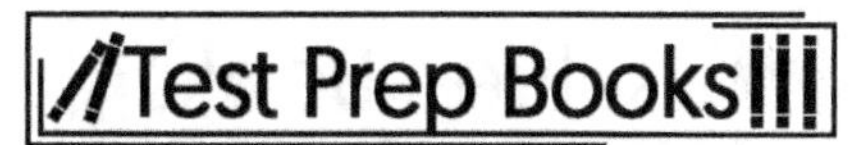

Magnesium Sulfate

Magnesium sulfate is a calcium antagonist that relaxes smooth muscle in the lung passages, leading to bronchodilation. Clinical studies indicate it can be used as an adjunct to Beta-2 agonist therapy during status asthmaticus. Intravenous magnesium sulfate is given slowly to prevent adverse effects, such as bradycardia and hypotension. The administration of magnesium sulfate is controversial due to varying clinical studies of effectiveness, but its use (inhaled or intravenously administered) may be considered as an adjunct treatment for the asthmatic patient.

Leukotriene Inhibitors

Leukotriene inhibitors target inflammation related to asthma. Typically used for the long-term control of asthma, this class of medication can be helpful for a minority of individuals with status asthmaticus. The primary leukotriene inhibitors used in the treatment of asthma are montelukast and zafirlukast. Adverse effects of leukotriene inhibitors include headache, rash, fatigue, dizziness, and abdominal pain.

Medication Monitoring

Beta-2 agonists used for pulmonary system support, such as albuterol and terbutaline, can cause side effects that include tremor, dizziness, and palpitations. Prolonged corticosteroid use can induce **Cushing's syndrome**, which includes the following signs and symptoms: fat loss from arms and legs, muscle weakness, anxiety, moon face, diaphoresis, fatty deposits around upper back, and abdominal weight gain. Corticosteroids should be weaned following a gradual titration, as abrupt discontinuation may trigger an adrenal insufficiency crisis. Theophylline, a methylxanthine, can cause arrhythmias and seizures. The WHNP must carefully monitor vital signs and provide patient education on maintenance, which should include taking the medication at regular intervals during the day.

Reproductive System Medications

Erectile dysfunction (ED) is a condition in male patients that prevents them from achieving or sustaining an erection during sexual intercourse. Many factors influence ED, including spinal cord injuries, psychological distress, diabetes, and medications such as beta-blockers. There are several medications that can treat ED. The **corpus cavernosa** is a region of erectile tissue that fills with blood during an erection. Medications that dilate the corpora cavernosa are used to treat ED. These medications are known as **PDE5 inhibitors**. A common PDE5 inhibitor is sildenafil (Viagra®). Viagra relaxes the blood vessel walls and increases blood flow to specific areas of the body. Due to blood vessel relaxation, Viagra can cause a sudden decrease in blood pressure. Common side effects include flushing of the skin and headache. Other PDE5 inhibitors used for the treatment of ED include vardenafil (Levitra®) and tadalafil (Cialis®).

PCOS is an endocrine hormone disorder that affects the reproductive system in females. PCOS is characterized by high levels of androgen hormones, dysfunction in ovulation, and cysts within the ovaries. Excess insulin is a possible factor for PCOS development. Increased insulin levels can lead to an increase in androgen production. Metformin (Glucophage®) is often used to treat PCOS. Glucophage decreases insulin resistance and can assist with weight loss and prevent the development of type 2 diabetes. Obesity is part of the metabolic syndrome that often accompanies PCOS. Common side effects of metformin include diarrhea, nausea, vomiting, and loss of appetite. Birth control medications that contain estrogen and progestin will reduce the production of androgen hormones. Blood clots are a possible side effect of oral contraceptives, and careful examination of the patient's health history should be considered. Excessive hair growth on the face and chest is a manifestation of PCOS. Medications such as spironolactone (Aldactone) help block the effects of androgen hormones on the skin. Aldactone is a potassium-sparing diuretic that prevents the loss of potassium from the body. Patients should be educated on avoiding potassium supplements and excessive ingestion of potassium-rich foods. Common side effects are fatigue, headaches, nausea and vomiting.

Side Effects

The administration of any drug is associated with the potential for adverse effects. The **adverse effects** of commonly prescribed drug classes are predictable in some situations. However, the route of administration, ethnic differences related to the pharmacotherapeutic reaction, and patient adherence and comorbidities can all affect the expression of the adverse effects in an individual patient. The WHNP will also assess possible drug interactions among the patient's prescribed drugs and all OTC drugs and herbal supplements. Continuing surveillance of the incidence of adverse effects is necessary. According to practice guidelines a new adverse effect should first be considered as an adverse drug reaction (ADR). **Hypersensitivity reactions** are most often time sensitive, which means that the timing of the reaction can be associated with the administration of the drug; IV administration results in the most rapid reaction. Drug-to-drug reactions commonly are delayed; they manifest themselves in changes in the patient's physical condition.

The WHNP is aware that **adverse drug reactions (ADRs)** are more likely with drugs that are lipophilic, due to the increased absorption rate. Some of these reactions are well documented, however, other reactions are less predictable and may result from an identified reaction among the patient's prescription drugs. Additional risk factors for ADRs include polypharmacy, genetic alterations in pharmacodynamics and pharmacokinetics, age, gender, and comorbidities. ADRs are categorized according to response time. Immediate adverse drug reactions (ADRs) occur within the first hour after administration of the drug. Delayed ADRs occur after the first hour. However, the expanded view of response time identifies six specific categories of reactions: rapid, first dose, early, intermediate, late, and delayed.

Rapid reactions that occur during or immediately following the administration of a drug are generally believed to be due to administration errors. For instance, the incorrect administration of a vancomycin infusion can result in "red neck syndrome," which is manifested by erythema, flushing, and pruritus of the upper body. First dose reactions occur with the initial dose of the medication and may or may not occur with repeated doses. Early reactions occur after the first few doses, and this effect can often be avoided if the therapy is begun with the lowest therapeutic dose and then titrated according to the incidence of demonstrated reactions. Intermediate reactions occur after the repeated administration of the drug and are most common in susceptible patients. For instance, hyperuricemia secondary to furosemide administration is an intermediate reaction that warrants close observation and intervention. Late and delayed reactions occur at various times following administration of the drug. In most instances, these reactions are predictable and can be controlled by removing the drug from the treatment plan or altering the dosage.

The FDA categorizes ADRs as serious when the outcome of the therapy is death or results in permanent disability, birth defects, or prolonged hospitalization. Reactions that meet any of these criteria must be reported to the FDA MedWatch program. More commonly, adverse reactions are designated as mild, moderate, or severe.

Patient Outcomes

Patient outcomes can be positively affected by clear communication between the patient and provider as to the goals of the drug regimen. There is also clear evidence that comprehensive communication increases the patient's health literacy, which can enhance the patient's level of adherence, which can improve patient outcomes. In contrast, the number of drugs that is included in the drug plan or the patient's lack of understanding of the possible actions and reactions associated with the prescription drugs are inversely proportional to the patient's level of adherence and resulting outcomes. Self-monitoring programs that use technology such as phone applications or paper and pencil instruments have demonstrated limited effect in changing patient adherence; however, there is evidence of positive outcomes with self-monitoring in patients who are taking prescription drugs for the first time. There is also a significant relationship between patient adherence and the expected adverse effects of the prescribed drugs.

WHNPs should understand that the patient outcomes rely on a complex combination of the patient's individual biological pharmacotherapeutic profile, degree of adherence with the plan, socioeconomic factors, and existing comorbidities. Much of the research on patient adherence focuses on economic factors, while many providers believe that the patient outcomes should be the top priority. Quality improvement activities at the administration level of a primary care practice can address many of these issues by standardizing the provider approach to the development of the therapeutic plan. Some of the issues addressed can include methods of education, monitoring procedures for drugs with known or high-risk for the development of adverse drug reactions, and examination of hospital readmissions following the administration of the target drug.

Drug Interactions

Drug interaction refers to the alteration in pharmacology (absorption, distribution, metabolism, elimination, efficacy, side effects, etc.) of a medication by various factors including disease conditions, prescription and OTC medications, and foods or nutritional supplements. These interactions may result in either an augmentation or decrease in the efficacy and/or toxicity of the respective medication. Drug interactions should be carefully reviewed to avoid serious life-threatening conditions.

Examples of different types of drug interactions and examples within each type are described below.

Drug-Disease Interactions

NSAIDS and Peptic Ulcers

NSAIDs including aspirin, ibuprofen, naproxen, and indomethacin can cause stomach irritation and can aggravate peptic ulcer symptoms. Therefore, NSAIDs should not be used by patients with peptic ulcers or GERD. If NSAIDs are used by patients with hyperacidity, gastro-protective agents, such as proton pumps inhibitors (e.g. omeprazole, pantoprazole, lansoprazole, etc.), should also be used.

Diuretics and Diabetes

Diuretics are used to treat hypertension and edema. Hydrochlorothiazide is a commonly prescribed diuretic that can cause glucose intolerance and hyperglycemia. Therefore, if a patient with type 2 diabetes is prescribed a diuretic, blood sugar control becomes difficult, so routine monitoring of blood sugar is required. If blood sugar is not properly controlled, dose adjustments of the anti-diabetic medication or alternative diuretics should be considered.

Drug-Drug Interactions

Warfarin and NSAIDs

Warfarin is a commonly prescribed blood thinner, indicated to prevent blood clots in various cardiovascular diseases. Patients on warfarin should not take other prescription/OTC/herbal medications without consulting with their prescriber and pharmacist. For example, commonly available OTC NSAIDs can cause an increase in the blood-thinning effect of warfarin and result in internal hemorrhage.

The following medications can interact with warfarin:

- Aspirin
- Acetaminophen (at high doses)
- Ibuprofen
- Naproxen
- Celecoxib
- Diclofenac

- Indomethacin
- Piroxicam

Oral Contraceptives and Antibiotics

Antibiotics can decrease the effect of hormonal oral contraceptives thus increasing the possibility of pregnancy even while taking the contraceptive. Non-hormonal back-up methods, such as condoms, should be used while a woman taking an oral contraceptive is prescribed an antibiotic. Other medications that can affect the efficacy of oral contraceptives include anti-fungals, a few anti-seizure medications, certain HIV medications, and a few herbal preparations, like St. John's Wort.

Nitroglycerin and Erectile Dysfunction Medications

Nitroglycerin is a vasodilator that is often used to treat episodes of angina. To prevent recurring angina, the extended-release capsules of nitroglycerin are taken daily, whereas in cases of non-frequent occurrence, sublingual tablets or sprays can be used. Medications to treat erectile dysfunctions, such as sildenafil, tadalafil, and vardenafil, should not be taken with nitroglycerin. These medications augment the vasodilatory effect of nitroglycerin and can lead to irreversible hypotension and fatality. Emergency care should be sought immediately if this combination accidentally happens. The symptoms of hypotension include dizziness, fainting, and cold, clammy skin.

Drug-Food and Drug-Nutrient Interactions

Statins and Grapefruit Juice

Statins (e.g., pravastatin, simvastatin, atorvastatin, and rosuvastatin) are used to treat hypocholesteremia. Patients taking this medication should avoid drinking grapefruit juice or consuming large amounts of grapefruit because this juice decreases the metabolism of statins, resulting in a buildup of statins in the body. The risk of serious side effects is increased when statin buildup occurs, with possible resultant muscle or liver damage. Pharmacists should counsel patients about avoiding grapefruit juice while on statins. Although increasing statin dosage may seem to benefit the patient, the liver can only process so much. Accumulation of a statin in the body can cause muscle damage, pain, and rhabdomyolysis—a serious and potentially lethal side effect. In rhabdomyolysis, the skeletal muscle is rapidly catabolized. Patients taking statins should undergo routine blood tests and notify their doctors immediately about symptoms of muscle pain or fatigue. Undetected and unmanaged rhabdomyolysis can result in death.

MAOIs and Tyramine

Monoamine oxidase inhibitors (MAOIs) are used to treat chronic depression that does not respond to other medications or treatments. Due to side effects and drug interactions, MAOIs are not commonly prescribed. Examples of MAOIs are phenelzine (Nardil®), selegiline (Emsam®), and tranylcypromine (Parnate®). MAOIs can cause serotonin syndrome. There are many medications and foods that can lead to severe side effects when combined with MAOIs. Foods like wine, cheese, certain meats, and pickled foods carry tyramine, which leads to spikes in blood pressure, if co-administered with MAOIs.

Drug-OTC Interactions

Antihypertensives and Decongestants

Pseudoephedrine and phenylephrine are used as decongestants in different OTC cough and cold medications. These medications have sympathomimetic effects and can cause elevated blood pressure. Therefore, if a decongestant medication is taken by patients on antihypertensive medication, it reduces the blood pressure control of the antihypertensive agent. Hypertensive patients should avoid taking OTC medications containing sympathomimetic agents.

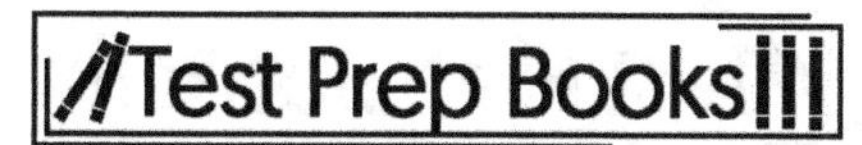

Antihistamines and Sedatives

OTC antihistamines, such as diphenhydramine and chlorpheniramine, are used to treat various allergic conditions. Antihistamines can cause sedation and drowsiness, which can potentiate the side effects of sedatives and hypnotics. Patients taking sedatives—such as diazepam, lorazepam, alprazolam, and midazolam—should be cautious when taking an OTC antihistamine.

Drug-Laboratory Interactions

Antibiotics and Bacterial Cultures

Treatment with certain medications can affect laboratory results. For example, the blood or urine sample collected from a patient taking an antibiotic for one infection might yield a false antibiotic sensitivity or culture report for a second infection. The lab work should, therefore, be scheduled after the wash-out period of the first antibiotic.

Contraindications

There are two kinds of contraindications for a pharmacotherapeutic intervention: absolute and relative. An **absolute contraindication** means that the administration of the drug or combination of drugs can result in life-threatening adverse effects that must be avoided. A **relative contraindication** means that the potential for adverse effects should be weighed against the expected therapeutic effect. An absolute contraindication can be related to the reaction of one or more drugs with another drug, or with certain patient populations, such as pregnant women, patients with renal failure, and people with other drug allergies. An example of an absolute drug-to-drug contraindication is that warfarin cannot be given with aspirin; one drug potentiates the effect of the other, resulting in an increased risk for bleeding.

Absolute contraindication for pharmacotherapeutic interventions in pregnant women is associated with teratogenicity, which is the risk for birth defects due to maternal exposure to the drugs. Patients with renal disease are at risk from the drug interactions because most drugs are excreted by the kidneys, and when there is any degree of altered renal function, the plasma concentration of the drugs, and therefore the risk of adverse effects, will be increased. Patients with identified allergies are at greater risk for hypersensitivity reactions to other drug therapies. Many of the recommended contraindications are contained in condition-specific protocols such as oral contraceptive use, smoking cessation, and obesity therapy. For example, absolute contraindications to oral contraceptive therapy include a known or suspected pregnancy or a history of thrombotic disease. Relative contraindications include the presence of hypertension and current smoking history. In children, there is an absolute contraindication for the use of aspirin in patients recovering from a viral infection due to the risk of Reye's syndrome, which is rare but often fatal.

Therapeutic Contraindications Associated with Medications

Alcohol

Alcohol should be avoided while patients are on prescription medications. Consumption of alcohol with medications can cause nausea, vomiting, fainting, loss of coordination, or extreme drowsiness. More severe reactions can lead to heart problems, internal bleeding, and difficulty breathing. Certain medications, when combined with alcohol, can cause toxicity. As alcohol is a strong CNS depressant, combining it with other depressants, like benzodiazepines or sleeping medications, can be dangerous and can cause respiratory failure. If alcohol is combined with a high dose of acetaminophen, there is potential for serious liver damage. Additionally, if alcohol is consumed while taking metronidazole, the patient can experience significant side effects including nausea, vomiting, abdominal pain, cramps, facial redness, headache, tachycardia, and liver damage.

Age

Age has a significant effect on the pharmacology of medications. Maturation during childhood causes various changes in body composition, accompanying growth and development. Therefore, newborns, infants, children, and adolescents often do not receive full adult dosages. As mentioned, medication doses should be appropriately calculated based on the age and weight of the child. There are many medications that are not approved by the FDA for children and yet are used "off label." Unexpected reactions can happen when medications are not studied in pediatric populations. For example, tetracycline is contraindicated in children because it can bind with the calcium in bones, modify bone cartilage, and cause growth retardation. Generally, if a physician prescribes a medication that is not approved for use in children, pharmacy technicians should consult with the pharmacist, who will rely on their professional judgment about how to proceed (i.e., dispense the medication or talk with the physician).

In elderly adults, there can also be significant changes in pharmacokinetics and pharmacodynamics of a medication. Geriatric populations often have comorbid conditions, including cardiovascular disease, diabetes, and renal insufficiencies. Aging can decrease the body's clearance of a medication, resulting in buildup and manifesting in unwanted effects. Routine blood work and dose adjustments may be necessary in the geriatric population.

OTC Medications

Some OTC medications impose significant risks with certain disease conditions. A few OTC medications can lead to an increase in blood pressure, so these may be contraindicated in patients with hypertension. The following medications are known to cause problems for patients with hypertension:

- NSAIDS (ibuprofen and naproxen)
- Decongestants like pseudoephedrine
- Migraine formulations with caffeine

Patients with high blood pressure should talk to a pharmacist or a physician before taking OTC medications or herbal supplements.

Patient Education

Facilitation of Learning

Facilitation of learning refers to the process of assessing the learning needs of the patient and family, the nursing staff, and caregivers in the community, and creating, implementing, and evaluating formal and informal educational programs to address those needs. Novice providers often view patient care and patient education as separate entities; however, experienced providers are able to integrate the patient's educational needs into the plan of care. WHNPs are aware that the patient often requires continued reinforcement of the educational plan after discharge, which necessitates coordination with home care services.

As facilitators of learning, WHNPs may be involved in a large-scale effort to educate all patients over 65 years of age about the need for both Prevnar 13 and Pneumovax 23 vaccinations to prevent pneumonia. In contrast, WHNPs may provide one-on-one instruction for a patient recently diagnosed with diabetes. The first step of any teaching-learning initiative is the assessment of the learning needs of the participants. Specific needs that influence the design and content of the educational offering include the language preference and reading level of the participants. WHNPs must also consider the effect of certain characteristics, identified in the Synergy Model, on the patient's capacity to process information. Diminished resiliency or stability, as well as extreme complexity, are examples of characteristics that must be considered in the development of the educational plan. WHNPs are also responsible for creating a bridge between teaching and learning in the acute care setting and the home environment. A detailed discharge plan, close coordination with outpatient providers, and follow-up phone calls to the patient may be used to reinforce the patient's knowledge of the plan of care.

Successful learning plans for staff members and colleagues also consider the motivation of the participants to engage in the process. Successful facilitators include a variety of teaching strategies to develop the content and evaluate learning to address adult learning needs and preferences, such as preferred language and reading level. Research indicates that when adults do not have a vested interest in the outcomes of the teaching/learning process, they may not participate as active learners.

The remaining element of successful facilitation of learning is the availability and quality of learning resources. There is evidence that individuals with different learning styles respond differently to various learning devices. The minimum requirements for successful facilitation of learning include the skilled staff to develop the educational materials, paper, a copy machine, and staff to interact with the patient in the learning session.

Barriers to the facilitation of learning must be anticipated and accommodated. Changes in the patient's condition commonly require reduction in the time spent in each learning session due to fatigue. Cognitive impairment can impede comprehension and retention of the information and will require appropriate teaching aids. The learning abilities of the patient's family members must also be assessed. Adequate instruction time might be the greatest barrier. Learning needs are assessed, and discharge planning is begun, on the day of admission; however, shortened inpatient stays require evaluation of the patient's comprehension of the plan of care.

Health Literacy

Health literacy refers to how capable patients are of understanding their diagnosis, treatment plans, prognosis, and follow-up health instructions. A high degree of health literacy is associated with the ability to make personal health decisions, higher confidence in personal health decisions, and higher compliance with medical instructions.

Teaching Methods

Patient teaching takes place in different settings and formats. The method of choice can be determined by a variety of factors, including learner preference, educator preference, the topic, the setting, and the availability of time and resources. Learning can occur with the help of audio, visual, written, or activity-based methods, and learners tend to fall on a wide spectrum of preference. Typically, individuals require several exposures to new information before it is retained. Additionally, factors such as age, level of education, language barriers, emotional state, desire to learn, pain level, disability, and many others can significantly impact the ability of an individual to take in and retain new information. Therefore, patient teaching requires individual consideration and benefits from the use of a variety of teaching methods over a span of time.

The following are some of the common methods used to facilitate teaching:

- **Written materials:** Written handouts, brochures, or pamphlets include information about various topics (e.g., disease, procedure, treatment, or medication). These are often accompanied by visual tools to support written information and are often more affordable and convenient for teachers. They can be reviewed repeatedly over time and taken from the care site to the patient's home.
- **Visual tools:** Charts, graphs, pictures, posters, and drawings can provide a visual way to convey a significant amount of information at once and can organize complex ideas. They can be reviewed repeatedly over time and are cost-effective resources. Some visual materials, like brochures, can be taken from the care site, while other materials, like posters, remain at the care site.

- **Audio and audiovisual materials:** Video clips, video programs, recorded interviews, podcasts, or recorded demonstrations can provide learners with opportunities to review information as often as needed and can also be a more interesting method of facilitating patient learning. This can be more costly for organizations to create and is also somewhat limited to individuals who possess the technology required to view the materials; it is also limited by a patient's comfort and desire to use the given media.
- **Discussion:** In-person, virtual, telephonic, email, support group, workshop, or classes provide an opportunity for two-way dialogue between learner and teacher. Discussions can be individual or group-based and can occur in a variety of settings. Teachers have an opportunity to provide learners with a variety of teaching methods to facilitate learning.
- **Demonstration:** Models and training equipment can be utilized in live or recorded sessions to supplement learning through visual representation of a process or procedure. This method is often accompanied by verbal discussion. Live demonstration can provide opportunities for repetition or focus on a specific portion of the demonstration. Patients can also sometimes have the opportunity to handle and practice with training equipment or models in order to increase comfort and decrease anxiety.

Teach Back Method

The **"Teach Back" method** is an interactive educational technique that fosters rapport, communication, and information sharing between healthcare providers and patients. It encourages the healthcare providers to explain medical diagnoses, prognoses, and plans of care to patients in clear, non-medical terms. Then, patients are asked to explain the medical situation and plan of care to the healthcare professional, utilizing their own understanding. This empowers patients to actively engage in their care plans and understand their health in a new way. It also allows the healthcare provider to determine whether or not the patient has an appropriate understanding of their health situation and how to manage care once they are out of the medical setting. Providers should remain calm, compassionate, and responsive during this process, even if the patient is unable to correctly teach back right away.

Patient Medication Education

Any time a new medication is administered, the WHNP should first educate the patient about the medication and any potential side effects. Providers should be able to relay how the medication works in the body, the intended effect of the medication and why it is being prescribed, and the potential adverse reactions. Patients have the right to be informed of their medications and to refuse them.

Another important aspect of medication education is explaining how to use a medication. For example, inhalers should be shaken and primed before use. The patient should be taught the proper technique for inhaling as they depress the canister. The patient should also be taught to rinse their mouth out afterward to avoid oral ulcers. Nitroglycerine is another great example. Patients should take one tablet of nitroglycerine and rest at the first sign of angina. If the symptoms are still present after five minutes, the patient should take another dose and call EMS. Then, they should wait five more minutes and take a third dose for a maximum of three doses. These are very complex instructions that the nurse is in the prime position to teach and have the patient repeat back to gauge understanding.

Stewardship

Stewardship can take many forms, including programs for common diseases like diabetes or harm-reduction programs that provide clean needles to reduce the spread of HIV. When following safe disposal practices, sharps should always be placed in red sharps containers. Never re-cap a needle used on a patient. A common example of safe drug management is **antibiotic stewardship**. Educating patients that only bacterial infections need antibiotics reduces antibiotic resistance and antibiotic-resistant super infections.

Regarding home medication management, providers should ensure patients know all their medications and the correct way to take them. This is especially true for patients with **polypharmacy** who are on multiple medications that are often taken more than once a day. Pill planners are an excellent tool for these patients because the planners allow them to sort their medications day by day. For disposal of at-home and over-the-counter medications, patients should discard the medications in specialized medication disposal bins often found at pharmacies. Unused medications should not be left in medicine cabinets, as children or other family members could misuse the medication. If a medication take-back option is not readily available, some medications can be flushed according to the FDA Flush List. If a medication is not on the flush list, it can be disposed of in a sealable container in the regular trash.

Pregnancy and Lactation Safety

During pregnancy, medications should be prescribed carefully, to prevent harm to the developing fetus. For some medications, there might not be enough data available regarding safety during pregnancy, and therefore, must be used cautiously after weighing the benefits versus the risks. Many medications are contraindicated during pregnancy, as they have **teratogenic** effects and can cause birth defects. If a patient is on a teratogenic medication prior to pregnancy, the medication should be stopped upon conception. A few examples of medications that are contraindicated in pregnancy include ACE inhibitors (e.g., ramipril, enalapril, lisinopril, etc.), ARBs (losartan, candesartan, irbesartan, etc.), isotretinoin, tetracycline antibiotics, hormonal therapies, and immunosuppressants (e.g. methotrexate).

Teratogens

A **teratogen** describes an environmental agent that can cause potential birth defects. One of the most sensitive times for a developing fetus is ten to fourteen days after conception, because this is when the prenatal fetus starts becoming more susceptible to these different teratogenic agents. During organogenesis, there are certain organs developing during certain periods of time. A teratogen can interfere with this development, resulting in structural and functional problems of the organs. The central nervous system is especially prone to the detrimental effects of teratogens because the central nervous system is the baby's brain and spinal cord.

Genetic predispositions carried by both the mother and infant can influence the type or degree of abnormalities caused by a teratogenic agent. For example, how the mother metabolizes a particular drug will determine the metabolites to which the baby is exposed, as well as the total interval of that exposure. The developmental stage a baby is in during exposure can also be a factor. Generally speaking, the fetus's genetic predisposition to a certain teratogenic agent tends to have an effect on how everything will turn out.

Some specific examples of teratogens include mercury, nuclear fallout radiation, potassium iodide, lead, alcohol, illegal drugs, prescription drugs, saunas, a disease affecting the mother, and even maternal psychological stress. While some of these agents are avoidable, there are others that are unavoidable, which could include anything required to treat a medical condition. Specialists can assess a baby's risk of being affected by teratogens after their exposure to certain environments.

Practice Quiz

1. A patient has brought in a prescription for Diazepam. Which of the following conditions is the most likely reason that the patient needs this prescription?
   a. Hypertension
   b. ADHD
   c. Epilepsy
   d. Depression

2. A patient overdosed on acetaminophen after retrieving it from their visitor's purse during visiting hours. While providing emergent care with the code response team, which medication should the WHNP order to counteract the effects of this poisoning?
   a. Atropine
   b. Acetylcysteine
   c. Naloxone
   d. Flumazenil

3. While providing patient education, the WHNP explains that the patient's medication dosage will need to be adjusted to find the most therapeutic level. What is this measured medication practice an example of?
   a. Medication compliance
   b. Medication reconciliation
   c. Medication titration
   d. Medication administration

4. Which of the following medications should not be taken in combination with nitroglycerin and what would be the result if they were taken together?
   a. Warfarin, excessive blood thinning
   b. Sildenafil, irreversible hypotension
   c. Allegra®, increased heart rate
   d. Sertraline, increased depression

5. An 18-year-old female presents with worsening wheezing, shortness of breath, and a cough over the past twelve hours. She has a history of asthma and has been using her albuterol metered-dose inhaler (MDI) every ten minutes for the past two hours. She's given supplemental oxygen, both albuterol and ipratropium (Combivent®) via nebulizer, and methylprednisolone IV in quick succession. Shortly afterwards, she complains of anxiety, develops hand tremors, and her pulse increases from 80 to 120 beats per minute (bpm). Which treatment is most likely responsible for her anxiety, tremors, and tachycardia?
   a. Supplemental oxygen
   b. Albuterol
   c. Ipratropium
   d. Methylprednisolone

See answers on the next page

Answer Explanations

1. C: Epilepsy is caused by overactive neuronal signaling in the brain, so a central nervous system depressant can calm such activity. Hypertension, ADHD, and depression do not improve with this type of medication, and it can be potentially harmful.

2. B: Choice *B* should be administered to the patient to counteract the effects of the acetaminophen overdose. Choices *A, C,* and *D*, while all antidotes for a variety of medications, would not prove effective in reversing the progression of acetaminophen poisoning.

3. C: Medication titration, Choice *C,* involves titrating the dosage to reach a therapeutic level, as it encourages careful consideration to achieve the maximum benefit without adverse reaction. Medication compliance, Choice *A,* involves patient agreement and fulfillment of medication intake. Medication reconciliation, Choice *B,* describes the process of creating a list of medications taken. Medication administration, Choice *D,* involves the practice of delivering medication for intake.

4. B: Sildenafil and nitroglycerin should not be taken together, as both cause blood vessel dilatation, leading to the potential of irreversible hypotension. The other listed combinations do not have documented direct effects when taken in combination with nitroglycerin.

5. B: The scenario depicts an episode of status asthmaticus. Common pharmacological agents used to treat this condition include albuterol (short-acting Beta-2 agonist), ipratropium (anticholinergic), and methylprednisolone (corticosteroid). Her new symptoms (anxiety, tremors, and tachycardia) are all common side effects which can be attributed to albuterol. Anticholinergics can induce side effects such as dry mouth, blurred vision, and constipation. Corticosteroids (if used for longer than two weeks) can have side effects such as weight gain, osteoporosis, thinning of skin, cataracts, easy bruising, and diabetes. She should be switched to the short-acting Beta-2 agonist levalbuterol because it's as effective as albuterol but without the alarming side effects.

Professional Practice Issues

Legal Issues

Professional Practice Regulations

All advanced practice registered nurses (APRNs) have advanced degrees, either master's or doctoral degrees, which prepare them for different areas of clinical practice. There are four different roles for ARPNs in the United States. Nurse practitioners (NPs) provide primary care services for all ages, although most NPs limit their practice to a specific patient population such as pediatrics, families, or geriatrics. Nurse anesthetists (CRNAs) provide anesthesia services in acute care institutions for general and obstetrical patient populations. Nurse midwives (CNMs) provide obstetrical care from conception to delivery of the infant in addition to gynecologic care for all women. Clinical nurse specialists (CNSs) provide care for a specific patient population in the acute care setting such as critical care, or for a specific disease or condition such as diabetes or wound care.

The practice of all APRNs is regulated by state boards of nursing, which provide the statutory limits of practice. Currently, all fifty states allow one of three forms of prescriptive practice by NPs: full, reduced, or restricted practice. **Full practice** means that the NP has permission to prescribe for, diagnose, and treat all patients without physician oversight. **Reduced practice** means that NPs can diagnose and treat patients; however, physician oversight is required for prescriptive practice. **Restricted practice** means that NPs require physician oversight for all areas of practice. Currently, NPs have full practice authority in twenty states, reduced practice in eighteen states, and restricted practice in twelve states.

This continuing inconsistency in NP practice guidelines from state to state is an area of concern for all NPs and for the professional associations representing them. Proponents of the full, unrestricted practice model cite research that supports the safety of NP practice and the positive level of patient satisfaction with all aspects of NP care. Opposition to the full practice model comes mainly from physicians' associations, which voice concerns about the disparities between physician education and NP education, especially in the area of pharmacology. However, increasing numbers of NPs are providing primary care, which increases the possible number of patients that can receive care in any single patient-centered medical home (PCMH). Additional assessment of APRN practice is carried out by the Joint Commission (formerly JACHO), research and regulatory agents such as state boards of health and nursing, the Agency for Healthcare Research and Quality (AHRQ), the National Committee for Quality Assurance (NCQA), and professional societies.

There are multiple educational maps that can lead to advanced practice. The most basic plan is completion of the baccalaureate degree in nursing, and then completion of the master's degree and possibly the clinically oriented doctoral degree in nursing. Currently, the DNP degree, or Doctor of Nursing Practice degree, is associated with APRN practice. However, other APRNs may chose the research-oriented doctoral degree of PhD. All APRNs also will complete additional clinical practice in the care of the specific patient population that is the focus of their practice. In many cases, professional organizations stipulate the curriculum hours that are needed to satisfy specialty certification requirements.

In 2008, the National Council of State Boards of Nursing along with several professional nursing associations announced the development of the APRN consensus model, which is designed to standardize the educational and practice regulations from state to state. The adoption of this model by all states will allow an APRN more mobility in the workplace. The model is based on the LACE criteria: licensure, accreditation, certification, and education. The map that identifies the "adoption score" of each state resembles the map that identifies current practice models. States that are in 100 percent compliance with the consensus model are commonly

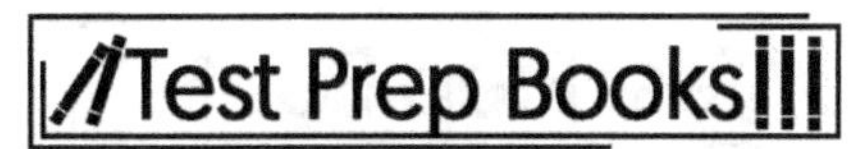

states with non-restricted practice models. The original 100 percent implementation target date for the model was 2015.

As of 2018 the process of adoption was continuing, but not yet complete. There are concerns about the model that relate to educational issues for different area of practice. The educational requirements of the model are based on the acuity of the patient, not the site of care. This means that an APRN who intends to practice in acute care will complete an educational tract for the patients that require acute care. If that same APRN is planning to care for a patient group that requires both acute care and primary, the consensus model requires additional education that possibly includes seven additional courses and more than 500 clinical hours. This represents a significant investment of time and money.

As mentioned, there are states that require physician oversight for APRN practice. A portion of these states require a formal collaborative practice agreement that explicitly states the APRN practice details for the duration of the agreement between the physician and the APRN. This identifies the assumption of risk by the physician because the agreement requires that the physician is responsible for everything that the APRN does in the clinical setting. Some of the agreements limit the number of collaborative agreements that the APRN can sign, and other states require physician review of the APRN's documentation. It is clear from this discussion that nurses who aspire to advanced nursing practice must become knowledgeable about each of the LACE criteria.

The wide variations in APRN practice and the slow pace of standardization is most likely due to public officials' misunderstanding of the patient benefits associated with APRN practice. However, physician's groups continue to be the strongest opponents with the loudest voices. Even when the number of APRNs in collaborative agreements with physicians in all care settings continues to increase, the message is the same; APRNs do not have the hours of clinical preparation in comparison with the physicians' clinical hours. Physicians' objections are not supported by the demonstrated benefits of APRN practice.

APRNs continue to improve patient satisfaction even with restrictions placed on the tests that can be ordered, the inability to refer patients for specialty care, or the inability to provide emergency services. Other variable permissions include procedures for controlled substances prescription, executing Do Not Resuscitate (DNR) orders, issuing handicapped parking stickers, prescribing physical therapy, and signing death certificates. Regardless of these impositions on patient care, two of the more successful practice areas for NPs are the retail health clinics and urgent care centers. The quality of care and the cost-effectiveness for patients and providers have been measured in the retail clinics. The cost-effectiveness of the clinics in states where NPs have unrestricted practice is greater than the cost-effectiveness of the same care setting in states where NPs have restricted practice. Interestingly, patient satisfaction remains high in both groups.

There are additional elements of the scope and standards of practice of APRNs that are no less important to the success of APRNs than the prescriptive practice issues. APRNs provide expert patient care by assessing and diagnosing the patient's health alterations, and then they plan and implement the care plan as developed by the patient and the APRN. Patient satisfaction is enhanced by the commitment of APRNs to health-promoting and patient education efforts, patient advocacy, patient autonomy, and quality assurance. This commitment also includes the pursuit of lifelong learning and the support for the advancement of the APRN practice model.

The price of healthcare in the United States has prompted analysis and comment from many authorities in and outside of the government. The one universal conclusion is that nurses are uniquely qualified to improve access to care and to improve the quality of care. In order to maximize this potential, all nurses will use the benefits of advanced education to interact collaboratively with all members of the interdisciplinary team and to actively participate in the redesign of the healthcare delivery system. APRNs are well positioned for this expanded role by virtue of their advanced educational preparation and their already well-established presence in all care delivery settings. In addition, a common theme in these analyses is the importance of nurses performing to the full extent of their educational preparation and experience. This means that the scope of practice for all APRNs must be standardized among all states and redesigned to promote expert professional practice. This redesign must also include reimbursement schedules for APRNs in every care setting.

Additional recommendations highlight the importance of interprofessional education that could alleviate current professional differences between APRNs and physician groups. There has been progress in redesigning nursing education models that increase access to seamless paths to advanced degrees. Advanced degree programs are more widely available and are admitting increased numbers of students, undergraduates can opt for fifth-year master's programs, and advanced baccalaureate courses can be applied to a master's degree. It is clear that nursing in general, and APRNs in particular, are part of the solution rather than the problem of healthcare redesign.

Professional Practice Evaluation

Personal and collective growth in the field of nursing requires ongoing evaluation of professional practice. This occurs on individual, group, organizational, and global levels throughout the field of nursing. Performing this necessary critique identifies strengths and weaknesses and allows for ongoing advancement of the profession.

General areas of evaluation can focus on many performance aspects. Aspects of professionalism (e.g., appearance, behavior, communication, and leadership style) can be addressed as well as the level of adherence to applicable standards or policies. Another performance category could be related to growth and development, including completed continuing education or advanced certification. Other areas of evaluation include engagement with professional organizations, committees, quality improvement projects, or community involvement. Additionally, contributions to the field of nursing or healthcare (e.g., professional writing or political involvement) can be considered.

On a personal level, WHNPs perform self-reflection and planning to determine how they feel about their performance and potential areas for improvement. They can formulate professional goals and plan the development necessary to achieve those goals. At a team or organizational level, nurses also receive feedback from peers and leadership. Peer feedback identifies how colleagues perceive the performance of their coworkers. Leadership feedback often provides a more global view of performance through comparison of personal performance to averages of larger groups (e.g., the unit, hospital, or region). Organizations also receive feedback in the form of surveys from employees as well as the organization's customers. Each level of evaluation provides opportunities to examine growth pathways and formulate development plans.

Upon identifying an opportunity for improvement, it is critical to follow up with a plan for development. Goals should be specific, time-bound, and identify resources necessary to achieve the goal. On an organizational level, this can include referencing education materials, enrolling in professional or organizational groups or counsels, or breaking goals down into smaller steps. Lastly, re-evaluation must occur at regular intervals to follow up on previous goals. This provides external accountability for completing the steps and achieving the stated goals.

Legal Liability

The WHNP must uphold and answer to certain legal rights and responsibilities within their profession. From simple tasks like managing a patient's property, to more complicated issues such as reporting abuse and neglect, the WHNP has a legal responsibility to act.

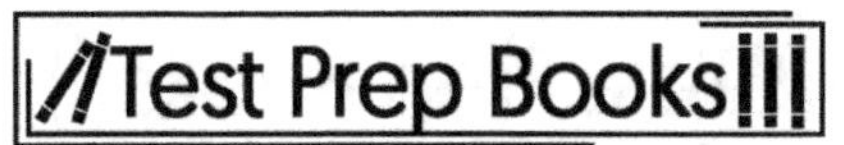

WHNPs need a knowledge of the common legal terminology in their practice. The following is a list of terms the WHNP should know:

- Common law: Based on legal precedents or previously decided cases in courts of law
- Statutory law: Based on a state's legislative actions or any other legislative body's actions
- Constitutional law: Based on the content of the Constitution of the United States of America
- Administrative law: Passed down from a ruling body, such as continuing education requirements mandated by each state's nursing association
- Criminal law: Involves the arrest, prosecution, and incarceration of those who have broken the law, including misdemeanors and felonies
- Liability: Involves accountability for one's actions from a legal standpoint
- Tort: Refers to nursing practice violations, such as malpractice, negligence, and patient confidentiality violations
- Unintentional tort: Examples can include negligence and malpractice in certain situations
- Intentional tort: Examples can include false imprisonment, privacy breaches, slander, libel, battery, and assault

Consent

Ideally, patients should always provide written consent for treatment. This should also include discussion between the healthcare provider and the patient about what treatment will entail, what the end goal is of treatment, the risks and benefits of the treatment, and the opportunity for the patient to voice any questions and concerns. Patient consent decreases liability for the healthcare provider and increases patient reports of empowerment. Patients also have the right to revoke previously given consent at any time.

However, problems with patient consent do exist. In many healthcare facilities, the consent process can be a rushed one; often, patients receive a large packet of paperwork in which the consent form is included. Many patients sign without reading, or do not understand what they are signing but complete the form out of fear, pressure, or to appear informed when they actually do not feel that way. Often, verbal exchange about the form or treatment does not occur. Legally, healthcare providers do not have to provide an explanation of information that is accepted as common knowledge. However, medical topics are often not part of the average person's body of knowledge, and this gap can be complicated to bridge without thorough communication. Healthcare providers can attempt to resolve these problems by taking the time to discuss the consent form with the patient, simplifying consent forms, and providing additional media (such as literature or video links) to patients, especially in the event of more complex procedures.

Informed Consent

An important part of the patient's bill of rights is **informed consent**. This means the patient has been adequately informed about their healthcare plan, whether that involves new medications, vaccinations, procedures, diagnostic screenings, and so on. The patient is granting their permission to go ahead with the care plan. It is up to the healthcare team to obtain this informed consent. This usually takes the form of a patient-signed document that goes in the permanent healthcare record.

Implied Consent

Implied consent does not involve the patient signing a document or even verbally granting permission, but rather it is assumed that any reasonable person would consent to the healthcare interventions being performed. The most common use of implied consent is in emergency situations, in which lifesaving interventions are necessary and there is not enough time to perform informed consent with the patient, such as cardiopulmonary resuscitation (CPR) after cardiac arrest.

Expressed Consent

This type of consent entails that the patient consent to a medical intervention either verbally, nonverbally through a gesture such as a nod, or in writing. This type of consent differs from informed consent in that there is not necessarily an education process that precedes it. This type of consent generally requires a witness.

Patient Incompetence

A patient who is unable to make their own informed decisions about their healthcare plan is termed incompetent. In the case of an incompetent patient, it may be necessary to use a proxy, such as a power of attorney, to make healthcare decisions for them.

Emancipated Minor

If a minor is legally emancipated, it means they are freed from having parental consent to certain things. The legal age for emancipation is generally sixteen. A patient may be medically emancipated if they become pregnant, thus freeing them to give consent with associated medical procedures and maintaining confidentiality of their records at that point.

Mature Minor

The mature minor concept applies to unemancipated minors and says that if a patient is deemed mature enough and the medical intervention is not especially serious, they may make their own decisions and give their own consent without parental consent.

Guardianship

Guardianship or conservatorship is a legal concept that protects a person who no longer has the ability to make sound decisions or to make those decisions known to others. Common medical diagnoses that are associated with incapacitation include dementia, brain injury, and irreversible coma. This relationship provides protection against fraudulent actions or undue pressure on the protected individual. This person does relinquish some personal freedoms in exchange for this protection, so the establishment of the guardianship is only considered when other protective measures have failed. Some of the personal decisions that are affected by this relationship include real estate transaction decisions, firearm possession, contractual negotiations, marriage, and end-of-life decisions.

Legal authorities encourage all individuals to execute a living will or advance directive that will be honored by the guardian in most cases, unless challenged by actions of the court. The guardian, who may be unknown to the ward, can be named in the advance directive. One of the criticisms of this relationship is the lack of stringent oversight of the guardians. In most jurisdictions, the performance of the guardian is reviewed once or twice per year, and further review is ordered only if complaints about the guardian's performance are submitted on behalf of the ward to the court.

The stated purpose of this relationship may be guardianship of the person or guardianship of the estate, or both. Those charged with guardianship of the person address all personal decisions related to choice of residence, medical care, and quality of life issues. Those charged with guardianship of the estate address all financial issues, including protection of property and assets. The ward retains possession of all financial assets; the guardian only manages those assets. The guardian acts on behalf of the ward only to the extent of the court order that establishes the relationship.

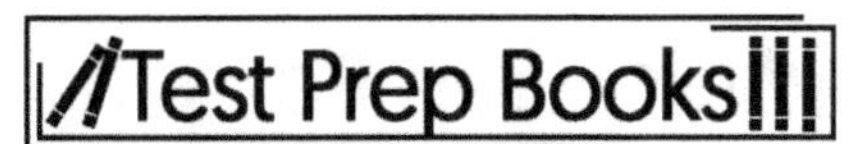

The individual rights removed by the initiation of the guardianship may be restored in the event that the court finds that the ward is no longer incapacitated; however, most commonly, the guardianship remains in place until the death of the protected person.

Guardianships involving minor children are often more complex and vary significantly from state to state. In many cases, the purpose of the guardianship is protecting parental rights and maintaining contact with the child's extended family. In this instance, the court will reassess the circumstances of the guardianship at appropriate intervals to protect the interests of the child.

Medical Directives

Advance Directives

An **advance directive** is a legal document that a patient draws up to ensure their wishes are honored even if they are unable to make their own decisions due to an incapacitating healthcare condition.

Living Will

A **living will** is a legal document that allows a patient to make clear their wishes regarding different end-of-life medical decisions should they become incapacitated in some way and unable to make these decisions. Part of a living will can name a person to make medical decisions for the patient, though a living will is not the same as a medical durable power of attorney.

Medical Durable Power of Attorney

A **power of attorney** document names a patient-appointed representative to make healthcare decisions on their behalf should they become incapacitated. The difference between this document and the living will is that the living will is more focused on **end-of-life care**, while the power of attorney can span a longer period and can end when the patient regains the ability to make their own decisions.

Patient Self Determination Act (PSDA)

The **patient self-determination act**, passed in 1990, mandates that healthcare facilities inform and protect a patient's right to make decisions about their care. This right extends even if they become incapacitated through advance directives such as the living will and power of attorney.

Documentation/Medical Records

Documentation Methods

The final step of assessment is the documentation of the findings. The WHNP is aware that safe patient care relies on accurate documentation that may or may not be shared in a larger provider network. Documentation is also required to meet reimbursement schedules for Medicaid, Medicare, and other private insurers. The assessment details, the subsequent interventions, and the patient's response to the interventions must be clearly evident and must be recorded in the appropriate EHR format.

A patient's chart is a legal record of assessments and care measures. Most facilities use an electronic health record, which with training provided during new employee orientation. Documentation may include timing related to observations, interventions, and patient responses. There are various charting systems used by patient care facilities to document patient data. Documentation requirements will be dictated by facility policy and regulatory guidelines. Two methods—**charting by exception** and **comprehensive charting**—are used.

Charting by exception requires that only vital signs and abnormal findings are documented. This charting method is somewhat controversial since a great amount of information about the patient is usually left out. It is sometimes argued that this is the safer way to chart, as only what is deviant from normal is noted, and thus, there is less room for documentation errors. The normal is assumed, unless otherwise noted. This method also saves time, as less information needs to be documented, leaving more time for patient care.

Some facilities prefer a comprehensive method of documentation, charting everything about the patient—normal and abnormal—in a very thorough manner. This way, when the patient's chart must be reviewed, especially in the case of a safety incident (e.g., a pressure sore develops or a patient falls), all details surrounding the event should be present in the medical record. This method is effective if all information is properly charted, although it can be quite time-consuming and take away from patient care time.

Documentation provides a defense for healthcare workers and patients in the case of patient incidents to show what was done for the patient. There is an adage that says, "If it wasn't charted, it didn't happen." The nurse needs to be mindful that the medical record is a legal document—a complete, thorough, and accurate documentation of care, according to facility policy.

Electronic Health Records

One way of improving patient outcomes is with the use of **electronic health records** (**EHR**s). EHRs help health care providers to access complete and accurate health information in a timely fashion. EHRs have also been shown to reduce (and even prevent) medical errors due to misinterpretation of handwriting. EHRs also allow built-in systems designed to prevent treatment errors. All documentation is typically added to an electronic health record (EHR), due to the need to maintain patient privacy and confidentiality. Anyone who accesses this information will be tracked and monitored. Most institutions will conduct routine audits to see who has been accessing which records and if they were authorized to do so. The use of paper records continues, but due to the sheer volume of information collected and the need to ensure the security of this record, this practice will soon be phased out. Basic standards of care require the EHR contains all pertinent information and that it is updated frequently as the plan of care changes. Basic demographic information, along with treatment protocols and correspondence, is readily available to be accessed by the necessary practitioners associated with the case. Further, the meaningful use of file sharing is expected. Meaning, one of the main stipulations of the use of the EHR is that the client and provider benefit from the use of the EHR in quantifiable and qualitative ways. For this reason, it is imperative that all healthcare providers periodically document in the EHR, addressing the client's progress throughout the treatment plan.

Downtime Procedures

Downtime procedures can vary from facility to facility, but the WHNP should be prepared for both planned and unplanned downtime. First, what is downtime? Considering healthcare predominantly uses electronic health records, downtime is any time that an aspect of the electronic health record system is not working. Downtime can be a planned situation during which staff is informed of a certain time frame where the system will be down for updates, repairs, or a reset. It can also be unplanned in the event of an IT malfunction, cybersecurity issue, or loss of power.

During downtime, the greatest concern is patient safety, as the safeguards in place through the electronic health record are no longer accessible. The WHNP's role in downtime procedures, both planned and unplanned, is to be prepared to access paper health records, understand the policy for paper documentation, and ensure no lapses in communication related to downtime. There will be minor setbacks with downtime procedures, but the goal of the nurse is to continue to provide safe, effective care to each patient.

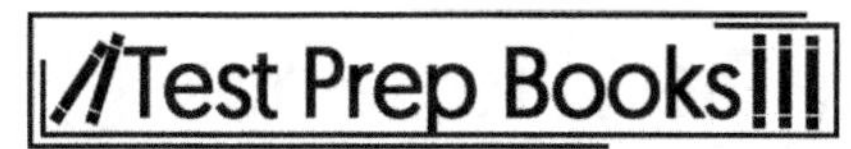

Coding Applications

Diagnostic Coding (International Classification of Diseases, Clinical Modification [ICD-CM])

The **International Classification of Diseases** (**ICD**) is a system of codes that classifies diseases and medical diagnoses. ICD codes are regulated by the World Health Organization and are used to communicate and file patient insurance claims for reimbursement. Each ICD code is unique and defines a specific disease process or medical illness. The most current ICD version is 10, with a newer version (ICD-11), replacing it in January of 2022. When submitting a claim, a procedural code must be included defining the services provided. Modification of codes is often necessary when multiple, complex procedures are performed for a particular disease process. Modifiers require supplemental information explaining why additional procedures, tests, or exams were medically necessary.

Procedural Coding (Current Procedural Terminology [CPT])

CPT is a standardized coding scheme that facilitates the reporting of medical, surgical, and diagnostic procedures for payment.

Modifiers

The WHNP understands that a **CPT modifier** refines the original CPT definition of the procedure to reflect some addition or alteration in the original category. Modifiers add details to the original CPT that more closely reflect the patient encounter, which increases revenue and decreases the potential for denial of services.

Upcoding

The WHNP recognizes that **upcoding** refers to the fraudulent practice of reporting a CPT that represents a higher level of care or more complex diagnosis than is supported by the patient's diagnosis or EHR and provider documentation. The level of service for evaluation and management of a single patient encounter is coded according to the complexity of the care. The WHNP understands that an example of upcoding could be using a level 5 code to report the care of a patient with a minor complaint for a brief encounter.

Downcoding

Providers that are responsible for billing and handling patient records need to be aware of how to properly use codes to submit claims to a patient's insurance or create bills for service. **Downcoding** refers to the process of assigning a low-level code to a medical service, lower than is accurate for the service that was provided. Insurance companies reimburse a healthcare facility at a lower rate when downcoding occurs. For example, a patient visits their healthcare provider for an annual physical. During the examination, multiple medical concerns are addressed, and the patient requires more services and tests than were originally intended. The patient's insurance denies the claims for additional services and only reimburses the care associated with a standard annual physical.

Bundling of Charges

Bundling of charges or episode-based payments is a reimbursement plan that reimburses providers for all episodes of care for an individual disease, diagnosis, or condition. For instance, the provider receives one payment for all outpatient and inpatient care for the patient with a total knee replacement, which contrasts with the traditional fee-for-service plan that includes charges and reimbursement for each care encounter or procedure. Proponents of the episode-based payment model view it as a cost savings measure that can contribute to improved patient outcomes, and positive provider and patient satisfaction. The potential cost savings are based on three assumptions: the contracted cost for episode-based care is less than fee-for-service cost for the same care; the savings that are generated are divided between the provider and the payer; and complications associated with the compensated illness or condition are not reimbursed. In addition, when hospitals participate in the episode-based payment model, providers who do not contract for bundled payment options that care for patients during a hospital stay receive fees for that care from the hospital, not the third-party payer.

Unbundling of Charges

When a claim is submitted to the patient's insurance, current procedural terminology (CPT) codes need to be entered for the services provided. When multiple CPT billing codes are used for one visit, this is termed "unbundling." Unbundling charges for each individual service leads to higher costs and larger reimbursements for the facility. Various CPT codes are inclusive, bundling services that properly account for the care provided. For example, a patient has a pelvic exam with a Pap smear and collection of tissue samples. Submitting a claim for all three individual services as opposed to an inclusive procedure would be considered **unbundling of charges**.

Healthcare Common Procedure Coding System (HCPCS Level II)

The **Healthcare Common Procedure Coding System** (**HCPCS**) is a code system used by medical providers to submit service claims to health insurers and Medicare. Level II HCPCS is a national procedure code set for healthcare providers, practitioners, and medical equipment suppliers to use when they file health plan claims for any patient supplies, medications, devices, transportation services, and other needed items or supplies. Unlike CPT codes that define which medical services were performed, HCPCS codes define which supplies, medications, or items were used.

Linkage of Procedure and Diagnostic Coding to Meet Medical Necessity Guidelines

Every service claim that is submitted to a patient's health insurance or Medicare must include a CPT code. Additionally, the CPT code must be linked to an ICD code, which defines the medical condition that necessitates the service. For example, a healthcare provider determines a patient has symptoms of a third-degree heart block and orders an electrocardiogram to confirm the diagnosis. The CPT code for the electrocardiogram may be 93000 but requires an ICD code to justify its need. The accompanying ICD code for this medical condition would be I44.2.

Mandatory Reporting

The WHNP's first responsibility for **reportable diseases** is to prevent them from occurring. Health promotion teaching aimed at prevention includes decreasing high-risk behaviors such as unprotected sexual activity, encouraging adherence to immunization guidelines, and decreasing the risk of environmental diseases by adequate protection against predictable risk factors such as mosquito bites and tick bites. If prevention is inadequate, the WHNP will be alert for early signs and symptoms of disease, in order to increase the opportunity for early intervention. In addition, when a patient presents with an infection, the WHNP will reinforce the need to complete all prescribed doses of the anti-infective agents in order to prevent re-infection. In contrast, if a patient doesn't have an infection, the WHNP will discuss the proper use of antibiotics with the patient. The WHNP will also provide prevention and treatment information for patients who are traveling to areas that might present additional risk for short-term or long-term infections.

WHNPs should be aware that immunization guidelines are not met with universal approval; however, most authorities believe that the immunizations are essential to the health of the individual and the community. Recently there has been a significant increase in the incidence of measles. Infectious disease professionals will determine the cause of outbreaks, and the WHNP will increase surveillance to monitor spread of the disease. Much of the reporting of infectious diseases is regulated by local and state health departments. WHNPs must be aware of the procedure for notifying the local board of health and for identifying the diseases that must be reported. EHRs can be programmed to identify and automatically report the occurrence of infectious diseases that are documented in the patient's EHR. On a community level, the WHNP must understand the emergency response protocols in the event of a large-scale catastrophe that

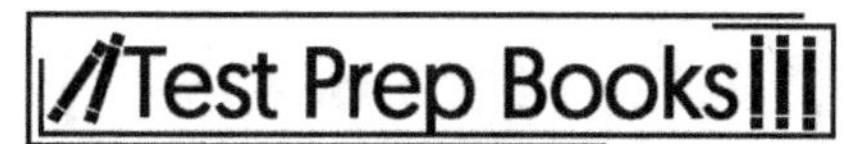

potentially can threaten large numbers of people. Appropriate liaisons with emergency response teams in the community must be maintained.

The provider, hospital, or laboratory are required to submit state-identified reportable disease information with personal identifiers to the local authorities to facilitate disease control. Reportable diseases are selected by surveillance case definitions that provide state and local public health officials with precise criteria to be used for these decisions. The local health authorities can voluntarily submit notifiable disease information without personal identifiers to the Centers for Disease Control (CDC). The formal report to CDC is submitted through the CDC's National Notifiable Diseases Surveillance System (NNDSS). The CDC also reminds providers that the reporting mechanism is not to be used in the diagnosis or the treatment of an infectious disease. The CDC aggregates national data related to the incidence of any one of approximately 120 notifiable diseases that are categorized as infectious, noninfectious, or as representing an outbreak due to a food source. These diseases are reported to protect the health of individuals and to defend against threats to public health.

Communicable Diseases

Entities must disclose information about **communicable diseases** to public health authorities to prevent the spread of disease in a community or nation. The information is usually reduced to the minimum of what is needed to protect the privacy of patients.

Vital Statistics

Birth records, birth rates, and death records are examples of **vital statistics** that must be disclosed to public health authorities for tracking and monitoring the population.

Abuse/Neglect

No patient should ever be abused or neglected. This should go without saying, but it is a patient right that is perhaps the most important. **Abuse** can be physical, emotional, sexual, mental, or financial. **Neglect** is when the patient's needs are being ignored, usually resulting in patient harm.

If the WHNP suspects abuse or neglect, they are mandated to report it to the appropriate entity. The appropriate supervisor should be notified, so the appropriate action can be taken to right the situation. There are also hotlines that can be called, such as the National Center on Elder Abuse (1-800-677-1116).

There are different types of abuse. **Physical abuse** involves injuries to the body from force, such as punching or kicking. If the WHNP notes various bruises or cuts in various stages of healing without explanation, it may be a sign of physical abuse.

Sexual abuse is when sexual contact is made without the consent of one party, including rape, coercion into doing sexual acts, and fondling of genitalia. The WHNP should look for unexplained bruising of or bleeding around the perineal area, new difficulty sitting or walking, or increased agitation as potential signs of sexual abuse.

Emotional or mental abuses are not quite as obvious as physical abuse as the damage inflicted is internal or hidden. Emotional and mental abuse is usually caused by verbal assault. The abuser may belittle and criticize the victim to the point that the victim feels worthless, insecure, and afraid. If the WHNP senses an uncomfortable relationship between an informal caregiver or family member and the patient, this should be monitored, investigated, and reported if abuse is suspected.

Financial abuse is a type of abuse in which the abuser limits the victim's access to money and financial information, sometimes stealing directly from the victim without the victim's knowledge. Being the caregiver of an older person grants a person special access to personal documents and financial resources; this privilege can be abused. If the WHNP suspects that checks and other financial means meant for the patient are being rerouted and misused by a caregiver, this abuse should be reported right away.

Negligence/Malpractice

An important part of professional nursing practice is understanding and operating within applicable laws and regulations. Nursing professionals are held to very high standards due to the delicate nature of the work they perform. Additionally, healthcare providers are subject to legal ramifications within their practice and must be aware of how to protect themselves from potential liability.

A foundation of nursing practice is to obtain and maintain nursing licensure as well as to follow the practice standards outlined by one's State Board of Nursing. The **State Board of Nursing** provides guidance for nursing education programs, state testing, provision of appropriate nursing care, and management of misconduct by licensed nurses. These provisions are outlined in the state's **Nurse Practice Act**, which outlines statutory laws governing legal nursing responsibilities.

There are many other legal materials that impact nursing practice as well. For example, common laws are previous legal decisions that set precedents for future proceedings. **Common law** can have significant influence on malpractice decisions and lawsuits involving patient rights. Additionally, the **Health Insurance Portability and Accountability Act** (**HIPAA**) legally governs the safe use of protected patient information. The **Patient Bill of Rights** is yet another binding document that outlines various protected rights for patients, including informed consent and the right to refuse. In non-hospital settings, nurses are protected by **Good Samaritan laws** to reduce legal liability for acts performed during emergencies. Also, nursing professionals are governed by The Centers of Disease Control and Prevention (CDC) health codes to protect and maintain public safety. These codes outline standards of mandatory reporting (e.g., cases of abuse and communicable disease) and standards of ensuring public safety (e.g., safety education and immunization).

In personal practice, WHNPs must consider how to protect themselves if they are required to defend themselves within the legal system. Patients and caregivers could potentially file lawsuits if they feel standards of care or patient rights were not upheld. Some of the more common issues brought against nurses can include any of the following: forced physical touch (assault), not performing standards of care (breach of duty), unlawful use of restraints (false imprisonment), privacy breach (HIPAA violation), not performing the typical standard of care action that would be reasonably expected (**negligence**), or being the direct cause of harm (proximate cause).

WHNPs can legally protect themselves in many ways. Proactive steps include maintaining all required licensure and training associated with state laws. Additionally, WHNPs can purchase malpractice insurance to financially protect themselves if they are involved with a legal case. WHNPs have a duty to understand and follow all laws pertaining to nursing practice in their state, and they also have a duty to uphold standards of care and patient rights as outlined by their organization. Accurate, concise, objective, and timely documentation practices also help to provide evidence of appropriate care. Lastly, developing and maintaining trusting relationships with patients and caregivers can help to lessen legal risks.

Adverse Event Reporting

Adverse event reporting can be commonly associated with legal formalities and repercussions, but it serves as a prominent resource for quality improvement measures when used correctly.

First, the WHNP must understand what defines an adverse event. An **adverse event** is a situation where an undesirable clinical outcome occurs related to the care provided, while not being related to the underlying disease process or condition. Types of adverse events in healthcare include medication errors, falls, equipment errors, and nosocomial infections.

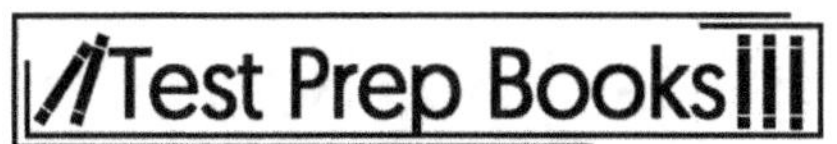

Next, the event must be properly reported, not only for the benefit of the patient affected by the adverse event, but also for future patient safety measures. For example, if a fall occurs related to an equipment error, reporting this adverse event can result in quality improvement measures such as in-services on equipment usage and fall prevention.

Never Event

"**Never events**" refer to errors in care that should never occur during a medical procedure, due to the catastrophic effects on patient safety and outcomes that the event could have. Additionally, these events can be costly for the healthcare facility. "Never events" include instances like performing an incorrect procedure on a patient, performing a procedure on the wrong patient, failing to take into account patient history such as allergies, the development of pressure ulcers on patients in care, and other situations that cause adverse outcomes, including death, to the patient. Associated costs with "never events" include time, labor, and money spent to correct medical errors, lawsuits, and future reimbursements lost due to tarnished reputation.

Risk Management

In a healthcare facility, human lives are the focus of services provided and risks are inherently present in the work. These risks include lawsuits, malpractice claims, financial loss, and harm (whether intentional or unintentional) to the patients. Effectively managing risk in order to reduce the probability of a negative outcome encompasses a number of theoretical and analytical steps.

Identifying potential causes of risk can come both from theoretical brainstorming, as well as reviewing concrete evidence. Key stakeholders can examine existing processes and hypothesize how they may present risk. Additionally, reviewing documented instances where risks came to fruition can bring attention to what the healthcare facility and providers should avoid. Documented instances can be those that occurred at another facility, which can serve as a learning lesson for the industry, or they can be instances that occurred internally, such as a filed patient lawsuit or complaint. Regular **risk assessments**, similar in nature to an audit, can pinpoint areas of risk. These should be system-wide and conducted at regular intervals, with extra assessments conducted any time a new system is implemented or a new healthcare regulation comes into effect.

Once potential causes of risk have been identified, stakeholders should objectively identify which have the possibility to cause the most overall harm, whether it is to the organization, to medical staff, or to patients. These should then be listed in order of urgency, and individual solutions should be discussed. The PDCA cycle of process and quality improvement can be a useful tool when determining an effective yet streamlined solution, as it encompasses many of the qualities that a risk-mitigating solution will need.

Finally, a system should be in place that allows all medical staff to voice areas of risk that they see on the job. As the front line in many of the processes that take place in a healthcare facility, medical staff are able to provide valuable insight regarding risk. Medical staff should feel comfortable reporting causes of risk in the workplace, and a standardized procedure for reporting risks should be in place. In the event that a negative outcome due to preventable or unavoidable risk does occur, it is important that all staff members know how to best respond to the event in order to mitigate its effects on the organization's reputation, business operations, staff members, and patients.

Legal Terms and Doctrines

The following is a list of common legal terms the WHNP should be acquainted with should they come up in their practice.

- **Subpoena duces tecum**: This Latin term translates to "under penalty you shall bring with you." This is a legal document ordering a person to come to court and bring any relevant documents to the case.
- **Subpoena**: This simply entails the person must produce evidence for a case.
- **Respondeat superior**: This Latin term literally means "let the master answer." This legal term refers to an employer being responsible for the actions of their employees, usually used in the case of tort.
- **Res ipsa loquitur**: In Latin, this term means "the thing speaks for itself." It applies to medical malpractice where negligence is implied when an accident occurs.
- **Locum tenens**: This phrase is Latin for "one holding a place" and in medicine usually refers to one physician filling the place of another.
- **Defendant/plaintiff**: A defendant is the person against whom the plaintiff is filing a complaint or suit. A patient would be the plaintiff, and the physician would be the defendant if the patient filed a lawsuit against the physician.
- **Deposition**: A deposition is a legal statement that is recorded outside of the court, usually an oral testimony that is written down as evidence.
- **Arbitration/mediation**: Both these terms refer to a way of settling legal disputes outside of court. Arbitration is a cheaper, faster alternative to settling disputes. An arbitrator, a third party, is selected to help resolve the dispute. They decide who to award, if anyone. If one decides to go the arbitrary route, the case may not be tried in court, since it is considered legally resolved. Mediation differs from arbitration in that it is more flexible, can occur before arbitration, is more informal, and the mediator simply facilitates communication between opposing parties in search of a resolution.
- **Good Samaritan laws**: These laws protect persons who choose to assist someone in need of emergency medical assistance outside of a healthcare facility. If an unintended consequence results, or the person's life is not saved, the person is protected if they had good intention and offered reasonable assistance.

Contracts (Physician-Patient Relationships)

- **Legal obligations to the patient**: Due to the sensitive nature of information exchanged between a doctor and their patient, confidentiality is an obligation that must be honored, or there will be legal consequences.
- **Consequences for patient noncompliance**: There are some cases in which a patient becomes noncompliant, or refuses to follow medical advice regarding their care. In some cases, the physician might feel the need to protect themselves from any potential legal consequences of the patient's noncompliance, telling the patient to seek a new provider. There may be documents that the physician can have the patient sign, indicating that they were advised one way and that they refused to follow medical direction, thus freeing the physician from any liability.

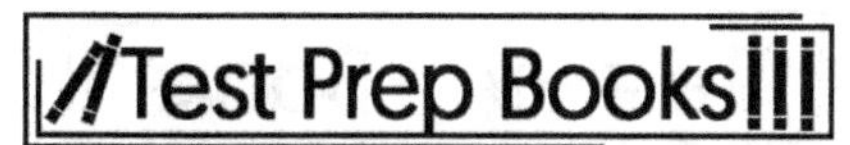

- **Termination of medical care**

  1. Elements/behaviors for **withdrawal of care**: The patient has the right to refuse to follow medical advice; however, they cannot hold the physician liable for any consequences they suffer, such as a medical emergency or worsening of their condition. Healthcare staff must respect the patient's right and always treat them with respect despite difference of opinions.

  2. Patient notification and documentation: It is important when terminating care of a patient to properly notify them and thoroughly document the case for legal protection.

- **Ownership of medical records**: Each state in the United States has different rules as to who owns medical records. In some states, the hospital and/or the physician has ownership; in other states, the patient owns the information; and in some states, there is no legal specification as to who owns medical records. Under HIPAA, all patients have a right to access their own medical record and may argue this legally.

Pharmaceutical Laws

E-Prescribing

The licensed provider can use a secure computer network to send medication prescription orders to participating pharmacies as allowed by federal and state laws.

Drug Schedules

The Controlled Substances Act (CSA) is a federal drug policy regulated by the DEA. Certain medications such as stimulants, narcotics, depressants, hallucinogens, and anabolic steroids have the potential for abuse and a likelihood of causing dependence. There are five schedules under the CSA. Schedule I drugs have a high potential for abuse with no medical necessity. Schedule V drugs have a low risk of dependence if managed appropriately. All prescriptions that include medications within the CSA should include the prescribing provider's DEA number for tracking and recordkeeping purposes.

Controlled Substances (Use and Abuse)

The provider will understand that:

- Pharmacies require either a handwritten and signed prescription, a faxed copy of a handwritten and signed prescription, or a prescription transmitted on a secure computer network in order to dispense controlled substances.
- Individual state laws may impose limits on the number of times that a prescription for a controlled substance can be written for an individual patient.
- Prescription authority is granted to licensed providers in accordance with federal and state laws and professional practice acts in the individual states.

Patient Confidentially

Patient privacy and **confidentiality** are constant concerns for all healthcare providers. Given the sensitivity of medical procedures, the healthcare team must maintain strict patient confidentiality. Under the Health Insurance Portability and Accountability Act (HIPAA), a patient's information is required to be protected and kept confidential regardless of the form, including electronic, written, and spoken communication. **Protected health information** (**PHI**) should be shared only on an as-needed and minimum necessary basis. When discussing patients or cases in settings where other personnel may overhear the conversation, the medical team should be careful not to include any PHI that may violate the patient's confidentiality. Additionally, when information is displayed electronically to families and visitors in waiting rooms, patient names should be avoided. HIPAA violations can have negative consequences for the providers and/or the facility.

Electronic Access Audit/Activity Log

Most of the patient's health information will be logged in an electronic health record (EHR). Anyone who accesses this information will be tracked and monitored. Most institutions will conduct routine audits to see who has been accessing which records and if they were authorized to do so.

Use and Disclosure of Personal/Protected Health Information (PHI)

- Consent/Authorization to Release: A patient is usually asked to sign a consent to release PHI before receiving treatment. This allows the healthcare provider to release their information for treatment, payment, and healthcare operations, abbreviated to TPO. Treatment is all care given to the patient by the healthcare provider; payment involves claims, billing, and collection by insurance companies; and healthcare operations involves educational purposes such as training new employees. Healthcare operations does not include using patient information for research; a different consent must be signed for that purpose.
- Drug and Alcohol Treatment Records: Certain patient health records regarding the treatment of drug and alcohol addictions are specifically protected by federal regulations. Violation of the confidentiality of these records could result in a criminal penalty to the offender. There are certain emergency situations in which this information may be shared as well as research purposes in which release of information is allowed.
- HIV-Related Information: HIV-related information is protected by law. Reports on diagnoses and treatments are to be kept private and confidential by healthcare providers. The reason this information is kept confidential is that persons with an HIV-AIDS diagnosis may face discrimination because of some people's unfair prejudices.
- Mental Health Records: Part of HIPAA provides special protection to mental health records. For example, though mental health information is largely grouped together with general health information about a patient, psychotherapy notes have special safeguards that keep them confidential. In the case of minors with mental health issues, there are specific guidelines that dictate who can be talked to about which issues, such as discussing a teen's medication regimen for mental illness with a legal guardian or parent.

Genetic Information Nondiscrimination Act of 2008 (GINA)

In 2008, Congress enacted GINA to prevent employers and health insurers from discriminating against people based on their genetic information. Genetic discrimination means to discriminate against a person based on defects or perceived defects in their DNA.

Public Policy

Healthcare Economics, Policy, and Organizational Practices

One of the leading goals of healthcare is to reduce medical costs. Hospital stays and readmissions are costly and can take a toll on healthcare debt. Healthcare economics is based on supply versus demand. Demand can refer to treatment and services that a large number of patients require. Supply is the available treatment and services that can be provided to the patients who need them. Practitioners should have a basic understanding of the healthcare market and how it affects patients.

Health insurance acts a third-party payer in the private sector. When no health insurance is available, the government is the responsible third party. Patients are often unaware of medical costs and will not seek follow-up treatment if faced with high medical debt. Part of the health history includes assessing the patient's occupation and concern with financial resources. Providers should be sensitive to these concerns when prescribing treatment. Patient compliance with treatment is often dependent on their ability to afford

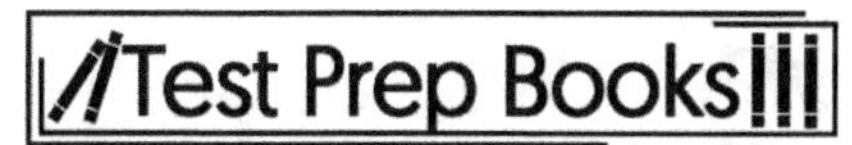

medications. Encouraging lifestyle modifications and regular wellness visits can limit complications or prevent the development of a costly disease process.

Healthcare policy follows a particular structure and process. At the state level, policymaking will vary by region. Appointed governors can set policy and issue regulations that eventually become state laws. Provider licensing, accreditation, and public health concerns are all managed by state entities. At the federal level, Congress has the responsibility to provide for the general welfare, collect revenue, and pay debts. The Department of Health and Human Services (HHS) is an entity with multiple branches that cover activities related to medical research, health insurance programs, substance use prevention, and infection control.

There are numerous healthcare organizations that promote, serve, and support the public. Among these organizations is the CDC. The CDC helps promote quality of life by preventing and controlling disease. The Centers for Medicare & Medicaid Services (CMS) ensures healthcare coverage is effective and up-to-date. The Food and Drug Administration (FDA) ensures the safety, security, and efficacy of medical drugs and devices. Substance Abuse and Mental Health Services Administration (SAMHSA) facilitates the recovery for current or at-risk patients struggling with substance use and mental illness. It is vital for providers to stay up-to-date on new policies, regulations, and approved treatment options.

Healthcare Accessibility

Healthcare accessibility means an individual can obtain timely attention for all their healthcare needs in order to realize optimal clinical and humanistic outcomes. There are three separate components to accessing healthcare:

- Entering the healthcare system, which generally requires some form of insurance coverage
- Having services available in the patient's geographic area
- Entering a caring relationship with a skilled provider

Each of these steps is a barrier to significant numbers of individuals, despite government plans like Medicare, Medicaid, veteran's health benefits, and the **Affordable Care Act** (**ACA**) plans.

As healthcare costs and insurance costs continue to escalate, fewer patients have insurance. Employers increase employee contributions to health insurance costs, elderly patients discontinue supplemental Medicare policies, and healthy young people pay fines that are less expensive than insurance coverage. As technology expands the available care options, more of the advanced procedures are provided only in large medical centers in major cities, making the therapies unavailable to large numbers of patients. In addition, acute care and even primary care services are not available in many rural areas. Individuals with insurance coverage may find that their choice of provider is dictated by the network restrictions of that policy, or they may find that their chosen provider does not accept their insurance coverage. Patients without insurance coverage have even greater difficulty accessing a primary care provider and may resort to using emergency services for routine healthcare needs. Accessibility for vulnerable populations such as the homeless who have a disproportionate incidence of mental illness is also a significant problem in the United States.

Efforts to address these disparities include incentive programs to provide primary care coverage for rural areas, expansion of outpatient primary care services for uninsured and under-insured patients, and increased preventive and health-promoting care for all patients. Lack of accessibility is associated with the increased costs of caring for patients with greater morbidity and more complications that require emergency services and hospitalization.

Ethical Principles

Healthcare providers routinely face situations with patients where they must analyze various moral and ethical considerations. Above all else, WHNPs have the responsibility to do no harm while serving as advocates, minimizing injury, and protecting the overall health and functioning of their patients. It is important to consider the patient holistically when applying these values, such as considering what the patient may view as a good quality of life, what family values the patient holds, other family members that may be affected (such as a spouse or children), legal considerations, and logistical considerations (such as how much time and medical resources are available). When patients are unable to make decisions autonomously or provide consent to treatment (as can be common in emergency cases), WHNPs should act from these responsibilities to make wise and compassionate decisions on the patients' behalf.

Dilemmas that can arise for healthcare staff include situations where the patient may have cultural or personal beliefs that prevent lifesaving treatment. For example, a female patient may not want to be treated by any male staff, or a patient that needs a blood transfusion may not accept this procedure due to religious beliefs. In cases where the patient is able to directly communicate their wishes, the WHNP may need to defer to the patient's wishes in order to preserve the patient's autonomy. This may mean providing alternative means of care (such as finding available female medical providers to assist with the female patient that does not want to be treated by male staff).

It may mean withholding treatment that the patient refuses. If the patient's life is in question and rapid medical action is necessary, healthcare staff must consider the patient's wishes in the plan of care. Ethical considerations like these will vary by case and patient and will depend on the severity of the case, the medical and personal history of the patient, and the judgment of the provider. In all cases, it is ideal if the provider and patient are able to communicate openly with each other about the case and potential medical options, and hope that the resolution is able to be for the greatest good.

Autonomy, Beneficence, and Non-maleficence

Advocacy is the promotion of the common good, especially as it applies to at-risk populations. It involves speaking out in support of policies and decisions that affect the lives of individuals who do not otherwise have a voice. WHNPs meet this standard of practice by actively participating in the politics of healthcare accessibility and delivery. They are educationally and professionally prepared to evaluate and comment on the needs of patients at the local, state, and national level. This participation requires an understanding of the legislative process, the ability to negotiate with public officials, and a willingness to provide expert testimony in support of policy decisions. The advocacy role of WHNPs has the potential to address the needs of the individual patient, society, and members of the nursing profession.

In clinical practice, WHNPs represent the patient's interests through active participation in the development of the plan of care and subsequent care decisions. Advocacy, in this sense, is related to patient **autonomy** and the patient's right to informed consent and self-determination. WHNPs provide the appropriate information, assess the patient's comprehension of the implications of the care decisions, and act as patient advocates by supporting the patient's decisions. Patient advocacy for acutely ill patients requires the WHNP to represent the patient's decisions even though those decisions may be opposed to those of the healthcare providers and family members.

WHNPs understand the complex care requirements of patients with multiple comorbidities. Therefore, they are often called upon to intercede on a patient's behalf to facilitate the delivery of adequate and appropriate care in both the acute care setting and the primary care environment. In addition, WHNPs understand the care needs of the greater community and serve as advocates for the provision of preventative interventions

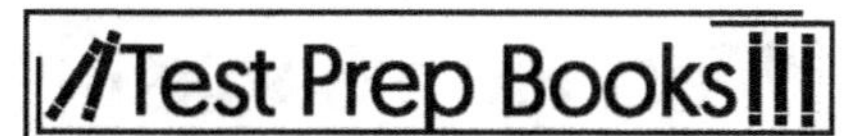

and policies that affect public health. WHNPs advocate for increased resources to address the needs of specific community populations. In this way, WHNPs practice **beneficence**, defined as doing good for another individual, including acting as an advocate, supporting the individual's autonomy, and working to ensure justice. Related to beneficence is the concept of **nonmaleficence**, which means non-harming, or inflicting the least harm possible to reach a beneficial outcome.

Professionally, WHNPs advocate for policies that support and promote the practice of all nurses regarding access to education, role identity, workplace conditions, and compensation. The responsibility for professional advocacy requires WHNPs to provide leadership in the development of the professional nursing role in all practice settings that may include acute care facilities, colleges and universities, or community agencies. Leadership roles in acute care settings involve participation in professional practice and shared governance committees, providing support for basic nursing education by facilitating clinical and preceptorship experiences, and mentoring novice graduate nurses to the professional nursing role. In the academic setting, WHNPs work to ensure the diversity of the student population by participating in the governance structure of the institution, conducting and publishing research that supports the positive impact of professional nursing care on patient outcomes, and serving as an advocate to individual nursing students to promote their academic success. In the community, WHNPs may collaborate with government officials to meet the needs that are specific to that location.

The role requirements for advocacy require WHNPs to maintain clinical expertise through continuing education (formal and informal), to actively follow and comment on legislative initiatives that affect at-risk populations, and to model the professional nursing role in practice.

Bioethics

Bioethics is defined by principles of theology, humanities, philosophy, medicine, and nursing. It addresses ethical dilemmas that result from the rapid expansion of medical technology. Bioethics attempts to answer "why" questions. Are there frequent instances of expensive duplication of services that did not improve patient outcomes? Bioethics is the conscience of providers. The principles of bioethics also provide a framework for the assessment of difficult healthcare issues, which include end-of-life decisions, treatment decisions for vulnerable populations, and scarce resource allocation. Recent additions to this list include the consideration of medical errors, confidentiality, and artificial intelligence. Each of these decisions relies on the principles of beneficence, nonmaleficence, autonomy, justice, and utilitarianism with respect to the allocation of scarce resources. WHNPs should understand that all care decisions involve an ethical component.

Treating a patient with sickle cell disease requires the use of donated blood, which is a scarce resource. The care of the patient with end-stage renal disease requires a discussion of organ transplantation, which is one of the more complex ethical decisions. Expert counseling skills are required to advise and comfort a family caring for an infant with genetic defects that are inconsistent with life. There is evidence that advancing technology is rapidly outpacing the ability of the bioethical framework that currently assists providers with making these tough decisions. Many believe that genetic engineering can be a source of abuse if not managed appropriately by ethical professionals. Others voice concerns about stem cell utilization, while at the same time others believe that denying the progress of stem cell research is unethical.

Communication technology presents another list of potential threats to ethical patient care, including loss of privacy, insecure data storage, increased patient access to information that may or may not be appropriate to their care, and disparities in online access to patient portals due to socioeconomic factors. Large data breaches put sensitive patient data at risk every day, with potentially devastating effects. Providers also deal with the consequences of misinformation because patients can access information, but they frequently do not understand the information. In the extreme this can lead to the use of unnecessary diagnostic testing to calm patient fears. The positive side of access to information is that it allows the patient to participate more actively in development of the plan of care, which is associated with more cost-effective outcomes and increased patient satisfaction.

WHNPs should understand that progress requires adaptation and accommodation of all treatment decisions that must be based on ethical principles that respect all individuals. Providers in larger acute care settings have ethical committees that can assist with these decisions. Providers in primary care must develop community resources, including patient advocacy groups that can provide similar assistance.

Justice

The concept of **justice** in the healthcare setting is associated with utilitarian decision-making, the issues related to accessibility, and the allocation of scarce resources. WHNPs should understand that primary care providers are "gatekeepers", and their clinical practice is influenced by all these responsibilities. This gatekeeper function does not always favor the individual, if the greatest benefit to the greatest number of people is related to an alternative solution, the WHNP must rely on that alternative action.

Healthcare justice has also been defined as distributive justice which is related to the justice of distributing scarce resources. There are three additional elements of distributive justice: equity, equality, and need. The provision of equitable healthcare focuses on eliminating the differences in the care provided to different patient populations by providing needed resources for all patients. Equality means everyone is treated the same. It is obvious that the resolution of some inequities is beyond the ability of the provider; however, when scarce resources are allocated by a provider, the decisions must be fair and equitable. The administration of justice in healthcare is an ethical responsibility that may also be a legal responsibility. This means that primary care providers understand the needs of their patients and their legal responsibilities for care.

The WHNP is aware that there are significant inequalities in the delivery of healthcare to vulnerable populations in the United States. Each of these groups has special needs that are not currently being addressed equitably. This list includes the chronically ill and disabled patients, low income and/or homeless individuals, rural-dwelling individuals including Native Americans, lesbian, gay, bisexual, transgender, and queer individuals, and the very young and the very old.

The risks differ among these populations, but the need for equitable access and delivery of services is common among these groups. For instance, homeless individuals are affected by the lack of financial resources, which increases their vulnerability to the onset of chronic disease. Residents of rural areas are increasingly without access to routine primary care such as obstetrical services. Healthcare access for these populations can be improved as greater numbers of APRNs are employed in all care settings. In addition, all APRNs are obligated and uniquely qualified to advocate for all of these individuals by active involvement in the efforts of professional associations at the local and national levels to affect changes in healthcare policy. These efforts potentially can improve access, increase cost-effectiveness of care, decrease the incidence and burden of chronic disease, and improve the quality of life and patient satisfaction.

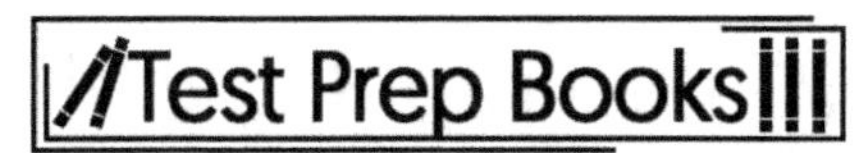

Safety

Communication

Therapeutic Communication

Overcoming barriers to communication requires practicing **therapeutic communication**. Therapeutic communication is a type of communication that assists the patient in the healing process rather than hindering it. There are a number of useful communication techniques the WHNP can employ to aid in therapeutic communication.

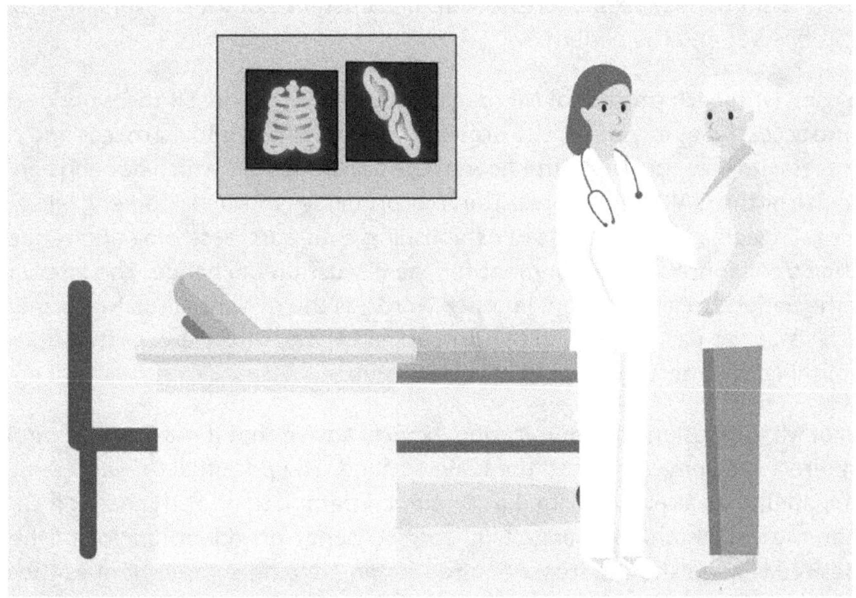

Sometimes, silence is the best way to get clarification from a patient, or simply asking them to clarify when one does not understand. WHNPs may offer themselves to support the patient without providing personal details, by sympathizing and saying, "Yes, I have been through something similar." The nurse may ask the patient to summarize their thoughts or identify a theme when stories go on at length. This helps redirect communication in a positive direction.

Asking the patient how certain events made them feel is a way to investigate the patient's emotional status. The WHNP may give information about their role and make observations, such as "I noticed you seem tense," to open the door to more fluent conversation. Giving the patient praise and recognition without overt flattery is a way to show support, such as complimenting a noticeable effort during a physical therapy session. The WHNP may want to determine the chronological order of events, which can be helpful for reporting information.

Employing therapeutic communication aids smooth collaboration and cooperation between members of the healthcare team. Incorporating smart, simple, therapeutic communication techniques and overcoming barriers to communication are important parts of achieving this goal.

Motivational Interviewing

Motivational interviewing (MI) is a communication technique that focuses on altering the patient's behavior. It is often used as a counseling tool for patients with substance use disorders, behavioral alterations, smoking, and obesity. There is a subset of skills used in MI that facilitate the progress in each of the MI phases. The OARS skills are a set of verbal and non-verbal interview techniques, which can be tailored to the specific needs of the MI process. The acronym OARS stands for open-ended questions, affirmations, reflections, and summaries.

Open-ended questions encourage two-way conversation because they are not generally answerable with a simple "yes" or "no." Questions beginning with the word "why" can potentially elicit a defensive patient response and should be avoided. Affirmations acknowledge the patient and convey a message of empathetic understanding. These statements can also build a patient's self-efficacy which positively affects motivation. Reflections, or reflective listening, improve the interviewer's understanding of the patient's narrative. Periods of reflection after the patient speaks slow the pace of the conversation so that it is not simply a series of questions and answers. Summaries provide a review of the substance of the conversation and an opportunity for closure by the interviewer and the patient.

The OARS skills are used with each process of MI to maximize the outcomes. If the work of the MI process is slowed down or is unsuccessful at any point, the provider returns to the initial process and reestablishes it. MI is not a linear process; it is responsive to the flow of the conversation, which depends on the skill of the interviewer and the use of the OARS techniques. The four processes of MI include engaging, focusing, evoking, and planning. Engaging is the process of establishing a rapport, assessing and reducing any defensive behavior, and creating a collaborative environment for the discussion of change. The interviewer is able to assess the focus of the patient's conversation, in other words, is the patient actually engaged in the work of MI. If the patient is resistant to participating in the process of MI, the interviewer often finds that empathy is effective in re-establishing the interviewer-patient relationship.

The second process of MI is focusing. Communication experts advise that it may take several sessions before the interviewer can direct the conversation to the issue at hand. The potential for success at this stage is enhanced when the patient has already reached a state of contemplation for the desired change. The process of evoking focuses on the discussion or "change talk" for two behaviors: identification of the specific steps necessary for the desired change and the steps required for an ongoing commitment to the changed behavior. There are two forms of change talk: preparatory refers to the desire to change, and mobilizing addresses commitment and action. The planning process may be optional, but when it is included in MI, it identifies the "how" for the planned change.

Shared Decision-Making

Shared decision-making is a patient care model that focuses on the patients' involvement in care decisions for every aspect of their own care, in partnership with the primary care providers. Although patients currently have access to vast amounts of information in many forms, the average patient continues to voice frustration with the perceived amount of personal input into the plan of care. The SHARE approach is a five-step program that was developed by the Agency for Healthcare Research and Quality (AHRQ) to give primary care providers the necessary tools to improve patient satisfaction through increased participation in decision-making. One of the key elements of this model is enhanced communication between the provider and the patient. Researchers found that providers wait an average of 17 seconds after their first question before asking their second question. Clearly, this does not provide the patient with sufficient time to participate in the care planning process. Providers are reminded to provide the patient with appropriate information sources and to then use "teach back" to verify the patient's understanding. In addition, providers should avoid the use of medical jargon, use skilled interpreters as necessary, and actively listen to the patient and family.

The initial step of the SHARE program is to engage the patients and encourage their participation in the process of shared decision-making. The patients should understand that their participation is voluntary, their families are welcome to participate as well, and their decisions will be based on their understanding of their

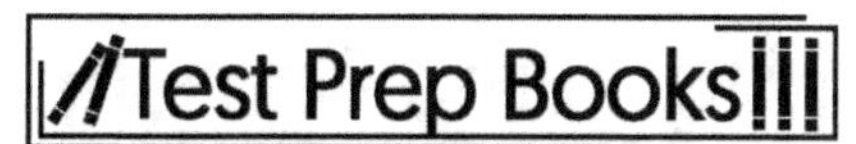

care options. Many providers first enroll patients in the electronic patient portals that can then be used as a recruitment delivery system for the SHARE program.

The second step of the SHARE program is to present the patient with all available evidence-based treatment options while recognizing that the choice of no treatment is also a viable option. The AHRQ provides extensive patient education resources for a wide range of clinical conditions. The provider is encouraged to present the information in several different forms to be sure to match the patient's learning style. The third step of the SHARE program asks the provider to identify the patient's values by using empathetic open-ended questions. This step also involves considering the potential differences between patient-centered outcomes and clinical outcomes. Providers must recognize that the patients' priorities are often not the same as the provider's priorities. The fourth step is to assist the patient in making the final choice of the available options.

Once the treatment decisions have been made, the provider will schedule follow-up visits to complete the treatment and to monitor the treatment outcomes. The final step is ongoing evaluation of the patient's treatment decisions with appropriate modifications as the patient's condition changes. There have been modest decreases in emergency room visits for patients who participated in shared decision-making and received information about acute coronary syndrome. Although shared decision-making is appropriate for all patients, in most cases, only the treatment outcomes and patient satisfaction have been measured.

Culturally Sensitive Practice

Culturally sensitive practice requires identification of the diverse patient populations, assessment of cultural issues that affect healthcare delivery to those individuals, educational interventions to increase cultural awareness of all providers, and adaptation of services to meet the distinctive healthcare needs of all individuals. In addition to ethnic and racial groups, the plan of care must also be adapted to meet the needs of disabled children and adults, and LGBTQI patients. The WHNP also recognizes that the essential components of patient adherence are closely related to the patient's cultural identity, which means that health beliefs, language preferences, and health literacy must be assessed for all patients. The recommendations for culturally sensitive practice are consistent with the national standards for **culturally and linguistically appropriate services (CLAS)** in healthcare.

The specific language and communication support criteria include support for limited English proficiency, accommodation for any additional communication deficits, provision of all patient information sources in the patient's native language at the appropriate reading level, and the provision of skilled, professional interpreters. The WHNP is aware that mandatory compliance is required for these support criteria by all federally assisted institutions to satisfy Title VI of the Civil Rights Act.

Culturally appropriate care is not one size fits all; therefore, the provider will assess the needs of individuals within and among cultural and ethnic groups by collecting real data that includes preferences for race, ethnicity, and language. It is important for the provider to know which diseases or conditions ethnic and racial groups are prone to. The white population is more prone to atrial fibrillation than people of other races, while the Hispanic population has high rates of obesity and diabetes. In individuals from Puerto Rico, there is an increased incidence of HIV infection and AIDS.

Obesity and type 2 diabetes are common in African Americans, and the death rate from HTN, stroke, HIV infection, and AIDS is higher than the rate in the non-Hispanic white population. Asian Americans have an increased incidence of tuberculosis, and hepatitis B infection occurs more commonly in recent immigrants to the United States. Asian Americans also have an increased rate of chronic obstructive pulmonary disease (COPD), although smoking rates among Chinese and Japanese Americans are lower than average. Native Americans have a high incidence of alcoholism; recent pharmacologic research indicates that altered metabolic pathways may contribute to this finding. As with the Asian American population, the WHNP will be aware of the frequent use of herbal preparations in the Native American population as well.

Patients may turn to alternative healers. Since it is important to know everything that a patient is taking, including herbs, the provider should be aware of these other healers. Cultural competence demands the provider not shame someone who has accessed alternative treatment. If the provider is culturally insensitive, the patient might not open up and reveal needed information. Caucasians may treat their conditions by taking colloidal silver or avoiding foods in the nightshade family, on the advice of an alternative practitioner. A Hispanic or Asian American person may take herbs prescribed by a healer. Given such historical abuses of experimental protocol as the "Tuskegee Study of Untreated Syphilis in the Negro Male," African Americans may have reason to mistrust allopathic medicine, and some may access traditional folk medicine remedies (as do whites, Hispanics, and other people). Bear in mind, these are far from rules, and people of any race may or may not turn to alternative or conventional treatments or carry fears about doing so.

At the organizational level, culturally competent care requires the recruitment and retention of a culturally diverse staff, the availability of professional interpreters that are well versed in the language and cultural preferences of the individual cultural groups, and coordination with traditional healers in the community. The development of a culturally competent staff relies on the provision of proper recruitment, career advancement opportunities, and educational interventions that support organizational standards for competent cultural practice by all providers. The skilled interpreters provide support for patient care staff, patients, and their families. Community liaisons provide important connections with faith healers, medicine men and other important individuals from ethnic and racial groups. These institutional efforts are also supportive of shared decision-making between the patient and the provider, and culturally sensitive practice by the individual providers.

Culturally sensitive practice benefits the patient and the healthcare institution. The focus on patient education allows the patient to put culturally or ethnically associated risk factors in perspective and to gain trust in providers who demonstrate cultural competence in care delivery. Providers have the satisfaction of delivering total care for their patients, and the ties to the greater community increase the availability of needed resources. Institutions benefit from staff and patient diversity and the potential increases in patient satisfaction.

Approach to Communication Barriers with Empathy and Compassion

Death and Dying

Not only will each individual respond differently to grief based on personality and relationship with the deceased, but also the response will differ based on their own spiritual beliefs and cultural influences. These beliefs and influences affect how a person thinks they should act during the mourning period, what to wear, what rituals need to be performed, and what happens after a person dies.

Each individual culture will not be discussed since there are many variations of how different people handle this process. It is not necessary for the WHNP to know each and every one, but rather have a general knowledge of differences and be respectful towards them.

Some cultures believe an outward show of emotion is appropriate and necessary. Sometimes, this entails an outward expression of weeping and wailing. Other cultures may be more conservative and think it is appropriate to be stoic, serious, and somber, without crying and losing one's composure. Some have specific rituals before and after the death, involving holy men, priests, or other clergy who prepare the person and/or the body for an afterlife. Some may not have any religious affiliation and may not believe in a life after this one.

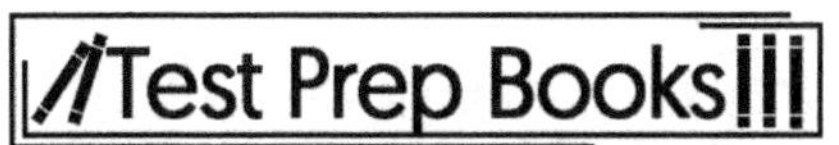

Regardless of what cultural and spiritual beliefs are present, the role of the healthcare team is to respect those wishes as much as possible. It is imperative that the team explore the resident and family's wishes in this respect, rather than overlooking or refusing to allow them. It is always appropriate to politely ask how best to respect the resident and family's wishes when performing tasks for the dying or deceased resident. For example, some family members may prefer to clean the body themselves after death, an important ritual to express grief and ensure proper care in their view.

Each member of the healthcare team, including the WHNP, needs to assess their own beliefs about death and dying. Self-knowledge on the subject is valuable as it may not be something one has consciously acknowledged. This self-assessment also helps reveal any unfair biases and prejudices towards cultures and people whose worldview is different than one's own. Discovering what one's own beliefs and others' beliefs are leads to a better understanding between groups. These groups can then begin to find ways to work together during the difficult end-of-life period.

Terminal Illness

Navigating the tricky area of communicating with a patient who is diagnosed with a **terminal illness** can present a real challenge to the WHNP. It is important to be honest with the patient. The WHNP should be an active listener, looking for opportunities to connect the patient with valuable resources and support. The WHNP should offer compassion but not false hope. The WHNP may want to say something meaningful or helpful, but this is not always the best option. Sometimes simply being present, offering a hug, or holding a patient's hand is better than any words. The WHNP should also look for opportunities to communicate with and support the family of the terminally ill patient. After the patient passes, they will need guidance to bereavement, loss, and grief resources.

Visually Impaired

A patient with a **visual impairment** will require adaptations to the WHNP's communications techniques to ensure a clear message is sent and received. The WHNP should identify themselves clearly when beginning their assessment. The WHNP should never treat the patient who has a visual impairment as if they have a deficit in intellect or as if they are deaf. The WHNP should check the environment to make sure there are no distractions, such as a loud TV, that may make it difficult to be heard. The WHNP should ask questions to ensure the message has been received and understood by the patient. Assessing the level of visual impairment will assist in knowing how much assistance the patient will need. Someone who is legally blind versus someone with complete vision loss from birth will have different needs for assistance.

Deaf and Hard of Hearing

When communicating with persons who are **deaf** or **hard of hearing**, an important first step is to assess the level of hearing loss. This will guide further communication. Depending on the amount of hearing loss, lip reading, visual tools, hearing aids, an increased volume of the WHNP's voice, or the hiring of a sign language interpreter may or may not be useful. The WHNP should directly face the person with a hearing impairment when addressing them so that understanding can be better assessed. The WHNP should not be in another room, have their back to the patient, or compete with a loud TV or other distraction while trying to communicate. The WHNP may ask the patient questions to ensure understanding of the message.

Non-English Speaking/English as a Second Language/Interpreter

In the case of a **non-English-speaking** patient, the WHNP should seek out translation services. This can come from a family member who accompanies the patient or possibly be provided by the facility where the WHNP works. Seeking educational materials in the patient's native tongue will be helpful in clearly communicating with the patient after they leave the facility.

Americans with Disabilities Act Amendments Act (ADAAA) Compliance

Passed in 2008, the ADAAA amends a previous act, the ADA, to better define what "disability" means for certain Americans as well as protecting and upholding the rights of those with disabilities in the United States. The ADAAA was a response to several Supreme Court decisions that were thought to have limited the rights of those with disabilities.

Illiterate

A person who is illiterate cannot read and/or write. It is not always apparent to a WHNP which patients may have this problem. There is a type of illiteracy called **health illiteracy** in which a patient is highly unfamiliar with medical information and is, therefore, unable to apply it to their own health and healthcare management. In illiteracy and health illiteracy, asking questions and listening for comprehension are both tools the WHNP can use to determine how well the patient understands their individual healthcare plan. If a patient cannot read or write, the WHNP can offer their health information to them in a different format. The WHNP can read through instructions for home care and ensure that a literate caregiver is accessible to the patient to assist them with written materials. Patients with low healthcare literacy tend to make their healthcare decisions based on emotions and practical considerations such as if they will be able to get a ride to the doctor. An example of emotional decision-making would be a patient who doesn't go to the doctor because he "doesn't like needles"; this is irrational, since not every doctor visit implies needles, yet it creates a barrier to successful healthcare. Identifying these barriers is the first step to overcoming illiteracy.

Intellectually Challenged

A patient who is **intellectually challenged** may need additional help communicating with the healthcare team. The WHNP will need to practice patience and allow extra time for communicating messages with and receiving messages from a person with an intellectual disability. The WHNP should work with caregivers to get helpful tips for working with a patient. Every patient is different, and a full-time caregiver or loved one will know what works best when trying to communicate with the patient. The WHNP should try to explain care in the simplest terms possible, avoiding complicated medical jargon. The WHNP should focus on the patient's strengths rather than pointing out and focusing on weaknesses. As with all communication, the WHNP should concentrate on being an active listener, open to receiving the patient's concerns and giving them time to voice them.

Age-Specific Therapeutic/Adaptive Responses

There are considerations to be made regarding the age of the person the WHNP is communicating with.

Geriatric

Geriatric refers to an older adult, a population of patients the WHNP may work with quite frequently. The WHNP should remember that active listening is as important as, if not more important than, speaking as far as communication goes. The WHNP should ask questions but listen intently to the answers to ascertain if the patient understands. The WHNP needs to remember that interrupting is rude and can compromise trust and good communication. The WHNP should take their time when giving instructions, ensuring understanding. It is not wise to use jargon, slang, or other language that the geriatric patient may not understand. If the patient needs to use new technology such as an online patient account, an assessment of Internet usage and proficiency would be useful.

Pediatric

There are a few tricks a WHNP should have up their sleeve when addressing a **pediatric** patient to make them feel comfortable and safe in a medical environment. The WHNP should address the child by name to create a tone of familiarity. Getting down to the child's level physically—in other words, squatting down to eye level—will help the child feel they are on the same level as their caregiver, rather than the WHNP towering over them. Smiling and exuding a positive attitude will create the right environment for the WHNP to care for the

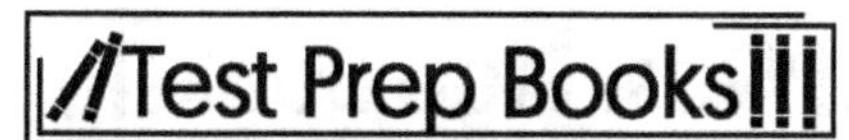

child. Making medical tools and equipment into toys when appropriate, such as gloves or tongue depressors, can help the child feel at ease. The WHNP should enlist the parents as team members in the child's care.

Adolescent

Communicating with teenagers can present its own unique challenges for the WHNP. No longer a child and not quite an adult, the **adolescent** must feel they are part of the care team and that they have a say in decision-making. It may be useful to conduct interviews with adolescents without their parents being present, if possible. This will help when trying to conduct a frank discussion on the patient's sexual activity as well as potential drug/alcohol usage. The assessment of an adolescent should include questions about mental health issues, such as depression and anxiety. The teen may feel more comfortable discussing these issues without their parent present, though the parent should be made a member of the team when addressing any issues that are discovered. Another important topic to approach with teens is stress, its causes, and coping mechanisms. In some cases, it is important to inform the adolescent which topics will remain confidential. This may encourage them to share more with the WHNP.

Nonverbal Communication

The WHNP not only communicates with their words but also with their body language. Knowing what one is communicating nonverbally and taking care to send the right message is vital to quality patient care.

Body Language

- Posture: Slouching indicates disinterest, fatigue, and disengagement. The WHNP should have erect posture, not only for the health benefit, but to show the patient they are engaged in their care.
- Position: The WHNP should be facing the patient, both their face and body. Not facing the patient indicates the WHNP does not care about sending a good message and that they do not care about their situation.
- Facial expression: It is not necessary for the WHNP to have a big, bright smile on their face at all times, but a pleasant expression that is responsive to the patient's own facial expression gives off a positive energy that the patient may find encouraging.
- Territoriality/physical boundaries: Different cultures have different boundaries that are considered acceptable. The WHNP should maintain a respectful distance from the patient, never too far away or too close for comfort. The patient's reaction is a good measure of whether the WHNP is at an appropriate distance.
- Gestures: Most people use hand gestures to help communicate a message. The WHNP may use hand gestures but must be aware of how much they are doing this. The WHNP should avoid overgesturing, as this will take away from their overall message.
- Touch: Therapeutic touch is appropriate in certain instances with certain patients. This could involve touching their hand, putting one hand on their shoulder, or even a hug. Caution should be used when employing therapeutic touch, as some patients might find this uncomfortable. The WHNP should use their best judgment on when this type of intervention is most appropriate and helpful.
- Mannerisms: Everyone has certain unique mannerisms, or a way they speak or gesture. The WHNP should be aware of their own quirks and idiosyncrasies if possible and make certain they do not interfere with the patient's care or cause offense.
- Eye contact: Good eye contact is crucial to good patient care. Not enough eye contact shows lack of interest and boredom; too much eye contact can be construed as weird and scary. The WHNP should

be aware of their eye contact and use it as a listening tool to properly tune in to the patient's message they are trying to send.

Interprofessional Practice

Interprofessional Roles and Responsibilities

The difficult part of coordinating care and ensuring consistency is the number of interprofessional roles and responsibilities within the healthcare team. Each individual healthcare professional working toward the goals stated in the patient's care plan introduces the possibility of unintended overlap and miscommunication. The nurse's role in preventing these discrepancies is to understand who does what and why. That may sound generic, but understanding the dynamics of the healthcare team can help prevent lapses in patient care as well as provide the patient with a better healthcare experience:

Doctors:

- Consists of medical doctors (MDs) and doctors of osteopathic medicine (DOs) Both MDs and DOs receive the same amount of training, but DOs specifically train with additional holistic models of care.
- Roles and responsibilities include diagnosing the patient, formulating treatment plans with additional diagnostics/therapies/medications, providing preventative healthcare, and providing information regarding healthcare decisions.

Advanced Practice Providers:

- Consists of nurse practitioners (NPs) and physician assistants (PAs)
- Advanced practice providers can function with the same roles and responsibilities as the doctors, but may require oversight depending on the state's scope of practice.
- Advanced practice providers receive less schooling and clinical training than a doctor.
- Nurses:
- Consists of registered nurses (RNs) and licensed practical nurses (LPNs, also sometimes referred to as licensed vocational nurses [LVNs])
- Roles and responsibilities of the nurse include performing routine patient assessments, administering orders from doctors or advanced practice providers, being a patient advocate, providing patient education, and coordinating care.
- The difference between RNs and LPNs is the level of education and treatments provided. The RN is able to perform more complex medical therapies, while the LPN provides more direct patient care.
- Nursing Assistants:
- Roles and responsibilities include duties assigned by the doctor/advanced practice provider or nurse that are within the state's scope of practice (e.g., bathing, feeding, and toileting).
- Medical Social Workers:
- Roles and responsibilities include providing counseling, providing referrals for community resources, being a patient advocate, and using tools to assess the patient's well-being.

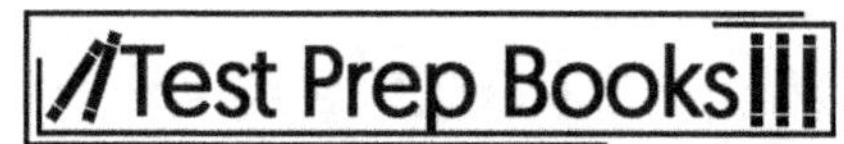

- Additional Interdisciplinary Team Members:
- Can consist of physical therapists, speech therapists, occupational therapists, respiratory therapists, dieticians, spiritual counselors/chaplains, healthcare specialists, or mental health counselors

Interprofessional Collaboration

The integration of physical and mental healthcare is an important aspect of the Medical Home, also known as the Medicaid health home model. The model shows collaborative care programs as an approach to integration in which primary care providers, care managers, and psychiatric consultants work together to provide care and monitor patient progress. These programs have been shown to be both clinically-effective and cost-effective for a variety of mental health conditions, in a variety of settings, using several different payment mechanisms.

Some of the benefits of **collaboration** include improved patient outcomes, decreased healthcare costs, decreased length of stay, improved patient and nurse satisfaction, and improved teamwork. Collaboration related to patient care has been widely studied and is considered as both a process and an outcome, which occurs when no single individual is able to solve a patient problem. Collaboration as a process is defined as a synthesis of diverse opinions and skills that is employed to solve complex problems. As an outcome, collaboration is defined as a complex solution to a problem that requires the expertise of more than one individual. This view of collaboration characterizes the process as a series of actions by more than one individual, which creates a solution to a complex problem.

Initially, all members of the collaborative team must identify their own biases and acknowledge the effect of these mental models on the decision-making process. In addition, members must also be aware that the complexity of the problem will be matched by the complexity of the mental models of the collaborative team members, which will influence the decision-making process. It is also essential for team members to recognize the elements of diversity in the group. For instance, while stereotyping is obviously to be avoided, there are gender differences that should be considered.

Research indicates that men tend to be more task oriented, and women tend to be more relationship oriented in the problem-solving process; this means that consideration of both points of view is necessary for genuine collaboration. Another requisite skill of the collaborative team is the development and usage of conflict resolution skills, which are required to counteract this common barrier to effective collaboration. Team members are required to separate the task from the emotions in the discussion. Effective collaboration also requires that members of the team display a cooperative effort that works to create a win/win situation, while recognizing that collaboration is a series of activities that require time and patience for satisfactory completion.

Common barriers to effective collaboration include conflicting professional opinions, ineffective communication related to the conflict, and incomplete assessment of the required elements of the care plan. Research indicates that physicians tend to stress cure-related activities while nurses tend to encourage care-related activities. This means that some resolution of these differences is required for effective communication. Although the Synergy Model defines collaboration as a necessary part of the process that matches the patient needs with the appropriate nursing competencies, it is also possible that the end product may be the best solution for the patient and at the same time be totally unacceptable to the patient. Collaborative team members should also be aware that while successful collaboration improves patient outcomes, research indicates that genuine collaborative efforts are rarely noted in patient care, often because the group is unable to integrate the diverse mental models of the group members.

Interdisciplinary Rounding

Interdisciplinary rounding can provide an opportunity for team collaboration. Much like a clear hand-off process, interdisciplinary rounds reduce patient care errors, decrease mortality rates, and improve patient outcomes. Interdisciplinary rounds are an excellent place to discuss social service needs, nutritional care services, and transportation needs with all teams coordinating care for the patient in a single setting.

The patient's service needs may vary in depth for the inpatient stay and at the time of discharge; however, there should be an evaluation of these needs and a coordination of care for those services in which there is a need. WHNPs document the action plan as it relates to services and requirements for the patient and collaborate with members of the interdisciplinary team to see that next steps are executed in a timely fashion. In many instances, rounding may not be possible due to the rapid pace and turnover of the medical environment, and thus, clear documentation will be needed to allow for synchronous care coordination.

Nurses, physicians, surgeons, nurse aids, physical and occupational therapists, mental health professionals, and medical assistants are just some of the members who may be collaborating on the care of one patient. Perception of power between these professionals can sometimes create a stressful environment that can also affect patient outcomes. Collaboration among team members is imperative so that patient safety does not become an issue. Collaboration involves joint decision-making activities between both disciplines, rather than nurses only following physician orders. Although each role may have a particular focus throughout the assessment and plan of care activities, they must jointly come together to formulate the best possible plan of care throughout the treatment period. Studies show that an attentive communication style between nurses and physicians has the most positive impact on patients.

Ongoing education of physicians and nurses may be a necessity to support a collaborative environment. In addition to continuing education and in-services, job shadowing can assist in promoting understanding and teamwork by exposing both the nurse and physician to one another's role.

Safety Huddles

A **safety huddle** is a short (ten- to fifteen-minute), interdisciplinary debrief of patient safety concerns that were faced yesterday and anticipated ones that may be expected on the current day. This is a way to improve communication between team members and raise awareness around areas of patient concern. It is not a forum to solve safety issues—that responsibility goes to managers or safety committees—but rather to make sure the healthcare team is on the same page regarding patients' safety. This opportunity for communication lessens the chances of near misses and patient harm. Huddles foster problem identification and team collaboration, thereby increasing patient safety.

Read-Back for Verbal Orders

Read-back occurs when staff reads back orders to ensure that there is a mutual understanding of the need. It is a sequential process that challenges individuals to include only pertinent and relevant data. The recipient of the information validates their understanding of the information. This clarification period gives the communicator an opportunity to clarify details if necessary or to take any essential action.

Ideally, verbal orders should only occur when the provider is physically unable to write out the orders due to an emergency or other extenuating circumstances. Verbal orders must be carefully read back to the provider to ensure accuracy. The verbal order process includes receiving, reading back, documenting, and executing the order. During the read-back, the nurse must repeat the order that was given as it is interpreted. The provider must then confirm the read-back with the nurse.

After the verbal order has been given, the nurse must document the date and time of the order as well as the provider's name. After the emergency situation has passed, the provider must review the verbal order for

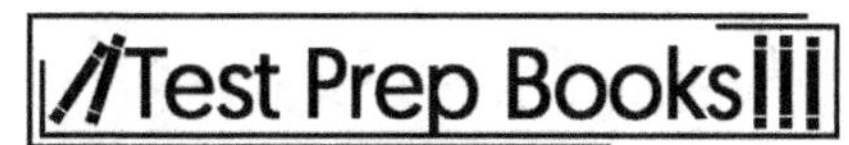

accuracy and sign the order, including the date and time. Verbal orders must be physically signed by the provider within 24 hours of being given to the nurse.

Care Coordination and Transition

Transitioning care refers to any context in which the patient's care level and/or specific caregiver changes. This could be as simple as a nursing shift change, where the nurse attending to a particular patient changes, or as complex as moving the patient from a healthcare facility to their place of residence when the patient requires in-home medical staff and equipment. Any time there is a change in care level, there is an opportunity for the quality of care to decline. This can be due to a lack of communication between healthcare providers, a lack of communication between healthcare providers and the patient, a lack of education provided to the patient about their care, a paperwork mix-up, or some other type of unintentional error. Therefore, standardizing transition procedures and documentation can be a critical and valuable component to quality patient care.

Initial patient boarding is an important moment of data collection. Whether it is the patient's first admission into the healthcare system or a transition into a new system, documenting as much information as possible about the patient's personal history, medical history, the condition that brought the patient into the facility, any documentation of advanced directives or medical proxies, and initial health assessments can be valuable as the patient's time in care progresses. A standardized electronic medical record that can be continuously accessed and updated by all healthcare providers who play a role in the patient's care can prevent complications that arise from lack of communication. Otherwise, comprehensive intake forms at each transition can help minimize the chance of the patient receiving inadequate or improper care.

Continuum of Care

Continuum of care refers to the healthcare team's ability to provide consistent services throughout the process of the patient's healthcare experiences. The healthcare team should be able to follow the patient throughout transfers of care and patient changes while providing the services needed over the patient's lifetime. There are multiple effective continuum-of-care models, but the main aspects include prevention, treatment, and maintenance.

Preventative healthcare can take the form of wellness checks, routine dental visits, and scheduled vaccinations, but the concept is evolving. It can mean education regarding heart health or weight management as well. Essentially, preventative healthcare is the attempt to prevent the need for further healthcare intervention.

This aspect of treatment is present in any healthcare environment, but it's most often found in EDs, urgent cares, specialty offices, and primary care provider offices. Treatment can take the form of medications, surgical interventions, therapies, or procedures.

The aspect of maintenance has the main goal of reducing the progression or symptoms of the disease process. Maintenance can include rehabilitation, therapies, medications, lifestyle changes, and education regarding compliance.

Quality Improvement

Quality improvement is a mechanism to continuously review and improve processes in a system, ensure that work is completed in the most cost-effective manner, and produce the best possible outcomes. Healthcare facilities are constantly aiming to drive down cost and increase reimbursements while delivering the highest quality of healthcare and utilizing analytical methods to achieve this. These analyses and implementations may be done by top administrative employees at the organization and be executed across the healthcare system, or within a particular department. Leadership support is always crucial for positive change to occur and sustain itself.

All processes should be regularly monitored for opportunities for improvement. Common opportunities include areas of reported patient dissatisfaction; federal, state, or internal benchmarks that are not being met; areas of financial loss; and common complaints among staff. While multiple opportunities for improvement may exist, focusing on one at a time usually produces the greatest outcome. When choosing a process to improve, it is important to select one that has the potential to be changed by the members involved (e.g., medical staff often do not have control over external funding sources). Processes where minimal resources are required for change, but that can produce positive end results, are also preferable to more costly improvements. Once the process has been selected, a group of stakeholders that are regularly involved in the process should map out each step of the process while noting areas of wasted resource or process variation. From here, stakeholders can develop a change to test.

PDCA Cycle

The **PDCA cycle** provides a framework for implementing tests of change. Plan, the first step, involves planning the change. This will include accounting for all workflow changes, the staff members involved, and logistics of implementation. It should also include baseline data relating to the problem. Do, the second step, involves implementing the change. During this step, data collection is crucial. For example, if a department believes that implementing mobile work stations will decrease nurses' wait time between patients, the department should keep a detailed record of the time spent with and between each patient. Check, the third step, involves checking data relating to the change with the baseline data and determining if the change improved the process. Act, the final step, involves making the change permanent and monitoring it for sustainability.

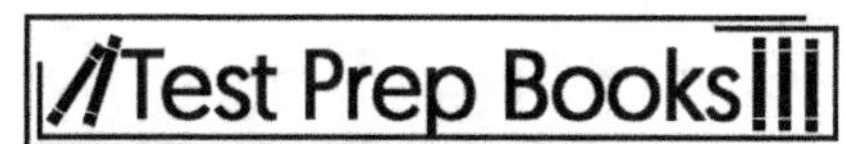

Systems Thinking

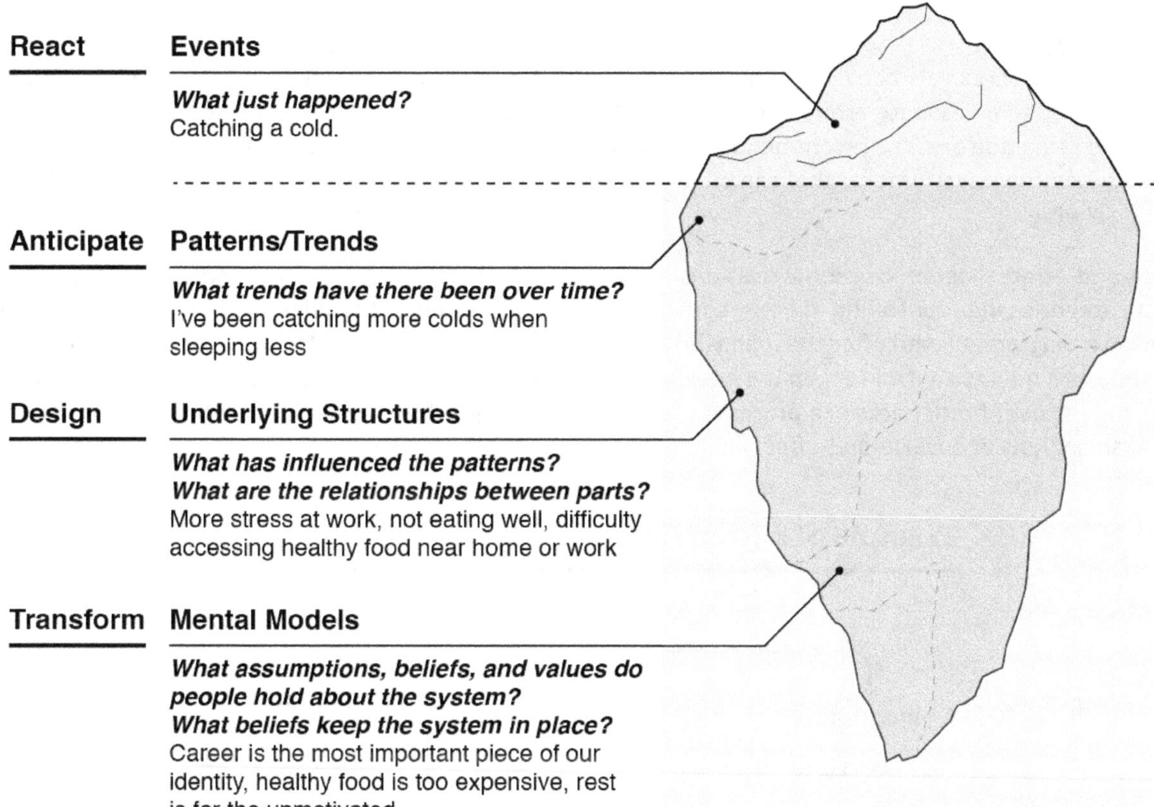

Systems thinking is defined as a link between individuals and their environment. For WHNPs, this refers to their ability to understand the influence of the healthcare environment on patient outcomes. Systems thinking is identified as the goal of all of the **Quality and Safety Education for Nurses** (**QSEN**) competencies, which are acquired by nurses on a continuum that ranges from the care of the individual patient to the care of the entire patient population. The QSEN competencies were originally identified to improve patient outcomes in response to extensive research that identified a significant difference between the care of patients and the improvement in patient outcomes resulting from that care. The nursing competencies include patient-centered care, evidence-based practice, teamwork and collaboration, safety, quality and improvement, and informatics. Successful interventions associated with each of these criteria for professional nursing practice require the ability to apply the systems thinking approach to care.

Competency related to systems thinking requires appropriate education and clinical experience, and is also identified as one of the nursing competencies in the **Synergy Model**. In that model, novice nurses view the patient and family as isolated in the nursing unit rather than being influenced by the healthcare system, while experienced nurses are able to integrate all of the resources in the healthcare system to improve patient outcomes. Several of the learning activities designed to improve nurses' ability to acquire systems thinking include creation of a grid that identifies the nursing competencies across the continuum from isolated, individual care to the level of care associated with systems thinking. There are assessment models that apply this exercise to specialty care units such as emergency care, long-term care, and outpatient care, which identify specific systems needs for these areas. Other exercises include tracking unit statistics for the QSEN competencies followed by the creation, implementation, and evaluation of a plan that applies systems thinking to address that competency. All of these activities help nurses integrate patient needs with all available resources in order to improve outcomes.

Root Cause Analysis

Root cause analysis can also be used as a learning exercise for systems theory because this process, which is commonly used to investigate errors, looks at all elements of an institution's relationship with the error. Case studies and reflection are also recommended as useful learning aids for systems thinking. In addition, there are valid assessment instruments that can be used to assess systems thinking skills acquired through these learning activities.

A **cause-and-effect diagram** can show relationships between factors and can organize potential causes into smaller categories in order to find out why something happened or how it could happen. It is also known as an Ishikawa diagram, named after the man who designed it, Kaoru Ishikawa. Although it was originally developed as a quality control tool, in the healthcare setting the diagram is used to discover the root cause of a problem, uncover bottlenecks in a process or identify where and why a process isn't working. This is called a root cause analysis or a cause-and-effect analysis.

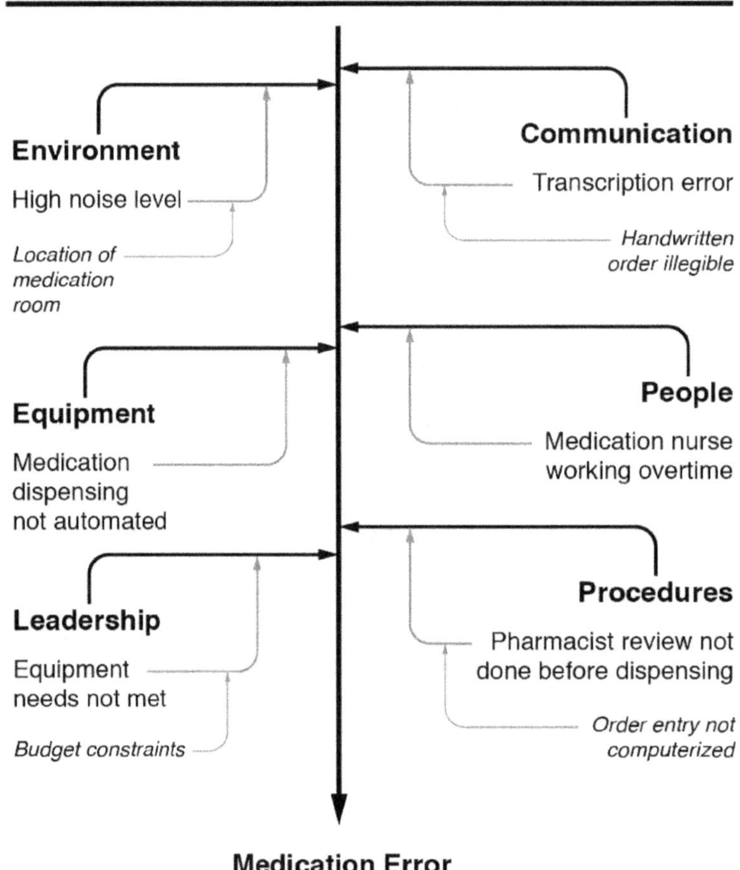

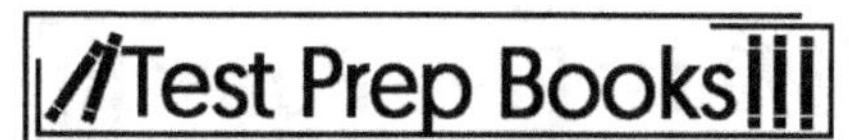

The root cause analysis (RCA) is used when there is an adverse event, a sentinel event, or close call in the medical setting. It can also be used when there is a concern about a process due to repeated errors, when there is a possibility of serious errors, and when there are high-cost errors. The RCA answers the following critical questions:

- What happened or is still happening?
- How did it happen?
- Why did it happen?
- How can we prevent it from happening again?
- What can we learn from this?

FMEA

Failure mode and effects analysis (FMEA) is a systematic method to discover all the ways something can go wrong in a process and then addressing each of those possibilities. The failure mode is the way something might fail. The effects analysis concerns the consequences of the failure. The overall goal of this system is to identify potential failures and prevent them from happening. FMEA is a team-based tool that includes the following:

- Identifying the steps in the process
- Failure modes (What could go wrong at each step?)
- Failure causes (How could the failures happen?)
- Failure effects (What would the consequences of each failure be?)

Once these have been identified, the next steps are to determine the likelihood of the failure occurring, the likelihood of catching the failure, and the severity of consequences if the failure occurred. Then the potential failures are ranked by risk level so the team knows which to address first.

The FMEA tool can be used at several different junctures, but is best used before a new process is launched to predict potential failure. It can also be used when an existing process needs improvement, when existing processes are being used in a new manner, or when an existing process is being modified.

Let's walk through an example. Say a provider initiates a new drug therapy for a patient. The steps in the process are identified. First, the provider initiates therapy; second, the administration of medication begins; third, the provider monitors the patient's initial response to the new medication; etc. Then potential failures for each step would be identified. So, for the first step (provider initiates therapy), possible failures could include that the order wasn't entered into the electronic health record (EHR) or that the provider did not check the five rights of medication administration. These possible errors would be identified for each step mentioned earlier. Then the team would identify how these mistakes could occur. Maybe the provider got called away to an emergency and could not enter the order, maybe the wrong patient was pulled up on the EHR and the order was entered under the wrong patient's record, or maybe the wrong medication was entered for the correct patient. Next the team would determine the consequences of each failure and rank them in order of severity. If the medication was not ordered, there would be a delay in care. If the medication was urgent, not administering it could have serious consequences. The same applies if the wrong medication or patient was chosen. Along with the severity ranking, the team would evaluate the likelihood of catching these errors before they happen. Lastly, strategies would be developed to prevent these errors from happening. Most EHRs have safety checks built in when prescribing medications. Nurses must scan the patient and the medication before administering. The five rights of medication administration are frequently reviewed on the unit. By breaking up a process into steps and then identifying and preventing potential pitfalls, the workplace and the patients become much safer.

Reflective Practice

Reflective practice refers to the act of looking back upon one's practice or work to understand a particular situation better and then using this reflection to improve their practice. Reflection can be more appropriate in certain situations, and understanding when and how to reflect is necessary for this practice to be successful. Reflective practice may also involve making changes to one's practice and then further assessing how those changes worked. In addition, reflective practice can be promoted by positive nurse leaders and mentors. Reflective practice can create better outcomes for patients when integrated into practice.

There are many situations when the WHNP may find that reflection is helpful and even necessary. Most commonly, reflective practice may be implemented following negative situations. If there are mistakes made during a procedure, complications following a procedure, or a patient expresses unhappiness with the care they have received, it can be beneficial to look back on what may have gone wrong. Identifying where a fallout may have happened and then considering how it could be avoided in similar situations in the future is a necessary form of practice improvement and education. This can also be done in positive situations. When the WHNP reflects on how actions taken in a situation were successful, those actions can then be further applied to promote more positive outcomes.

Once the WHNP has reflected upon how a particular situation proceeded, the WHNP can then take action to potentially implement changes for future situations. After these changes are implemented, reflective practice is further used to determine the successes and/or failings of said changes. The WHNP may reflect on whether the changes made a difference in outcomes, and if these outcomes were better or worse than before the change was implemented. Here's an example of this: when a nurse reconstitutes a medication, he notices that the pressure in the bottle causes some of the medication to spray out when drawn up, leading to waste and the patient not receiving all of the medication. The nurse might try a new method of mixing and drawing up the medication, such as first drawing air out of the bottle to reduce the pressure. The nurse should then reflect on whether or not his new technique prevented medication waste. The nurse may even employ the knowledge and experience of those in leadership or mentor roles to help solve this problem. When nurse leaders and mentors promote a nonjudgmental environment that allows for constructive feedback and quality improvement, they can play a vital role in promoting reflective practice in the nursing profession.

Reflective practice is not always purely an individual action; it can involve the entire healthcare team. Often after a particularly difficult situation with unclear outcomes, the team may come together to debrief on what went well, what could have improved, and what to do moving forward. These can be especially common following situations involving close teamwork and high levels of stress, such as codes or procedures with unexpected complications. However, reflective practice can also be applied to day-to-day activities and changes. Reflective practice can be an important part of quality improvement measures within a unit.

Resource Management

Coordination

Resource coordination occurs at the federal and state levels, at the care organization level, and at the provider and patient level. The goal at each level is the same: for all patients, provide comprehensive, cost-effective, timely, and individualized care that results in positive patient outcomes. Poor resource management is associated with duplication of services, lengthy wait times for care delivery, and decreased patient satisfaction. The purpose of the patient-centered medical home (PCMH) is to provide access to primary care and specialty providers, timely completion of preventive, diagnostic, and therapeutic services, and the ongoing evaluation and revision of the plan of care.

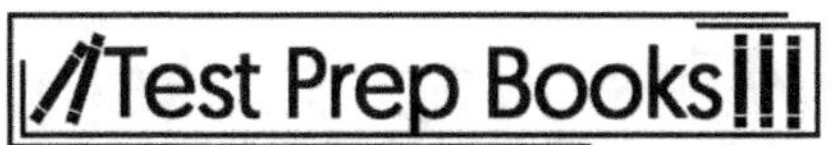

Care coordination in this model also requires the expertise of certified medical assistants who might manage insurance claims and reimbursement, provide patient care, or manage the agency's calendar. Coordination of services in the primary care setting also addresses support for patients' self-care management for specific patient populations such as patients with chronic illnesses such as diabetes, modifiable risk factors such as obesity and smoking, and special needs such as pregnancy. Improved self-management skills are associated with improved outcomes. The patient portal can be used for patient-provider messaging, coaching, and e-visits to monitor the patient's progress when face-to-face visits are not required. The downside of the electronic patient interfaces is that the technology remains inaccessible to many patients, either because of the inability to negotiate the websites or the lack of internet access.

The use of the electronic health record (EHR) is an important element for the coordination of care at the agency level. The EHR is regulated by the Office of the National Coordinator for Health Information (ONC). Currently, most providers choose onsite architecture for the EHR; however, cloud-based systems are increasingly available. There are several ONC-approved software providers for the onsite management of the EHR, such as Epic, Cerner, and MEDITECH. This expensive but necessary technology can be configured to meet all the coordination needs of the provider, including data that support reimbursement and regulatory requirements and enhanced patient interactions that can track the progress of clinical therapies such as hypertension or blood glucose management.

Cost-Effectiveness

Cost-effectiveness compares the effectiveness of the patient outcomes with the costs associated with the outcome. Consumer groups collaborated with physician's groups to establish the Choosing Wisely initiative which calls attention to the wide-spread use of low-value interventions in primary care. One of the initial targets of this initiative was the identification of low-value interventions used to treat patients that were covered by Medicare. Currently, the database contains more than six hundred recommendations from physician's groups that are updated as the guidelines as necessary. The Choosing Wisely website also includes a patient database that prepares patients to ask all the right questions when considering treatment options.

A national study recently identified three common low-value treatments that should be reconsidered by providers. These treatments include spinal injections to treat lower back pain, imaging for non-specific lower back pain, and head imaging for non-specific headache complaints. Low-value interventions are more commonly prescribed for patients with insurance coverage, or by providers that are concerned about litigation or in agencies with reimbursement plans that support utilization.

Providers and patients should understand the process of **cost-effectiveness analysis** (CEA) that calculates the effectiveness of an intervention relative to the costs of the intervention. Additional cost versus effectiveness information is provided by comparative effectiveness research (CER), which generates outcome comparisons for two or more interventions for a specific disease. The information obtained from these analyses provides patients and providers with evidence-based options. CER can address, for example, hypertension, diabetes care for patients receiving chemotherapy, and myocardial infarction drug therapy. There are procedural questions surrounding the use of observational studies in CER; however, there is also agreement that randomized controlled trials (RCT) studies are expensive and unnecessary.

Quality Patient Outcome Measures

WHNPs should understand that the patient outcomes rely on a complex combination of the patient's individual biological pharmacotherapeutic profile, degree of adherence with the plan, socioeconomic factors, and existing comorbidities. Much of the research on patient adherence focuses on economic factors, while many providers believe that the patient outcomes should be the top priority. Quality improvement activities at the administration level can address many of these issues by standardizing the provider approach to the development of the therapeutic plan. Some of the issues addressed can include methods of education, monitoring procedures for drugs with known or high-risk for the development of adverse drug reactions, and examination of hospital readmissions following the administration of the target drug.

WHNPs promote best patient outcomes by providing education to patients and families by utilizing best practice guidelines and using these in the nursing process. Ultimately, the purpose of education, care bundles, core measures, and guidelines is to promote the best possible patient outcomes. Patient outcomes are identified as high priority by nurses, physicians, patients, families, professional organizations, and governing bodies. One of the quality objectives of the Affordable Care Act (ACA), enacted in 2010, is fewer avoidable hospital readmissions. Avoidable hospital readmissions are considered negative outcomes for all parties involved, but especially for the patients. The Institute for Healthcare Improvement (IHI) is a worldwide driver of healthcare improvement and best patient outcomes. The IHI's work focuses on improvement capability, person- and family-centered care; patient safety; and quality, cost, and value. These focus groups are all aimed to improve patient outcomes.

The **Centers for Medicare and Medicaid Services** (**CMS**) was formed in 1977. CMS provides value-based incentives to providers and institutions by tying reimbursement to better patient outcomes. Conversely, CMS withholds reimbursement to institutions and providers if a patient is readmitted to the hospital within thirty days of discharge if the readmission is related to the same problem causing the initial hospitalization. For instance, a patient is admitted to the hospital with CHF exacerbation, treated, and released. Two weeks later, the patient is readmitted with CHF exacerbation. Neither the hospital nor the physician is reimbursed for care related to the readmission.

TJC created the **Surgical Care Improvement Project** (**SCIP**) with the goal of substantially reducing negative patient outcomes (surgical mortality and morbidity), specifically surgical site infection (SSI) and venous thromboembolism (VTE).

Patients at Risk for Readmissions

One of the healthcare team's primary goals is to prevent the need for patient readmission and to recognize those patients that are at a higher risk of readmission. **Readmission** is defined as the readmission of a patient to an acute care facility with the same chief complaint within thirty days of discharge. While not all readmissions can be avoided, there are some steps the healthcare team can take to recognize risk factors and provide the necessary resources.

Certain Disease Processes

Disease processes with complexities (especially progressive diseases) increase the need for readmissions, even with adequate treatment and education. These disease processes can include CKD, heart failure, COPD, sepsis, CVA, and MI.

Patient Demographics

Patient demographics that increase the likelihood of a readmission include advanced age, male gender, and lower-income individuals. The patient's education level can also be an issue regarding comprehension of medical treatment.

Inadequate Healthcare

Inadequate healthcare refers to gaps in interdisciplinary communication and poor discharge instructions. If the patient is discharged without proper follow-up, extensive discharge information, and a clear understanding of the path forward, the likelihood of readmission is high.

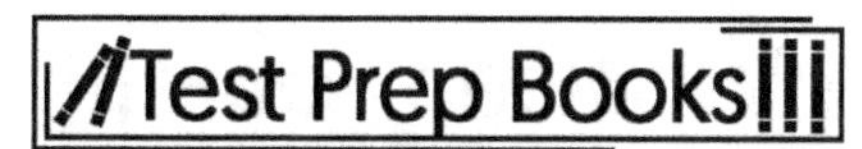

Noncompliance

Lastly, patient noncompliance with the medical treatment plan increases the likelihood of readmission. The nurse can assist in the prevention of noncompliance by thoroughly reviewing the importance of each aspect of the treatment plan (e.g., taking furosemide as ordered to prevent another heart failure exacerbation).

Patient Satisfaction

Patient satisfaction is a highly valued benchmark of healthcare quality. Data relating to patient satisfaction can be collected internally by a healthcare organization or through external institutions that focus on healthcare quality. In the business of healthcare, patient satisfaction often serves as the "demand" in a supply and demand economy. Higher patient satisfaction scores are associated with better patient health outcomes, and consequently associated with happier patients, patients who are more likely to return to and recommend a particular healthcare organization, higher quality of medical staff that the healthcare organization retains, increased level of outside funding that the healthcare organization receives, and fewer medical malpractice suits. Patients report higher satisfaction when they receive care that they find to be tailored to their needs, care that is safe yet efficient, and care that is accessible. In this regard, healthcare delivery requires a nuanced level of customer service; however, rather than delivering a tangible manufactured product, medical staff deliver a product that affects the patient's ability to live well and their long-term physical, mental, and emotional state.

All medical staff are able to provide exceptional patient service by being welcoming and concerned about the patient, allowing space for the patient to voice their concerns and fears, treating the patient like a person rather than a medical case, respecting the patient and showing concern for the patient's family, and being reliable and punctual in their interactions with the patient. Many burdensome aspects of care that could be looked at negatively, such as patient wait times, can be alleviated by simple communication that explains the reasoning behind the issue. Communication and transparency are simple tools that often serve as the key players in managing patient expectations. Medical staff can also maintain communication with the patient after discharge, such as through an online patient portal, to ensure adequate care continues through the patient's full recovery and make the patient feel valued.

Evidence-Based Practice

Evidence-based practice (**EBP**) is a research-driven and facts-based methodology that allows healthcare providers to make scientifically supported, reliable, and validated decisions in delivering care. EBP takes into account rigorously tested, peer-reviewed, and published research relating to the case, the knowledge and experience of the healthcare provider, and clinical guidelines established by reputable governing bodies. This framework allows healthcare providers to reach case resolutions that result in positive patient outcomes in the most efficient manner. This, in turn, allows the organization to provide the best care using the least resources.

There are seven steps to successfully utilizing EBP as a methodology in the nursing field. First, the work culture should be one of a "spirit of inquiry." This culture allows staff to ask questions to promote continuous improvement and positive process change to workflow, clinical routines, and non-clinical duties. Second, the **PICOT framework** should be utilized when searching for an effective intervention, or working with a specific interest, in a case. The PICOT framework encourages WHNPs to develop a specific, measurable, goal-oriented research question that accounts for the patient population and demographics (P) involved in the case, the proposed intervention or issue of interest (I), a relevant comparison (C) group in which a defined outcome (O) has been positive, and the amount of time (T) needed to implement the intervention or address the issue. Once this question has been developed, staff can move on to the third step, which is to research. In this step, staff will explore reputable sources of literature (such as peer-reviewed scholarly journals, interviews with subject matter experts, or widely accepted textbooks) to find studies and narratives with evidence that supports a resolution for their question.

Once all research has been compiled, it must be thoroughly analyzed as part of the fourth step in the process. Analysis of data ensures that the staff is using unbiased research (stringent methodology, statistically significant outcomes, and reliable and valid research designs) and that all information collected is actually applicable to their patient. The fifth step is to integrate the evidence to create a treatment or intervention plan for the patient. The sixth step is to monitor the implementation of the treatment or intervention and evaluate whether it was associated with positive health outcomes in the patient. Finally, practitioners have a moral obligation to share the results with colleagues at the organization and across the field, so that it may be best utilized (or not) for other patients.

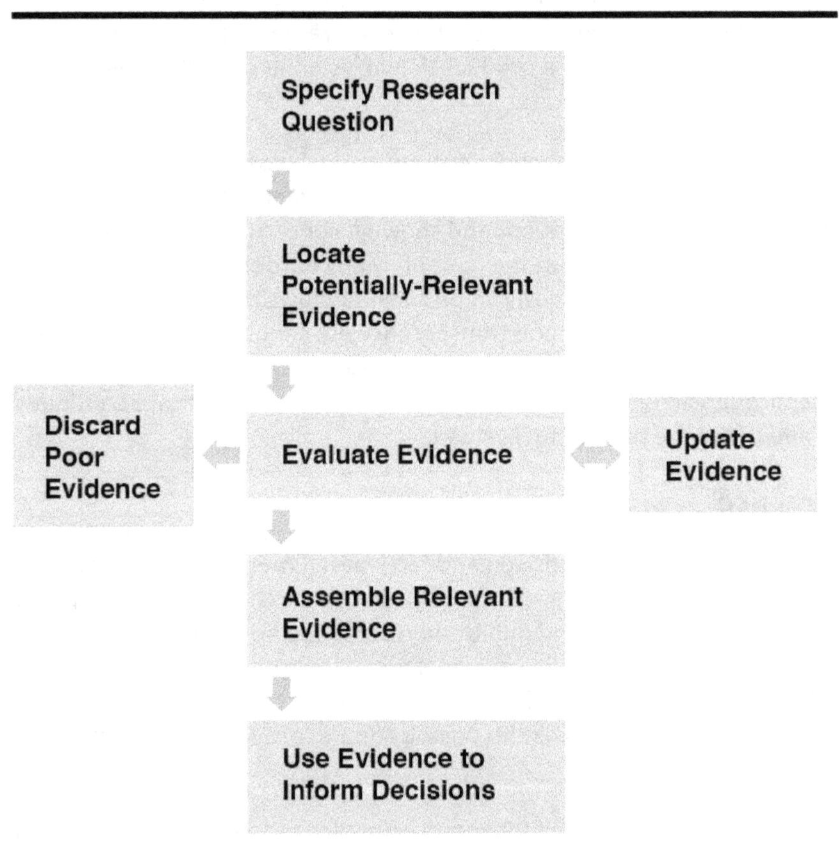

Best Practice

Best practices refer to a set of procedures that are generally accepted to be the most effective method of accomplishing a specific goal. These are shaped by evidence-based practice, professional expertise, and patient or client input. Organizations should follow established best practices in an industry in order to maintain high-quality standards. If an organization is underperforming in an area, researching established best practices for that area and implementing change to reflect best practices is likely to result in improved quality.

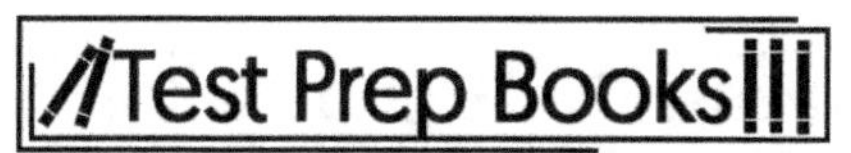

Care Bundles

A **care bundle**, developed by the Institute for Healthcare Improvement, is a succinct set of evidence-based practices to improve patient care for common treatments that pose risks. One example is a central line bundle that has five steps to prevent catheter-related bloodstream infections. Bundles are helpful because they pull together multiple ways of performing a task into one evidence-based process to promote uniformity. The goal of the bundle is to provide the highest possible patient care and outcome.

Bundles have specific formats that are slightly different from checklists and algorithms. Bundles have a stepwise approach in which each step must be completed before moving to the next to achieve the optimum outcome. They are based on Level 1 evidence-based practices, which compare randomized controlled trials to ensure the nurse is using the best data to perform the procedure. Additionally, bundles provide black-and-white, yes-or-no distinctions that leave no gray area up for interpretation. Lastly the bundle must be completed by one healthcare team in one setting. Care bundles are to be repeated as needed until the service is no longer required.

Another example of a bundle is the ventilator bundle, which was created to prevent ventilator-associated pneumonia, a common hospital-acquired infection. Through research, it was found that doing the following four interventions may prevent or delay the onset of this type of pneumonia:

- Administering deep vein thrombosis prophylaxis
- Administering gastric ulceration preventative medications
- Elevating the head or bed to between 30 and 45 degrees
- Assessing whether the patient can breathe on their own daily

Legislative and Licensure Requirements

Similar to the procedural scope of practice for advanced practice nurses, there are legislative and licensure requirements for the use of evidence-based practice (EBP) and research. As with the procedural scope of practice, each state board of nursing will have specific guidelines for EBP and research practices. The nurse must understand the similarities and differences between EBP and clinical research. While both serve as pivotal tools in the improvement of safe, effective patient care, the actual processes and end results are different.

Evidence-based practice looks towards evidence seen in clinical practice to make informed decisions on patient care. Evidence-based practice puts the gathered information into practice. Research focuses more on validating the current nursing practice and gathering information that is already in practice.

Research Terminology

Reliability

Reliability of research articles can be assessed by reviewing the consistency and repeatability of the data. The studies encountered should be able to be reproduced in further trials with similar and consistent results. Reliability does not always equate with validity in the sense that, while a study may be able to repeat the results, that does not necessarily mean that they are accurate. Reliability when the results are also accurate and valid will increase the trustworthiness of the results and study. Valid results should also be reliable and replicable to ensure that the study achieved accurate findings.

Critically Appraising Literature

When performing a literature review, it is important to be able to identify what sources have the most useful information related to a current problem. Not all sources are trustworthy, and not all trustworthy sources are relevant. It is up to the researcher conducting the literature review to determine which sources contain the most useful, credible data. When critically appraising literature related to healthcare and disease prevention, it is important for each source to be free of errors that might steer the course of further research in the wrong direction. Literature should be appraised based on credibility, relevance, and date of publication.

The most **credible literature** comes from academic sources that have been peer reviewed by professionals before publication. For disease prevention, scientific and healthcare-related medical journals are the best source for finding data and articles that have been well researched and cross-examined by multiple parties. Information that has already been confirmed by those in the same industry will have the least chance of containing misleading errors or too much unrelated or opinionated information. The relevance of the literature also needs to be compared with the problem that is being researched. Before conducting research, it is important to set goals and write questions that need to be solved to help the situation. The most relevant data is the data that directly solves these goals and answers the questions that have been laid out in relation to the current problem.

Literature that includes too little or too much data that may be hard to interpret should be avoided. Also, it is important to pay attention to when the literature was published to avoid using data that may be out of date or proven to be ineffective. The most recent articles are the most helpful because they contain the most up-to-date data collection methods and pertain to more modern health problems than those published before newer advancements in modern science were made.

Peer Review Methods

Peer review methods refer to the processes of assessing the validity and use of clinical articles, journals, studies, or nursing practices. The intent behind peer review is to ensure the integrity of the science behind the article or study and to ensure that practice is evidence based. The hope is to minimize harm from inaccurate or deceptive information. Peer review can be used in the academic setting and within the professional setting using several different methods.

Two forms of peer review within the academic setting are meant to emphasize anonymity. One is "single anonymized," where the author does not know who will be reviewing their article or study. This prevents the author from leaning the article's bias in favor of the reviewer and allows the reviewer to feel more comfortable providing negative feedback. The other is "double anonymized," where both the author and reviewer are anonymous in the review process to prevent bias in either direction. While these methods can be useful in reviewing academic articles and studies, it is important for nurses to be aware that the American Nurses Association does not consider anonymized peer review to be the standard of practice within the professional setting as it does not allow for accountability for either party.

Peer review methods that provide more transparency are open peer review and transparent peer review. Within open peer review, all parties are known to one another and accountability from all parties is encouraged. However, this method may discourage some reviewers from providing negative feedback. In order to encourage unbiased feedback, transparent peer review may be employed, in which the reviewer may choose whether or not to have their identity known. These methods can be applied both in the academic setting and within professional practice. A mentor may use open peer review with a mentee to provide feedback to ensure that their practice is evidence-based. On the other hand, a nurse may use transparent peer review when submitting a quality improvement form regarding an incident that had a negative outcome when it might not be appropriate or possible to provide negative feedback to a specific individual.

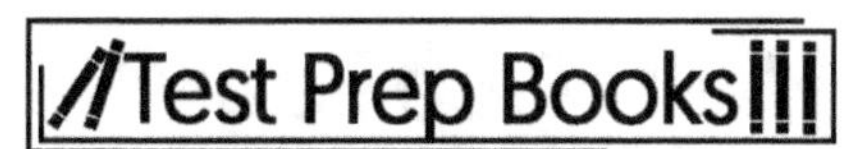

Validity

External Validity

External validity illustrates how well inferences from a sample set can predict similar inferences in a larger population (i.e., can results in a controlled lab setting hold true when replicated in the real world). A sample set with strong external validity allows the researcher to generalize or, in other words, to make strongly supported assumptions about a larger group. For a sample to have strong external validity, it needs to have similar characteristics and context to the larger population about which the researcher is hoping to make inferences. A researcher typically wants to generalize three areas:

> Population: Can inferences from the sample set hold true to a larger group of people beyond the specific people in the sample?
>
> Environment: Can inferences from the sample set hold true in settings beyond the specific one used in the study?
>
> Time: Can inferences from the sample set hold true in any season or temporal period?

If results from the sample set can't hold true across these three areas, the external validity of the study is considered threatened or weak. External validity is strengthened by the number of study replications the researcher is able to successfully complete for multiple settings, groups, and contexts. External validity can also be strengthened by ensuring the sample set is as randomized as possible.

Internal Validity

Internal validity illustrates the integrity of the results obtained from a sample set and indicates how reliably a specific study or intervention was conducted. Strong internal validity allows the researcher to confidently link a specific variable or process of the study to the results or outcomes. The strength of a study's internal validity can be threatened by the presence of many independent variables. This can result in confounding, where it's difficult to pinpoint exactly what is causing the changes in the dependent variables. The internal validity can also be threatened by biases (sampling bias, researcher bias, or participant bias) as well as historical, personal, and/or contextual influences outside the researcher's control (natural disasters, political unrest, participant death, or relocation). Internal validity can be strengthened by designing highly controlled studies or experiment settings that limit these threats.

Significance

Significance in research is vital to explain the purpose of the study as well as who the study is pertinent to and why. Without a statement of significance, there would be no direction or purpose to the research criterion. The significance should also address the importance of the study information and why it is necessary to conduct additional research. The significance statement should cover the "who, what, where, and why" of the study to ensure that the purpose is clear to find reliable and accurate results. Addressing the potential impacts of the study can also help it reach the target audience and ensure that the data is used correctly.

Research Utilization

Nursing research is a crucial component of EBP, high quality healthcare delivery, and positive patient outcomes. Effective nursing research creates and compiles bodies of knowledge relating to all clinical and non-clinical aspects of nursing. Nurses who play a role in nursing research are typically advanced-level, senior practitioners who have the necessary experience to contribute further to existing bodies of nursing knowledge through personal expertise, the ability to run or be involved in conducting research trials, and in accurately collecting and analyzing data.

Nurse researchers typically have advanced educational degrees, such as a master's or doctorate degree, and may work in specialized fields as a nurse practitioner. However, as entry-level nurses spend more time and gain more exposure to different aspects of the field, they should keep in mind that a nurse researcher is a highly skilled and rewarding career path that is critical to the development and advancement of the nursing field. High quality nursing research shapes the scope of clinical education for entry-level and experienced nurses; influences healthcare policy at the local, state, and federal levels; and enhances standard operating procedures within a healthcare organization. Together, these allow for organizations to deliver the highest level of care to patients who need them at the lowest costs.

Nurses who choose to pursue research as a career can expect to become involved in different aspects of research design and the research process. Nurse researchers will need to pass training modules that review the legalities and ethics of working with human populations in research, which is a different avenue than treating patients for disease or injury. Nurse researchers can expect to learn how to write research proposals, which serves as a large component of applying for funding, in addition to becoming familiar with seeking out viable funding sources. Depending on the end goal of the study, nurse researchers may learn how to design objective study trials, collect data through laboratory work or through sample surveys, conduct and interpret statistical data analysis, and write conclusive discussions about their findings.

Upon completion, nurse researchers can expect to be involved in the publication process, where a formal manuscript detailing the design and findings of the research study are submitted to scholarly journals. Journals often require extensive revisions and editing, so nurses should be prepared to follow up with their manuscripts. Most research projects include collaboration with doctorate-level researchers from other disciplines who share a vested interest in the topic or have skills to contribute to the project. For example, health research teams often include a biostatistician whose primary contribution is to compile, analyze, and interpret collected data. Entry-level nurses, interns, or students may choose to assist with simpler, but necessary, tasks such as survey administration or data entry. Recruiting individuals to help with these sorts of tasks can provide a great support to the research team.

The National League for Nursing (NLN) is an organization in the United States that promotes research activities through networking, support, guidelines, and funding. The NLN publishes research priorities every four years. Current priorities include further investigating evidence-based practices, promoting research exposure to student learners in order to set the foundation for health promotion and disease prevention, and evaluating best practices relating to end-of-life and other life transitional care for both patients and their families. The NLN's website, www.nln.org, is an excellent resource for current nurses to find continuing education opportunities and explore research tools to support and enhance their career paths.

Research Process

The **research process** in nursing is similar to the research process in any workplace, with the goal of finding and accumulating information in attempts to further knowledge. The importance of routine research within healthcare cannot be overstated. With evolving technology and improvements in care processes, protocols are almost constantly changing. For the nurse to stay up to date in the constantly evolving healthcare system, using the proper form of research is essential. Just as important as the concept of research itself, is the correct practice and use of the research. Credibility is of utmost importance in clinical research. The following is a review of the procedural process of nursing research:

1. Select the specific topic: While this step sounds relatively straightforward, the research team will need to understand the importance of selecting an appropriate topic. While there are plenty of issues that warrant discussion, not all issues are appropriate for a research topic. The research team needs to be sure that the topic selected has an attainable solution or outcome. The topic will also need to be specific enough to be measurable.

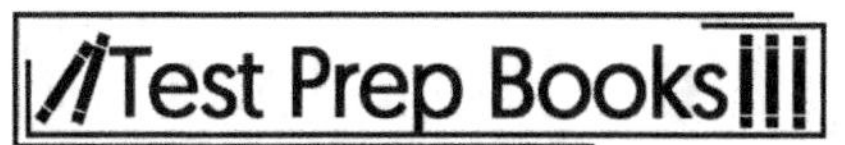

2. Find additional background information on the specific topic and formulate hypotheses: This stage can be known as the pre-planning phase, as the research team will be looking for general background information to formulate hypotheses. The point of this phase is to further assess the quality of the topic selected for a research project.

3. Design framework for research: This stage can be known as the planning phase. The research team will focus on finding the appropriate forms of data collection and establishing specific roles for the extraction of the data. The goal is to find data specific enough to answer the research topic/question while maintaining practical and ethical values.

4. Utilize approved resources for detailed data collection: Data collection is the meat and potatoes of the research process. It is the unrefined collection of data that is related to the research topic. The importance of data collection is to obtain unbiased information from credible sources. Most facilities/agencies will have a resource library that can be freely used, but access to multiple credible sources is the best research practice.

5. Organize data collected and evaluate findings: Separating the data into quantitative and qualitative sections can help with the organization and evaluation of data. Using visuals for the quantitative data (based on numbers/measurable) and using direct quotes for the qualitative data (interpretive/subjective) can help the research team organize the information to closely assess the general findings.

6. Analyze and interpret data collected: Analyzing the data and interpreting the results is rarely the form of closure to the research topic. This stage usually brings clarity on the need for further research on the topic, research on an additional topic, or revision of the entire research plan. This stage allows the research team to review the interpreted data with the hypotheses.

7. Properly cite any sources: Properly citing sources is not only giving credit to the original author but also avoiding plagiarism. Giving credit to the original source—whether it's a demonstration of the research or written literature—also allows the audience to follow the research.

Clinical Inquiry

Clinical inquiry is an ongoing process that evaluates and challenges clinical practice in order to propose the needed change. Clinical inquiry has several components or attributes, including critical thinking, clinical reasoning, clinical judgment, critical reasoning and judgment, and creative thinking. The process is viewed as the critical structure for the establishment of evidence-based practice and quality improvement efforts. In the Synergy Model, professional nurses employ clinical inquiry to innovate and facilitate interventions that are appropriate to patient care needs. Clinical inquiry is a rigorous process that requires attention to the rules of nursing research, such as attention to sample size, and a correct match among the data, the study design, and the statistical measures.

When used to implement evidenced based practice, clinical inquiry can result in replacing an outdated, even counter-productive nursing intervention with an intervention that effectively addresses the needs of the patient. Nurses who are involved in this form of clinical inquiry are viewed as evaluators and innovators in the Synergy Model. Matching patient needs with nursing competencies means that professional nurses are responsible for challenging all nursing interventions to be sure that they represent current best practice standards. As innovators, nurses are in the best position to research, implement, and evaluate alternative care practices.

Nurses acquire clinical inquiry skills on a continuum that is based on education and clinical experience. As is the case with the other nursing competencies included in the Synergy Model, this progressive development is consistent with Benner's Novice to Expert model that views the development of nursing expertise as a progressive process that requires ongoing education and clinical experience. Novice nurses are able to implement clinical innovations developed by others, identify their own learning needs, and enlist the aid of other nurses to identify critical needs of the patient. Experienced nurses are able to question the adequacy of interventions and challenge the "we have always done it this way" philosophy that is the most common rationale for many nursing interventions. They are also able to assess the utility of alternative interventions. The Synergy Model views the practice of expert nurses as the point at which clinical inquiry and clinical reasoning become inseparable elements of clinical practice. Expert nurses are able to predict changes in the patient's condition that require revision of the plan of care, and they are also able to develop and implement alternative approaches to address those changes.

Dissemination of Findings

Public funds are the most common source of research funding, which means that researchers are obligated to design studies that provide valid results that are applicable to some form of patient care and to disseminate the results appropriately. Common barriers to nursing research efforts include inadequate funding, limited access to appropriate patient populations, and lack of institutional support for research initiatives. The rapid expansion of new knowledge from multiple sources can also inhibit the assimilation and application of new care interventions by expert nurses.

In addition, the final step of the clinical inquiry process, knowledge translation or dissemination, may be the most important step. Knowledge translation refers to the complex process of synthesizing the research findings, disseminating those findings to others, and integrating the findings into clinical practice. Barriers to this process include lack of rigor in the original research design with respect to sample size, data interpretation, and the applicability of the research findings. The failure of nursing researchers to access all possible modes of the dissemination of study results has also been identified as a significant barrier to the application of new interventions. All of these system-wide and individual barriers potentially limit the use of innovative patient care interventions.

Practice Quiz

1. The hospital where the WHNP works has been experiencing an increase in patient readmissions. How can the WHNP become involved in addressing this issue?
    a. Provide detailed written discharge instructions for patients.
    b. Create an improved, standardized discharge education process with the interdisciplinary team.
    c. Conduct a root cause analysis on reasons for readmission.
    d. Reiterate the importance of medication adherence to the patients.

2. The WHNP is doing an admission assessment with a patient who speaks Farsi. The patient speaks some English but is not fluent. The patient's husband is fluent in English and says that he will translate for her. What is the best response by the WHNP?
    a. "Thank you. That will be very convenient, and I appreciate your help."
    b. "It's better if we speak English. I think she'll be able to understand, and I want her to be able to reply to me directly."
    c. "I'm concerned that you might not be able to translate the complex medical terms I'm going to be using, so I think we should use a translator."
    d. "The hospital does not allow me to use family members as translators. We will use an approved translator, but you are more than welcome to participate."

3. Which of the following correctly identifies a critical distinction between the two concepts of advocacy and moral agency?
    a. Advocacy is legally binding.
    b. Moral agency requires accountability for right and wrong decisions.
    c. Advocacy is implied in the paternalistic view of patient care.
    d. Moral agency only refers to support for at-risk populations.

4. Which of the following ethical principles is MOST closely related to advocacy?
    a. Distributive justice
    b. Beneficence
    c. Nonmaleficence
    d. Fidelity

5. When can a minor give consent for their own care?
    a. All minors under the age of 18 can give consent for their own care.
    b. Only emancipated minors can give consent for their own care.
    c. Only minors between the ages of 16 and 18 can give consent for their own care.
    d. Minors can only give consent for care in the presence of a guardian or parent.

See answers on the next page

Answer Explanations

1. C: The WHNP should conduct a root cause analysis to determine the reasons for increased readmission rates prior to taking any interventions. This will then allow the WHNP to collaborate with other healthcare professionals to decrease readmission rates. Choice *A* is helpful but does not address the root cause. Choice *B* is also helpful, but this cannot be done until the root cause is addressed. Choice *D* is also incorrect as the nurse does not know whether the cause of readmissions is due to medication compliance. However, this is an important idea to discuss during discharge teaching.

2. D: Bilingual family members should not be used for translation of nursing communication. However, they should be respected and included in the conversation. Choice *A* is incorrect because the husband should not be relied upon as a translator. Choice *B* is incorrect because the patient is not fluent in English and may not be able to express herself fully. Choice *C* is incorrect because it is disrespectful to the husband and does not convey that use of a hospital-approved translator is required.

3. B: Moral agency refers to decision-making that includes accountability for right and wrong decisions by the moral agent. Advocacy is an ethical principle that is not legally enforced. However, many argue that paternalism is contrary to advocacy because of the assumption that the "system" knows what is best for the patient without concern for the patient's wishes. Moral agency is not restricted to a specific population; however, the nurse will assess the ability of all patients to make informed decisions.

4. A: Distributive justice refers to the allocation of scarce resources, and advocacy is support for policies that protect at-risk populations. The WHNP understands that scarce resource allocation may be sub-standard in certain populations. In nursing, nonmaleficence refers to the act of inflicting the least amount of harm possible in order to reach a favorable result. Fidelity refers to faithfulness but does not specifically address resources or the patient population.

5. B: An adult must be present to make decisions regarding a child's medical care unless the child is an emancipated minor. Emancipated minors are individuals under the age of 18 who are legally independent of any biological or non-biological guardians. Because of this, they can declare decisions about their healthcare without the input of another person.

Practice Test #1

1. A 47-year-old woman has been recommended to undergo hormone replacement therapy (HRT) to address symptoms of menopause. She asks the WHNP if there are any cancer risks associated with starting this therapy. The WHNP understands which statement to be true?
   a. HRT use can lower the risk for ovarian cancer.
   b. The risk of lung cancer increases with long term use of HRT.
   c. HRT can increase the risk for breast cancer.
   d. Estrogen may have a role in preventing pancreatic cancer.

2. The WHNP is caring for a 24-year-old woman in her first trimester of pregnancy who has been experiencing moderate vaginal bleeding. The WHNP understands that which of the following factors is true regarding first trimester spontaneous abortions?
   a. Young maternal age increases the risk.
   b. Type 2 diabetes is a common cause.
   c. Moderate exercise increases the risk.
   d. Chromosomal abnormalities are the most common cause.

3. A patient is being seen for the treatment of breast cancer. Which of the following is considered a positive prognostic factor?
   a. The tumor is 6 centimeters.
   b. The cancer is node-positive.
   c. The tumor is hormone receptor-negative.
   d. The cancer cells are low grade.

4. The WHNP is providing care for a 73-year-old female patient with advanced stage breast cancer who is currently inpatient for treatment of dehydration and diarrhea. The WHNP enters just after the patient's family has left from a visit. The patient states, "I know my daughters keep telling me to keep fighting, but I am so tired of being sick all the time. I wish I could just be done with all these treatments." Which of the following would be the most appropriate response by the WHNP?
   a. "You are doing a great job. You will get through this! Keep fighting."
   b. "This must be very challenging for you. Have you talked to your family and doctor about your feelings?"
   c. "Are you having thoughts of harming yourself?"
   d. "I know this is difficult. You should consider what your family is saying."

5. Which of the following is the first line of treatment for chronic neuropathic pain?
   a. Calcium channel alpha-2-delta ligands
   b. Opioids
   c. Nonsteroidal anti-inflammatory drugs
   d. Nonopioid analgesics

6. An adolescent male presents with severe left testicle pain following a soccer game. The patient endorses nausea and vomiting. The left testicle is red, swollen, and edematous. The cremasteric reflex is absent. Which part of the treatment plan should the NP perform first?
   a. Perform a doppler ultrasound.
   b. Call 911.
   c. Perform manual reduction.
   d. Order pain medications.

7. Which statement about chlamydia is correct?
    a. Men are more often asymptomatic than women.
    b. Antibody testing is the most reliable indicator of the presence of the condition.
    c. Routine testing is generally not necessary for men.
    d. The degree of risk for complications in women is similar to a UTI.

8. A 57-year-old woman wishes to discuss breast cancer prevention with the NP. She is concerned because her 49-year-old sister was recently diagnosed with breast cancer. The patient herself is nulliparous, has enjoyed good health, and has a reassuring physical examination, including normal vital signs and no abnormalities on breast imaging. A history of which of the following is a contraindication for raloxifene (Evista®)?
    a. Osteoporosis
    b. Uterine fibroids
    c. Venous thromboembolism (VTE)
    d. Type 2 diabetes mellitus

9. High blood sugar stimulates the kidneys to do which of the following?
    a. Produce less urine
    b. Concentrate the urine
    c. Retain more sodium
    d. Produce more urine

10. The WHNP is providing education to a patient with a history of PE who is prescribed Warfarin and asks about consuming foods high in vitamin K. Which of the following statements by the WHNP is the most appropriate response?
    a. "It is important to avoid foods high in vitamin K because they can interfere with the effectiveness of Warfarin."
    b. "You should consume foods with vitamin K consistently to maintain a balanced diet while on Warfarin."
    c. "It is important to maintain a consistent intake of vitamin K to avoid sudden changes in Warfarin's effectiveness."
    d. "You should completely eliminate foods high in vitamin K from your diet to ensure the optimal effects of Warfarin."

11. A WHNP is meeting with a 37-year-old female with newly diagnosed breast cancer prior to initiating chemotherapy. The WHNP understands which of the following to be true about discussing fertility preservation?
    a. Most women over 35 years of age prefer to focus on initiating treatment instead of prioritizing future fertility.
    b. Pre-cancer fertility preservation counseling has little effect on the patient's quality of life post-treatment.
    c. Pre-treatment fertility counseling can decrease decisional regret post-treatment.
    d. Emergent treatment takes precedence over discussions of fertility.

12. Which of the following is NOT a congenital heart defect found in the tetralogy of Fallot?
    a. Pulmonary valve stenosis
    b. Ventricular septal defect
    c. Atrial septal defect
    d. Hypertrophic right ventricle

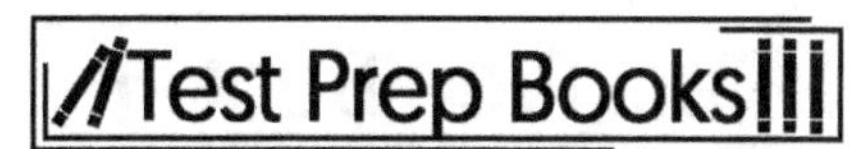

13. T. F. is a 52-year-old female preparing to undergo a core needle breast biopsy. The WHNP understands that this procedure will involve which of the following?
    a. Removing the entirety of the tumor to clear margins
    b. Using a small needle to remove fluid for testing
    c. Using a large needle to aspirate bone marrow for testing
    d. Using a needle to remove tissue for testing

14. Which alteration can result in abnormal increases in the plasma concentration of a drug?
    a. Induction
    b. Inhibition
    c. Desensitization
    d. Absorption

15. Which hormone in the female reproductive system is responsible for progesterone production during pregnancy?
    a. FSH
    b. LH
    c. hCG
    d. Estrogen

16. Which of the following clinical manifestations are indicative of iron-deficiency anemia?
    a. An inflamed and sore tongue
    b. Hyperactivity
    c. Bradycardia
    d. Fingernail clubbing

17. The WHNP is caring for a patient who identifies as transgender. Which of the following interventions is the most appropriate?
    a. Avoid using pronouns when addressing the patient.
    b. Use gender-neutral terms when addressing the patient.
    c. Use the patient's chosen name and pronouns.
    d. Encourage the patient to speak with the provider regarding transitioning.

18. Mammograms have high sensitivity and low specificity. What does that mean?
    a. Most cases of cancer are identified by mammograms with few false positives.
    b. Mammograms can confirm that cancer is not present, but false negatives are common.
    c. The patient's individual cancer characteristics do not affect the mammogram.
    d. Half of the women who have regular mammograms will have a false positive in ten years' time.

19. The nurse practitioner is reviewing labs for a 70-year-old female. Her TSH comes back at 9.0, and Free T4 is low. The NP diagnoses her with hypothyroidism and starts her on Levothyroxine. Given the patient's age, what should the NP consider when choosing the medication dose?
    a. Levothyroxine can cause anticholinergic effects.
    b. Levothyroxine can cause cardiac side effects.
    c. Levothyroxine can cause hepatic side effects.
    d. Levothyroxine can cause renal side effects.

20. Which statement made by a woman with gestational diabetes indicates to the nurse that more teaching is needed?
    a. "I need to monitor my weight."
    b. "I need to watch what I eat."
    c. "I need to stay off my feet as much as possible."
    d. "I need to see my obstetrician regularly."

21. What test is often used to determine if a patient has peripheral arterial disease?
    a. Echocardiography
    b. CT scan of the leg
    c. Electrocardiogram
    d. Ankle-brachial BP index

22. Which of the following should the nurse prioritize when providing education about breastfeeding to expectant parents?
    a. The use of pre-recorded video demonstration
    b. The use of practice dolls
    c. The use of written step-by-step instructions
    d. The use of verbal discussion

23. A patient has had three separate blood pressure readings of 138/88, 132/80, and 135/89, respectively. The WHNP categorizes the patient as which of the following?
    a. Prehypertensive
    b. Normal
    c. Stage 1 hypertensive
    d. Stage 2 hypertensive

24. A nurse is administering a blood transfusion to a patient. An hour after initiation of the transfusion, the patient experiences oxygen desaturation, fever, and hypotension. Transfusion-related acute lung injury (TRALI) is suspected. Which other clinical finding assists in the diagnosis of this condition?
    a. Hypertension on routine vital signs
    b. Sinus bradycardia on an electrocardiogram
    c. Pulmonary infiltrates on a chest x-ray
    d. Jugular venous distention upon assessment

25. Blood product administration can cause which electrolyte imbalance?
    a. Hypocalcemia
    b. Hyponatremia
    c. Hypokalemia
    d. Hypophosphatemia

26. Owing to the role of prostaglandins in the pathophysiology of dysmenorrhea, which medication would most be most appropriate when treating this painful condition?
    a. Dexamethasone
    b. Ibuprofen
    c. Fluoxetine
    d. Venlafaxine

27. Psychosis is a common side effect of which of the following?

    I. Schizophrenia

    II. Methamphetamine, cocaine, or LSD use

III. Bipolar Disorder
IV. HIV antiviral medications

a. Choices II and IV
b. Choices I and II
c. Choices I, II, and III
d. All of the above

28. A 60-year-old female with essential hypertension presents with the following blood pressure readings from the last three visits: 168/90, 172/86, 165/88. She is currently taking Lisinopril 20 mg daily. What adjustment should the nurse practitioner make to the treatment plan after evaluating this data?

a. Switch to Losartan 20 mg
b. Increase Lisinopril to 40 mg
c. Increase Lisinopril to 80 mg
d. Switch to Hydrochlorothiazide (HCTZ)

29. Where does sperm maturation take place in the male reproductive system?

a. Seminal vesicles
b. Prostate gland
c. Epididymis
d. Vas deferens

30. Which technique is most appropriate when inserting a urinary catheter into a patient to help in the prevention of CAUTIs?

a. Sterile
b. Clean
c. Sanitary
d. Aseptic

31. Which of the following is associated with the fetal effects of the Zika virus?

a. Microcephaly
b. Premature birth
c. Cerebral palsy
d. Congenital hip defects

32. Which of the following is an indication for the placement of a vena cava filter to prevent pulmonary embolism (PE)?

a. Pregnancy
b. Documented recurrent PE
c. Active smoking history
d. Age > 65 years

33. Which of the following correctly identifies one of the characteristics of the S_2 heart sound?

a. The sound is heard most commonly in elderly patients.
b. A split S_1 in well elderly patients is more common than a split S_2 sound.
c. The sound is heard best at the left second intercostal space close to the sternum.
d. It requires immediate additional diagnostic testing if present.

34. A 64-year-old woman presents for her annual well-woman exam with concern for pelvic pressure, 20 pound unintentional weight loss, anorexia, and early satiety. She first noticed these symptoms about two months ago. Vital signs are within normal limits. She is ill-appearing, and physical examination reveals a unilateral adnexal mass that is mildly tender to palpation. These findings are concerning for what diagnosis?
   a. Uterine leiomyomata
   b. Endometriosis
   c. Endometrial cancer
   d. Ovarian cancer

35. Which of the following creates sperm?
   a. Prostate gland
   b. Seminal vesicles
   c. Scrotum
   d. Seminiferous tubules

36. A 34-old pregnant patient who is 36 weeks' gestation presents with severe upper abdominal pain, nausea, vomiting, and headache. She reports feeling generally unwell and fatigued for the past few days, and her prenatal care has been unremarkable until now. The WHNP assesses the patient and considers the possibility of HELLP syndrome after reviewing the patient's lab work. Which of the following laboratory findings is most consistent with a diagnosis of HELLP syndrome?
   a. Elevated liver enzymes, low platelet count, and evidence of hemolysis
   b. Normal liver enzymes, elevated white blood cell count, and low platelet count
   c. Elevated liver enzymes, normal platelet count, and evidence of hemolysis
   d. Low liver enzymes, low platelet count, and evidence of hemolysis

37. WHNPs should understand that the lipid-soluble drugs dissolve across the capillary membrane. Which of the following is an additional advantage of lipid solubility?
   a. Lipid-soluble drugs are the only substances that can passively diffuse across the blood-brain barrier.
   b. Lipid solubility is associated with 100 percent absorption rates.
   c. Lipid-soluble drugs cross the cellular membrane by passive diffusion.
   d. The first-pass effect decreases lipid solubility.

38. The WHNP is talking with a patient who is receiving treatment for breast cancer. The patient mentions to the WHNP, "My family and friends keep trying to get in touch with me, and I just don't want to see anyone. I don't really care about anything like I used to." Which of the following is the most appropriate response by the WHNP?
   a. "This is something that everyone goes through."
   b. "That must be difficult. Have you talked to anyone else about how you are feeling?"
   c. "Maintaining support systems is really important, so you should really keep contact with your family and friends."
   d. "I know how you feel. I have experienced that feeling, too."

39. A patient with breast cancer is being evaluated for follow-up after receiving chemotherapy. Which statement made by the patient would be most concerning?
   a. "I have been walking for 30 minutes a day, three times a week."
   b. "I cannot stand the taste of meat since starting treatment."
   c. "I was feeling a little nauseated this week, but ginger tea really helped!"
   d. "My friend recommended I go to acupuncture therapy, so I started that this week."

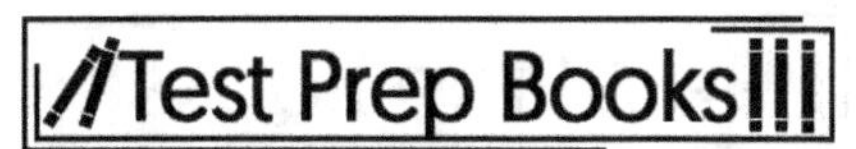

40. Which set of laws was enacted in order to prevent healthcare facilities from turning away patients that needed life-sustaining care, regardless of ability to pay?
    a. The Patient Protection and Affordable Care Act of 2010
    b. The American Health Care Act of 2017
    c. The Emergency Medical Treatment and Labor Act of 1986
    d. The Medicare Introduction Act of 1965

41. Which of the following embolism prophylactic procedures would be contraindicated in a patient with known deep vein thrombosis?
    a. Heparin administration
    b. Enoxaparin administration
    c. Early ambulation
    d. Sequential compression device use

42. The WHNP is caring for a patient with suspected HELLP syndrome. The patient asks the WHNP to explain the complications associated with this diagnosis. Which of the following statements correctly identifies the complications of this syndrome?
    a. The syndrome creates a state of hypercoagulation that can result in infarction of the hepatic vasculature.
    b. Liver dysfunction is reversible with correction of the coagulation defects.
    c. Cerebrovascular effects are rare.
    d. The "complete" form of HELLP is manifested by red cell hemolysis, elevated liver enzyme levels, and low platelet levels.

43. The muscular tube that connects the outer surface to the cervix in a woman's birth canal is referred to as which of the following?
    a. The uterus
    b. The cervix
    c. The vagina
    d. The ovaries

44. What is the most effective intervention to prevent a surgical site infection (SSI)?
    a. Administering prophylactic antibiotics prior to surgery
    b. Maintaining a sterile technique during surgery
    c. Performing hand hygiene before and after patient contact
    d. Drawing a complete blood count on the patient prior to surgery

45. A patient with iron deficiency anemia is unsure which foods to consume to support an improvement in health status. Which food option should the WHNP explain would provide the least support for this condition?
    a. Beans
    b. Spinach
    c. Cheese
    d. Raisins

46. Urinary incontinence is a very disruptive symptom. What can help reduce the incidence of incontinence for patients?
    a. Bladder training
    b. Wearing incontinence briefs or pads
    c. Drinking caffeinated drinks only in the morning
    d. Using a straight catheter to fully empty the bladder

47. Which of the following is the most common type of vulvar cancer?
    a. Melanoma
    b. Adenocarcinoma
    c. Transitional cell carcinoma
    d. Squamous cell carcinoma

48. Which of the following manifestations would the WHNP expect to observe in a patient with a serum potassium level of 2.5 mEq/L?
    a. Palpitations
    b. Paresthesias
    c. Decreased deep tendon reflexes (DTRs)
    d. Prolonged P-R interval

49. When discussing breast cancer prevention and screening with a female patient who has regular periods, what is the recommended timing for breast self-examination?
    a. As the menstrual period is ending
    b. In the middle of the menstrual cycle
    c. At the beginning of the menstrual period
    d. On the same day each month

50. The WHNP percusses the patient's lungs during a focused assessment. Which sound aligns with a normal finding?
    a. Tympany
    b. Hyperresonance
    c. Dullness
    d. Resonance

51. The primary cause of catheter-associated urinary tract infection (CAUTI) is which of the following?
    a. Urinary retention when the catheter becomes blocked
    b. Immune system compromise in acutely ill, hospitalized patients
    c. Trauma to the urethra from catheter insertion
    d. Bacteria that ascend either on the surface or in the lumen of the catheter

52. Which of the following describes the pain resulting from a sprained ankle?
    a. Visceral pain
    b. Referred pain
    c. Somatic pain
    d. Radicular pain

53. A WHNP is providing care to a patient who is 24 weeks pregnant. The patient suddenly reports excruciating localized uterine pain and has dark red vaginal bleeding. The WHNP suspects abruptio placentae. Which subsequent complication is the WHNP most concerned with?
    a. Idiopathic thrombocytopenic purpura
    b. Disseminated intravascular coagulation
    c. Uterine atony
    d. Pulmonary embolism

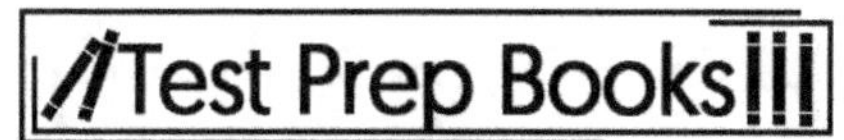

54. The WHNP is reviewing the history of a patient who is being evaluated for ovarian cancer. Which of the following risk factors is unrelated to the incidence of ovarian cancer?
   a. Infertility treatment
   b. Hyperthyroidism
   c. Tubal ligation
   d. Tamoxifen use

55. A WHNP is reviewing the chart of a patient with ovarian cancer who is in DIC. Which lab value is indicative of this?
   a. Increased fibrinogen level
   b. Increased platelet count
   c. Increased thrombin time
   d. Decreased D-dimer assay

56. The WHNP is doing a pain assessment on a patient who had hip replacement surgery two years ago. The patient describes their pain as a dull ache deep in the affected hip. It is improved with movement but gets worse with cold. It does not radiate, burn, or sting. The patient has been experiencing this pain daily for six months despite medical assessment and various pain relief modalities. The patient is most likely experiencing which type of pain?
   a. Acute pain
   b. Neuropathic pain
   c. Visceral pain
   d. Chronic pain

57. Which of the following terms refers to severe bronchoconstriction with wheezing that does not respond to the usual bronchodilation treatment?
   a. Delirium tremens
   b. Status asthmaticus
   c. Pulsus paradoxus
   d. Febre rubra

58. The WHNP is caring for several post-surgical patients. The WHNP knows that which patient is likely to be at highest risk for surgical site infection (SSI)?
   a. A 40-year-old vegetarian in good health with a BMI of 20, post-op day two from cholecystectomy
   b. A 65-year-old with hypertension and hypercholesterolemia and a BMI of 26, post-op day one from ovarian cyst removal
   c. An 85-year-old smoker with diabetes, malnutrition, and a BMI of 15, post-op day three from a lung lobectomy
   d. A 25-year-old with a BMI of 30, post-op day three after a cesarean section

59. After the removal of a breast tumor and surrounding lymph nodes, a patient begins to develop swelling and enlargement of her left arm. The WHNP recognizes that this is likely lymphedema. What can the patient do to minimize the lymphedema?
   a. Use compression on the affected limb
   b. Use the left arm less so that it can rest
   c. Use hot compresses
   d. Use cold compresses

60. What is the most common bacterial cause of pneumonias in patients?
   a. *Streptococcus pneumoniae*
   b. *Klebsiella pneumoniae*
   c. *Chlamydophila pneumoniae*
   d. *Mycoplasma pneumoniae*

61. What is the correct order of the three stages of prenatal development?
   a. Embryonic, germinal, fetal
   b. Germinal, embryonic, fetal
   c. Germinal, fetal, embryonic
   d. Fetal, germinal, embryonic

62. A patient has received general anesthesia for a surgical procedure. After surgery is initiated, the patient develops malignant hyperthermia. Which clinical value is consistent with this complication?
   a. Heart rate of 54 beats/min
   b. Temperature of 38.2 °C (100.7 °F)
   c. Potassium level of 3.2 mEq/L
   d. CO_2 level of 47 mmHg

63. The 36-year-old patient's current orders include levothyroxine 88 µg PO daily. Which assessment by the WHNP prompts patient education regarding levothyroxine administration?
   a. The patient reports that they take their medication in the afternoon, 30 minutes after consuming lunch.
   b. The patient reports that they take their medication at night, at least four hours after their last meal.
   c. The patient reports that they take their medication in the morning, 30 minutes before their first meal.
   d. The patient reports that they take their medication in the morning, 2 hours before consuming their first meal.

64. A 41-year-old woman presents to her primary care provider with concern for a vulvar enlargement on the side of her vulva that she first noticed three days ago. She states that it is not painful, but she reports a sensation of pressure when sitting and during sexual intercourse. She denies fevers, drainage, or abnormal uterine bleeding. Vital signs are within normal limits. Physical examination reveals a 2 centimeter mass at the left inferior aspect of the vulva with no drainage, fluctuance, or purulence. Which of the following is the most appropriate management?
   a. Reassurance and monitoring
   b. Incision and drainage
   c. Oral antibiotics
   d. Excisional biopsy

65. A 59-year-old woman presents to her OB/GYN provider complaining of painless vaginal bleeding. She experienced menopause at age 52 and has no history of abnormal pap smears. What diagnosis should the provider suspect until proven otherwise?
   a. Endometrial cancer
   b. Cervical cancer
   c. Endometriosis
   d. Sexually transmitted infection (STI)

66. Which of the following causes of thrombocytopenia is considered an immunological cause?
   a. Folate deficiency
   b. Drug side effects
   c. Acute respiratory distress syndrome
   d. Viral infection

67. Which of the following is the typical order in which people experience the stages of grief?
    a. Acceptance, Bargaining, Anger, Depression, Denial
    b. Denial, Anger, Bargaining, Depression, Acceptance
    c. Anger, Denial, Bargaining, Acceptance, Depression
    d. Depression, Denial, Bargaining, Anger, Acceptance

68. Which of the following is consistent with the physical assessment of the abdomen?
    a. Inspection is most accurate with direct visualization.
    b. Palpation should be avoided if the patient is complaining of pain.
    c. Percussion begins in the lower left quadrant and proceeds clockwise.
    d. Auscultation should precede palpation and percussion.

69. When taking a history from a pregnant woman with placenta previa, the WHNP would expect the patient to report which of the following?
    a. Maternal age of twenty-eight years
    b. First pregnancy
    c. Previous C-section
    d. One previous vaginal delivery

70. The WHNP is developing a teaching plan for a patient with newly diagnosed type 2 diabetes. Which of the following symptoms of hyperglycemia would be included?
    a. Tremors, fatigue, dizziness
    b. Excessive urination, excessive thirst, confusion
    c. Anxiety, blurred vision, headache
    d. Slurred speech, sweating, fainting

71. Which of the following most accurately describes a criterion for the diagnosis of primary amenorrhea?
    a. Absence of menses by one year after thelarche
    b. Absence of menses for over six months in a previously menstruating patient
    c. Absence of menses by age 15 with presence of secondary sexual characteristics
    d. Absence of menses by age 14 in the absence of secondary sexual characteristics

72. Which of the following conditions is an autosomal dominant disorder?
    a. Hemophilia
    b. Cystic fibrosis
    c. Polycystic kidney disease
    d. Thalassemia

73. A pregnant woman receives a prenatal pelvic exam early in her pregnancy. During the course of a normal pregnancy, when is the second pelvic exam typically performed?
    a. Late first trimester
    b. Second trimester
    c. Third trimester
    d. Postpartum

74. Which of the following statements made by a patient undergoing treatment for ovarian cancer indicates a possible need for additional teaching?
   a. "I stopped my morning walks so I wouldn't be so tired."
   b. "I have been eating with plastic utensils."
   c. "I have been trying to eat a small amount of food every hour or so."
   d. "My skin has been drier, so I have been using lotion in the morning and at night."

75. The WHNP is caring for a patient who is being treated for chronic pain. The patient says, "My pain medicine doesn't work anymore. I woke up twice during the night in such pain." The patient is most likely describing which event associated with pain therapy?
   a. Addiction
   b. Habituation
   c. Dependence
   d. Tolerance

76. A 38-year-old G1P1 woman presents with complaints of urinary urgency, frequency, and nocturia that began four months ago. She has been treated with antibiotics on two separate occasions, but her symptoms have returned each time. Her last menstrual period (LMP) began three weeks ago, and she notes her cycles are regular. She is monogamous with her husband, but she has had dyspareunia since the birth of her child last year. Vital signs are unremarkable. A clear-catch urinalysis is negative for blood, leukocyte esterase, or nitrites. Suprapubic palpation elicits minimal tenderness, and on cystoscopy, the NP notes small petechial hemorrhages when the bladder is distended. What is the most likely diagnosis?
   a. Urge incontinence
   b. Urinary tract infection (UTI)
   c. Bladder carcinoma
   d. Interstitial cystitis

77. A postoperative patient is bleeding profusely from their surgical incision. The patient's blood pressure is 89/50 mmHg and heart rate is 112 beats/min. Which priority intervention will the WHNP perform to maintain organ perfusion?
   a. Apply pressure to the surgical incision.
   b. Elevate the patient's lower extremities.
   c. Prepare to administer a blood transfusion.
   d. Initiate an additional peripheral intravenous line.

78. Which action should the WHNP omit from the treatment plan for a patient struggling with hemorrhoids?
   a. Witch hazel
   b. Hydrocortisone cream
   c. Stool softeners
   d. Low fiber diet

79. The WHNP is assessing a new 64-year-old female patient whose HbA1c is 5.7 percent and who has a BMI of 30. Which type of hypoglycemic agent is most appropriate for this patient?
   a. Biguanides
   b. Sulfonylureas
   c. Meglitinides
   d. Alpha-glucosidase inhibitors

80. Which of the following is NOT considered a teratogenic agent?
    a. Saunas
    b. Computers
    c. Potassium iodide
    d. Maternal stress

81. A laboring patient is found to have a low platelet count of <75,000/mm^3. This puts the patient at serious risk of bleeding. What actions should the patient avoid in order to reduce the risk of bleeding?
    a. Using a soft toothbrush
    b. Implementing a bowel regimen
    c. Walking in bare feet or open toed shoes
    d. Using only electric shavers

82. Which of the following statements correctly identifies the function of tamoxifen in the prevention of breast cancer?
    a. Tamoxifen reduces the risk of invasive breast cancer by 50 percent in postmenopausal women.
    b. Tamoxifen is more effective in premenopausal women.
    c. Tamoxifen is more effective as primary prevention and is not used in advanced disease.
    d. Tamoxifen is more effective against progesterone-positive tumors.

83. The WHNP is caring for a patient who is 36 weeks pregnant with manifestations of abruptio placenta. Which of the following statements is consistent with the use of the Kleihauer-Betke test?
    a. The test is a highly sensitive indicator of the onset of preterm labor in pregnant patients with trauma.
    b. The test measures the amount of fetal blood in the maternal bloodstream, which guides RhoGAM dosing.
    c. The test is only used in the assessment of Rh-negative patients who present with abruptio placenta during a second pregnancy.
    d. Based on the amount of fetal blood that is transferred to the maternal circulation, the test is predictive of the degree of separation of the placenta.

84. A 35-year-old patient with metastatic breast cancer reports numbness in her feet and new urinary incontinence. The WHNP suspects which of the following?
    a. Spinal cord compression
    b. Bladder infection
    c. Peripheral neuropathy
    d. Bone metastasis

85. The WHNP would expect a patient with urinary retention to report having experienced which of the following types of urinary incontinence?
    a. Stress incontinence
    b. Urge incontinence
    c. Overflow incontinence
    d. Functional incontinence

86. A 50-year-old female is newly diagnosed with hypothyroidism and started on levothyroxine. What is the appropriate interval for follow-up?
    a. Four weeks
    b. Six to eight weeks
    c. Six months
    d. Twelve months

87. Which of the following is a potential side effect of long-term first-generation antipsychotics use?
   a. Serotonin syndrome
   b. Muscle laxity
   c. Tardive dyskinesia
   d. Increased libido

88. Recent evidence-based practice and dissemination of findings guidelines have recommended limiting the conditions that are treated with proton pump inhibitors (PPIs). Therapy with PPIs is recommended for the continued management of which condition?
   a. Peptic ulcer disease that has been treated
   b. H. pylori infection that is asymptomatic
   c. Barrett esophagus that has been treated
   d. GERD that is asymptomatic

89. Which of the following is NOT identified as one of the five P's of the sexual history?
   a. Pills—the use of recreational drugs
   b. Prevention of pregnancy
   c. Prevention of sexually transmitted infections (STIs)
   d. Past history of STIs

90. A 26-year-old pregnant patient who is 34 weeks' gestation presents with a severe headache, blurred vision, and sudden weight gain. The WHNP also notices swelling in the patient's hands and face. The WHNP assesses the patient and considers the possibility of preeclampsia or eclampsia. Which of the following clinical features would indicate that the patient's condition has progressed from preeclampsia to eclampsia?
   a. Elevated blood pressure and proteinuria
   b. Severe headache and blurred vision
   c. Generalized swelling and sudden weight gain
   d. Seizures in the absence of a pre-existing seizure disorder

91. What is one way a woman may present differently than a man when experiencing a myocardial infarction (MI)?
   a. Symptoms beginning days to weeks before actual attack
   b. Profuse sweating
   c. Crushing chest pain
   d. Elevated serological markers

92. A patient is taking 50 mg of spironolactone daily. Which of the following drugs is contraindicated for the patient at this time?
   a. Simvastatin 40 mg PO daily
   b. KCl 20 mEq/L PO BID
   c. Clorazepate 3.75 mg PO
   d. Metronidazole 500 mg in 100mL D_5W IV over 60 minutes

93. A 19-year-old woman presents to urgent care and is visibly worried. She reports that she had unprotected sexual intercourse with her boyfriend two days ago. Her LMP began two weeks ago, and her cycles have always been regular. She states that she is under a great deal of pressure in college, as final exams are coming up, and she does not wish to become pregnant. Which of the following contraceptive options is most appropriate for this patient?
   a. Copper intrauterine device (IUD)
   b. Hormonal IUD
   c. Combined hormonal contraceptive
   d. Nonoxynol-9 gel

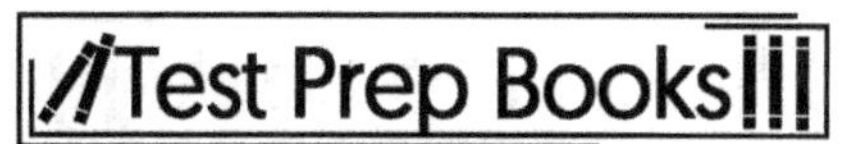

94. Sierra works in a manufacturing plant on the assembly line, a job that requires a moderate amount of movement from her upper body. She has recently transitioned into survivorship after experiencing breast cancer and a mastectomy. She is very excited to return to work and her specific job responsibilities, but still feels some tenderness and tightness across her chest, in her armpit area, and down one arm. Which of the following would assist in Sierra's transition back to work?

a. A blood thinning prescription medication
b. A new role at her place of employment
c. Occupational therapy three times a week
d. Night shift work, since less people are around

95. What are two sex hormones produced by the adrenal glands that play an important role in reproductive processes?

a. Cortisol and follicle-stimulating hormone
b. DHEA and androstenedione
c. Aldosterone and sodium
d. Ovary hormone and vas deferens hormone

96. The nurse is preparing to remove a patient's indwelling urinary catheter after abdominal surgery. The patient asks the WHNP to leave the catheter in because he is afraid it will hurt too much to get up to void. What is the best response to the patient's request?

a. "You can keep the catheter. It will be much less painful for you than getting up to void, and it's important that we control your pain."
b. "I will send a request to the physician to keep the catheter in and see what he says."
c. "I need to remove the catheter. I'm sorry if it hurts, but you will need to use the bedside commode to void."
d. "Leaving the catheter in puts you at greater risk for a UTI. It's also very important to get up and void on your own after surgery. But I will make sure to manage your pain."

97. A WHNP is performing a primary survey on a pregnant patient who sustained a traumatic fall. The patient is supine, the airway has been cleared, and intravenous access has been established. The patient suddenly verbalizes lightheadedness, heart palpitations, and the blood pressure is 84/48 mmHg. Which initial action does the WHNP take?

a. Order a fluid bolus.
b. Reassess the patient's airway.
c. Turn the patient to the left lateral position.
d. Contact the attending physician.

98. The WHNP is reviewing insulin management with a patient recently diagnosed with type 1 diabetes. Which of the following patient statements indicates that the teaching has been effective?

a. "I know that my insulin starts to work about two hours after I inject it."
b. "I know I have to be sure that my meal is ready to eat before I inject the insulin."
c. "I hope that someday I can use another kind of insulin that can be used with an insulin pump."
d. "I have to watch for the symptoms of hypoglycemia about five to six hours after I take my insulin."

99. Which of the following clinical manifestations indicates a possible lower GI bleed?

a. Hematochezia
b. Hematemesis
c. Melena
d. Diarrhea

100. Which of the following is NOT one of the categories for notifiable diseases?
    a. Outbreak
    b. Infectious
    c. Noninfectious
    d. Reproducible

101. Which of the following is NOT an indication to place a urinary catheter?
    a. Chronic wounds in the perineal area with urinary incontinence
    b. Recent hip surgery
    c. Urinary retention
    d. Strict intake and output measurement on a critical patient

102. A patient begins having a seizure. The patient's seizure lasts for four minutes and then recurs a few minutes later. What is this condition called?
    a. Grand mal seizure
    b. Serial epilepsy
    c. Tonic-clonic seizure
    d. Status epilepticus

103. According to the TNM model for tumor grading, which of the following definitions most closely describes a tumor classified as *TX*?
    a. The primary tumor cannot be assessed.
    b. The number of tumors cannot be determined.
    c. It is unknown if the tumor is malignant or benign.
    d. There is no evidence of a primary tumor.

104. A WHNP is caring for a 44-year-old woman with breast cancer who has received 4 cycles of paclitaxel chemotherapy. The patient notes that she has noticed tingling in her hands and feet beginning with her last cycle. Which of the following interventions should be discussed with the patient?
    a. Vitamin E supplements to prevent further neuropathy
    b. Application of a lidocaine cream to decrease discomfort
    c. Close inspection of hands and feet for burns, cuts, and abrasions
    d. Rest and avoidance of unnecessary walking

105. Which of the following is a type III immune-mediated adverse drug reaction?
    a. Ig E-mediated, immediate-type hypersensitivity
    b. Antibody-dependent cytotoxicity
    c. Immune complex hypersensitivity
    d. Cell-mediated or delayed hypersensitivity

106. The WHNP is providing community education on the connection between sexually transmitted infections and other ailments. In advocating for testing, which disease does the nurse explain is often associated with chlamydia and gonorrhea?
    a. Rheumatoid arthritis
    b. Celiac disease
    c. Pelvic inflammatory disease
    d. Systemic lupus erythematous

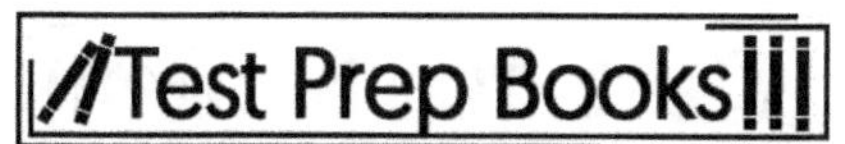

107. Which of the following screening tests is specifically designed to assess potential alcohol abuse in the ADULT patient?
   a. DAST-20
   b. TAPS
   c. CRAFFT
   d. CAGE B

108. What is an employer with more than fifty employees required to do for a nursing mother employee under the Fair Labor Standards Act (FLSA)?
   a. Provide a private bathroom for a mother when it is their normal break time.
   b. Provide a private non-bathroom space for the mother during their normal break time.
   c. Provide a private non-bathroom space for the mother as frequently as needed.
   d. There is no space requirement for accommodation if the mother has a car in the parking lot and breaks are provided when necessary.

109. A 34-year-old G0P0 woman presents to the clinic with complaints of cyclical pelvic pain and pressure. Upon further discussion, she also describes heavy menstrual bleeding and mentions that she and her husband have been trying to conceive for the past year but have thus far been unsuccessful. Her LMP began ten days ago. Physical examination reveals a healthy-appearing patient without visible abnormalities on speculum exam. Subsequent bimanual exam reveals an enlarged, mildly tender uterus with an irregular contour. What is the most appropriate initial diagnostic study for this patient's most likely diagnosis?
   a. CT scan of the abdomen and pelvis
   b. Urine pregnancy test
   c. Transvaginal ultrasound (TVUS)
   d. Endometrial biopsy

110. A 24-year-old obese female presents with acanthosis nigricans, hirsutism, oligomenorrhea, and an inability to conceive. The nurse practitioner suspects polycystic ovarian syndrome (PCOS). Which of the following is the patient at an increased risk of developing?
   a. Type 2 diabetes
   b. Endometriosis
   c. Cervical cancer
   d. Hypertension

111. Paula has a routine cervical exam which shows the presence of abnormal cells on her cervix. A biopsy shows that she has stage one cervical cancer. Paula has surgery to remove all of the cancerous cells, and her medical team feels she has a very good prognosis due to early detection. However, why will Paula need to continue to be monitored with follow-up visits?
   a. She appears to have a genetic predisposition to reproductive cancers.
   b. She is of child-bearing age and hopes to become pregnant.
   c. Cancerous cells can spread before becoming detectable.
   d. She is nearing menopause.

112. The WHNP is preparing a female patient for a general pelvic examination. Which position is the most appropriate for this procedure?
   a. Supine
   b. Fowler's
   c. Sims
   d. Lithotomy

113. The WHNP in the emergency department is caring for a 14-year-old boy with testicular torsion. The prehospital provider reported a TWIST score of 5; however, at the time of the patient's arrival in the ER, the urologist established a TWIST score of 6. The WHNP understands that which of the following is the recommended treatment plan for this patient?
   a. The patient most probably has an alternative condition causing his symptoms.
   b. The patient will need an immediate ultrasound to confirm the diagnosis.
   c. The patient requires immediate surgical intervention.
   d. The treatment recommendations are the same for scores of 5 and 6.

114. While doing an assessment on a patient with limited mobility, the WHNP notices that the patient's right leg has become swollen and red. The patient also reports increased pain in the leg. Which of the following additional assessment data would require priority intervention?
   a. The patient's left leg also appears swollen.
   b. There is a small wound noted to the patient's right great toe.
   c. The pulse in the right foot can only be found with a doppler.
   d. The patient complains of sudden shortness of breath.

115. An 8-month-pregnant woman presents to the ED with eclampsia. Which IV medication will be given to prevent seizures?
   a. Magnesium sulfate
   b. Sodium chloride
   c. Dextrose in water
   d. Potassium supplement

116. Which pH imbalance is the patient experiencing with the following ABG results: pH 7.51, PaCO2 72 mm/Hg, HCO3 41 mEq/L.
   a. Metabolic acidosis
   b. Fully compensated metabolic alkalosis
   c. Respiratory alkalosis
   d. Partially compensated metabolic alkalosis

117. Which drug increases Parkinsonian manifestations?
   a. Metoclopramide
   b. Cyclosporin
   c. Rapid-acting insulin
   d. Nicotine

118. Under the Pregnancy Discrimination Act of 1978, which of the following statements is TRUE?
   a. An employer can refuse to provide a pregnant woman with reasonable accommodation if she is unable to do her job and approaches her manager to that effect.
   b. An employer can ask a pregnant interview candidate when they are due and how much time they will plan to be off of work after the baby arrives.
   c. An employer must give a woman a comparable position to the one that she held prior to her maternity leave (if the company does so with employees on short-term disability).
   d. An employer can discriminate against an employee who has undergone an abortion if this act is against their personal convictions.

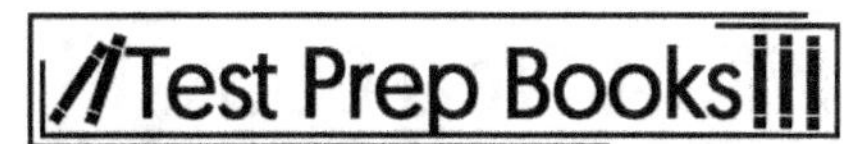

119. Noreen is a social worker who has a ten-month-old son. He has been a poor sleeper, and Noreen has not been able to sleep well since he was born. In addition, Noreen finds herself unable to fall asleep unless she is near him. She regularly wakes up in a panic, wondering if the baby is okay. She anxiously fears that something terrible will happen and is always identifying potential dangers and ways to protect her baby from them. She has a supportive husband, but Noreen does not want anybody besides her or her husband to take care of their son. She refuses to enroll him in daycare, instead working evening hours when her husband is at home. This further compounds her sleep deprivation, and she must nap occasionally during the day when she can no longer physically stay awake. What does Noreen seem to be experiencing?

a. Generalized anxiety disorder
b. Postpartum anxiety disorder
c. Social anxiety disorder
d. Circadian rhythm sleep disorder

120. A 23-year-old female was started on Fluoxetine for anxiety eight weeks ago. She returns to the office for evaluation of the effectiveness of the medication. Which screening tool should the NP use to assess the effectiveness of treatment?

a. PHQ9
b. MOCA
c. GAD7
d. CAGE

121. A WHNP is providing education regarding the HPV (human papillomavirus) vaccine. The WHNP notes that HPV is a risk factor for which cancers?

a. Liver cancer and non-Hodgkin lymphoma
b. Gastric cancer and gastric mucosa-associated lymphoma
c. Lung cancer and Kaposi sarcoma
d. Oropharyngeal cancer and cervical cancer

122. What is the pathway of oxygenated blood from the lungs?

a. Lungs to the left atrium, through the mitral valve into the left ventricle, pumped into the aorta upon contraction, then dispersed to tissues via a network of arteries and capillaries
b. Lungs to the right atrium, through the mitral valve into the right ventricle, pumped into the aorta upon contraction, then dispersed to tissues via a network of arteries and veins
c. Lungs to the left atrium, directly to the right aorta, then dispersed to tissues via a network of arteries and capillaries
d. Lungs to the left atrium, through the septum valve, stored in the left ventricles, then dispersed to tissues via a network of arteries and capillaries

123. Drugs from which of the following categories are NOT common to the initial treatment of HTN?

a. Loop diuretics
b. Angiotensin II receptor blockers
c. Angiotensin-converting enzyme inhibitors
d. Long-acting calcium channel blockers

124. Which of the following is the body cavity that contains the urinary bladder, urethra, and ureters?

a. The thoracic cavity
b. The pelvic cavity
c. The abdominal cavity
d. The spinal cavity

125. The WHNP is caring for a patient who has a complete placenta previa and is twenty-two weeks pregnant. She asks the WHNP to explain the action of betamethasone. Which of the following statements is consistent with the action of this medication?

a. The medication reduces newborn infections if the membranes rupture prematurely due to the placenta previa.
b. Prolonged gestation is more effective than treatment with betamethasone for lung maturation.
c. The therapy eliminates the occurrence of respiratory distress syndrome in the newborn.
d. Betamethasone is a tocolytic agent that can be used long-term to stop preterm labor.

126. The WHNP is caring for a patient who is at risk of developing a deep vein thrombosis. The WHNP knows that all of the following are factors that contribute to the development of a venous thrombosis EXCEPT:

a. Endothelial injury
b. Increased arterial blood flow
c. Blood stasis
d. Hypercoagulability

127. A WHNP is providing care to a patient diagnosed with a deep vein thrombosis to the right lower extremity. Upon assessment, the patient verbalizes dyspnea and has an oxygen saturation of 88%. Which other clinical finding best supports the diagnosis of a suspected pulmonary embolism?

a. Pleuritic pain
b. Temperature of 99.8 °F (37.6 °C)
c. Right calf erythema
d. Heart rate of 102 beats/min

128. If a person with AB blood and a person with O blood have children, what is the probability that their children will have the same phenotype as either parent?

a. 0%
b. 25%
c. 50%
d. 75%

129. A 60-year-old female patient who has been diagnosed with breast cancer and is undergoing chemotherapy is experiencing side effects such as nausea, fatigue, and hair loss. The patient has two adult children who are actively involved in providing care and emotional support. Which of the following actions best demonstrates patient and family-centered care for this patient?

a. Providing the patient with a pamphlet about chemotherapy and its side effects and encouraging her to read it
b. Asking the patient's children to leave the room during her physical examination to maintain patient privacy
c. Encouraging the patient's children to participate in care, such as accompanying her to chemotherapy appointments
d. Deciding on the patient's chemotherapy regimen without involving her or her family in the decision-making process

130. Which of the following is consistent with the recommended management for pregnant women and women with a history of gestational diabetes mellitus (GDM)?

a. 75 g oral glucose tolerance test (OGTT) ≥ 150 mg/dL at one hour is positive for GDM.
b. Women with GDM should be tested for diabetes every 5 years for life.
c. Women with GDM should be tested for diabetes 6 to 12 weeks postpartum.
d. The OGTT should be done at 36 weeks of gestation in patients not previously diagnosed with diabetes.

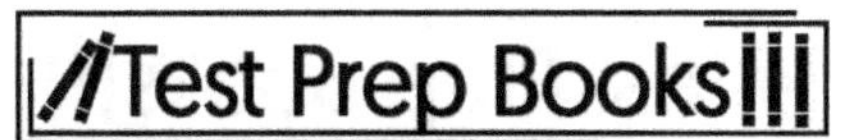

131. The WHNP is performing a follow-up assessment on a patient who underwent a total pelvic exenteration two months ago. The patient tells the WHNP, "I'm having doubts about the choice I made. I don't feel I will ever be able to have sex with a partner again." Which of the following is the best action by the WHNP?
   a. Encourage the patient to discuss future reconstructive surgery.
   b. Assure the patient that sex with a partner can resume in a few months.
   c. Redirect the patient to appreciate the medical benefit of treatment.
   d. Prepare the patient for a pelvic exam.

132. A 50-year-old female patient with a history of uncontrolled hypertension is observed to be restless and anxious. Her blood pressure readings over the past 24 hours have ranged from 185/95 mm Hg to 210/110 mm Hg. The patient reports a severe headache and has been complaining of blurred vision. Recognizing these signs and symptoms, the WHNP understands that the patient may be experiencing which of the following conditions?
   a. Hypertensive urgency
   b. Hypertensive emergency
   c. Acute heart failure
   d. Acute stroke

133. The WHNP is developing a teaching plan for a patient with newly diagnosed type 2 diabetes. Which of the following symptoms of hyperglycemia would the WHNP include?
   a. Tremors, fatigue, dizziness
   b. Excessive urination, excessive thirst, confusion
   c. Anxiety, blurred vision, headache
   d. Slurred speech, sweating, fainting

134. Which racial or ethnic group demonstrates a higher than normal incidence of lactose intolerance?
   a. Arab Americans
   b. Asian Americans
   c. Native Americans
   d. African Americans

135. A 63-year-old G2P2 postmenopausal woman presents for her annual visit. She has no complaints and has generally enjoyed good health. Her previous pap smear last year was normal, and she has never had an abnormal pap test. Her last colonoscopy two years ago revealed a benign 3 millimeter polyp, and her last mammogram results from two years ago were classified as Breast Imaging Reporting and Data System (BI-RADS) 1. She denies any family history of breast or other gynecologic cancers. Which of the following is the most appropriate screening test at this time?
   a. Pap test
   b. Screening mammogram
   c. Colonoscopy
   d. Dual-energy X-ray absorptiometry (DEXA) scan

136. What laboratory test is used to monitor the effectiveness of a patient receiving Coumadin (warfarin) therapy?
   a. Platelet count
   b. Hemoglobin count
   c. Prothrombin time (PT)
   d. Activated partial thromboplastin time (aPTT)

137. The WHNP has been teaching a patient with HIV-1 about her condition. Which patient statement indicates that the patient understands the course of his disease?
   a. "I do not need to start treatment until I develop symptoms."
   b. "I am going to die young."
   c. "With treatment, I cannot transmit the virus."
   d. "With treatment, it's possible to have a healthy life."

138. A 21-year-old woman presents to the emergency department (ED) complaining of fever, chills, and pelvic pain. She experienced similar but milder symptoms last week and was treated with nitrofurantoin for a suspected UTI; however, her symptoms have worsened despite this treatment. Vital signs include blood pressure 118/76 mmHg, heart rate 104 beats per minute, respirations 18 per minute, and temperature 39.3 °C (102.7 °F). Blood work reveals leukocytosis, and urinalysis reveals mild pyuria with negative leukocyte esterase or nitrites. On physical examination, there is no costovertebral angle tenderness, but the provider notes suprapubic tenderness and a positive chandelier sign. What is the most likely diagnosis in this patient?
   a. Pelvic inflammatory disease (PID)
   b. Pyelonephritis
   c. Acute appendicitis
   d. Uncomplicated cystitis

139. Which patient is at the highest risk for spinal cord compression?
   a. 54-year-old female with stage IV breast cancer
   b. 72-year-old male with stage III colon cancer
   c. 55-year-old female with stage II bladder cancer
   d. 74-year-old male with stage III prostate cancer

140. Which of the following statements by a patient with type 2 diabetes indicates that more teaching is needed?
   a. "My pancreas produces insulin, but my body isn't able to use it effectively."
   b. "I need to maintain an ideal body weight."
   c. "I need to cut down on carbohydrates in my diet."
   d. "I will need to take insulin for the rest of my life."

141. Which of the following statements regarding the grading system for cardiac murmurs is correctly stated?
   a. A 2/6 murmur is a soft sound with no palpable thrill.
   b. All 3/6 murmurs are moderately loud and are associated with a palpable thrill.
   c. A 4/6 murmur is loud but still requires close contact between the skin and the stethoscope for an accurate diagnosis.
   d. A 5/6 murmur is audible with only the bell of the stethoscope with no palpable thrill.

142. Which of the following lifestyle modifications would address the major cause of most aortic aneurysms?
   a. Low-fat diet
   b. Smoking cessation
   c. Exercise program
   d. Meditation

143. The WHNP is providing care to a patient with testicular cancer who is receiving chemotherapy. The patient tells the nurse, "I don't have any libido and I feel it's affecting my partner. I don't know what to do." Which of the following is the best response by the WHNP?
   a. "This is an expected side effect of chemotherapy."
   b. "Are you thinking about stopping treatment?"
   c. "Have you spoken to your partner about your feelings?"
   d. "Your partner should be more supportive of your treatment."

144. Which of the following is the gold standard for diagnosis of endometriosis?
   a. Transvaginal ultrasound (TVUS)
   b. Exploratory laparotomy
   c. CT scan of the pelvis
   d. MRI of the pelvis

145. What is the most common cause of edema caused by venous insufficiency?
   a. Deep vein thrombosis (DVT)
   b. Obesity
   c. Pregnancy
   d. Old age

146. The WHNP is caring for a patient with a suspected ectopic pregnancy. The patient asks the WHNP to explain how her smoking history is related to this condition. Which of the following statements correctly identifies the relationship between smoking and the development of an ectopic pregnancy?
   a. Smoking decreases the oxygen saturation of the fetal circulation, which compromises the process of implantation.
   b. Smoking alters progesterone levels, which interferes with the transfer of the fertilized ovum to the uterus.
   c. Smoking alters the endometrial lining, making it an inhospitable environment for the fertilized ovum, thereby preventing implantation.
   d. Smoking damages the cilia in the fallopian tube, which decreases motility and alters the movement of the fertilized ovum.

147. Wasting of muscle, bone deformities and tenderness, and joint pain or swelling are commonly due to which of the following nutritional deficiencies?
   a. Zinc and B12
   b. Folic acid and Vitamin C
   c. Vitamin C and Vitamin D
   d. Ferritin and niacin

148. Dabigatran (Pradaxa®), rivaroxaban (Xarelto®), and apixaban (Eliquis®) are recently introduced oral anticoagulants. Which one of the following choices is correct?
   a. The half-life of Warfarin is shorter than all of the newer anticoagulants.
   b. The "bridging" of the new drugs takes less time.
   c. The newer drugs do not require monitoring.
   d. Warfarin has fewer drug–food allergies than the newer drugs.

149. A 29-year-old patient has undergone a C-section and has returned to the unit. The nurse knows that he will oversee all of the following except which duty?
   a. Maintaining a clean dressing daily
   b. Monitoring for infection
   c. Applying prescribed medications
   d. Re-suturing if the incision opens

150. During which trimester are fetuses most vulnerable to developmental delays from chemotherapy that the mother is undergoing?
   a. First
   b. Second
   c. Third
   d. All of the above

151. The WHNP is caring for a patient with a history of STDs who presents with right upper quadrant pain. The nurse understands that this pain may be associated with Fitz-Hugh–Curtis syndrome. Which of the following statements is consistent with the pathophysiology associated with this disorder?
   a. This inflammatory process of Glisson's capsule results in adhesions.
   b. It is an abnormal autoimmune response to the antimicrobial treatment of PID.
   c. It is an infection of the liver that manifests in the tertiary stage of syphilis.
   d. The syndrome is most often associated with severe pelvic pain.

152. Which of the following interventions are NOT meant to reduce atelectasis following abdominal surgery?
   a. Incentive spirometer
   b. Bracing with a pillow to cough
   c. Early ambulation
   d. Enoxaparin therapy

153. When do treatment-related secondary cancers tend to develop?
   a. During the first six weeks of treatment
   b. During the first year of treatment
   c. Within one month after initial exposure
   d. Within several years after initial exposure

154. After receiving chemotherapy to treat testicular cancer, with which secondary malignancy is the patient at a higher risk of being diagnosed?
   a. Melanoma
   b. Leukemia
   c. Prostate cancer
   d. Rectal cancer

155. A 25-year-old G0P0 woman with no significant medical history complains of bilateral nipple discharge. She takes no medications. Physical examination reveals milky white discharge expressed from both nipples on palpation. Vital signs are within normal limits. A urine pregnancy test is negative. What is the most appropriate imaging study for this patient?
   a. Transvaginal ultrasound (TVUS)
   b. Diagnostic mammogram
   c. Breast ultrasound
   d. MRI of the brain

156. A 65-year-old female with a medical history of myocardial infarction and stroke presents with an INR of 1.3. After assessing the patient's diet and medications and finding no causes for this lab result, the NP adjusts her dose of warfarin. She returns three weeks later with an INR of 2.8. How should the NP interpret these results?
   a. The treatment was effective, and the medication dose should remain the same.
   b. The treatment was ineffective, and another course of treatment should be considered.
   c. The patient should be referred to a hematologist.
   d. The results are inconclusive, and more testing will need to be conducted.

157. The WHNP is caring for a patient with low-flow priapism. The patient also has a history of sickle cell disease, and the WHNP understands that this disease is a significant risk factor for priapism. Which of the following statements identifies the pathology of this relationship?
   a. Sickle cell disease results in decreased free hemoglobin, which leads to vasodilation in the penis.
   b. Hemolyzed red cells decrease nitric oxide stores, resulting in vasodilation and priapism.
   c. Sickle cell is an autoimmune defect associated with altered arterial pressure in the penis.
   d. Prophylactic use of sildenafil effectively reduces the recurrence of priapism in this population.

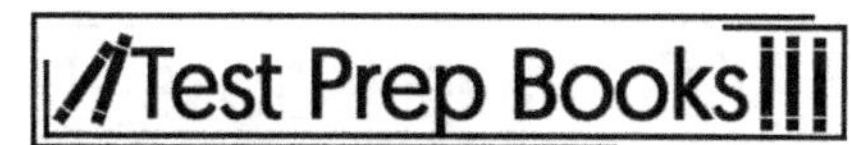

158. Which of the following correctly defines reduced practice?
   a. Physician oversight is required for all aspects of APRN practice.
   b. APRN practice is unrestricted except for physician oversight of documentation.
   c. Physician oversight is required only for prescriptive practice.
   d. There are no restrictions on APRN practice.

159. Which of the following is NOT included in the Post-Exposure care of a healthcare worker following occupational exposure to the HIV virus?
   a. Post-exposure anti-viral therapy is contraindicated if the exposed person is pregnant.
   b. HIV testing will be repeated at 6 weeks, 12 weeks, and 6 months at a minimum.
   c. The exposed person should avoid blood or tissue donation, breastfeeding, or pregnancy for 6 to 12 weeks after exposure.
   d. Renal and hepatic studies and a CBC will be done at baseline and repeated frequently.

160. A 30-year-old female presents to follow-up on her Type 2 diabetes. She has made significant changes to her diet and has begun exercising. She is currently taking Metformin 1000 mg twice a day. Her HbA1C comes back at 5.5. After evaluating this HbA1c, how should the nurse practitioner alter the current treatment plan?
   a. The Metformin dose should be increased.
   b. The Metformin dose should remain the same.
   c. The Metformin dose should be decreased.
   d. The Metformin dose should be discontinued.

161. Which statement about prenatal development is MOST accurate?
   a. Nutrition hasn't been shown to play a significant role in ensuring the well-being of a fetus.
   b. Maintaining a healthy weight while carrying an embryo decreases the possibility of negative risks.
   c. Substance use during pregnancy isn't known to result in any long-term problems for infants.
   d. The developmental stage of a baby has no bearing on an infant's susceptibility to teratogens.

162. A 28-year-old pregnant patient who is 32 weeks' gestation presents with painless vaginal bleeding that started suddenly about an hour ago. The bleeding is moderate, and the patient reports no abdominal pain or contractions. The patient's prenatal care has been unremarkable thus far. Which of the following conditions should the WHNP suspect based on the patient's symptoms?
   a. Placental abruption
   b. Placenta previa
   c. Uterine contractions due to preterm labor
   d. Placenta accreta

163. A 23-year-old woman presents to the clinic complaining of vaginal discharge and irritation. Physical examination reveals thin, watery discharge without blood or purulence. The NP obtains a sample for analysis. Which of the following is part of the Amsel criteria for diagnosis of bacterial vaginosis (BV)?
   a. Positive nitrites on urinalysis
   b. Clue cells on microscopy
   c. Vaginal fluid pH less than 4.5
   d. Cervical erythema

164. All EXCEPT which of the following are components of Virchow's triad?
   a. Heart disease
   b. Hypercoagulability
   c. Endothelial injury/dysfunction
   d. Hemodynamic changes such as stasis or turbulence

165. A 24-year-old patient is seeking a long-acting reversible contraceptive. After discussion of the benefits and drawbacks of each option with her gynecologist, she states that she would prefer the implantable rod known as Nexplanon®. Which additional counseling must the gynecologist provide?
  a. The implantable rod may stay in place for up to five years.
  b. The implantable rod is not a highly effective contraceptive.
  c. The patient will still be at risk for STIs even with this contraceptive.
  d. The patient may experience breast pain or mood swings with this contraceptive.

166. What is the purpose of the Wells score?
  a. Assess the risk potential for venous stasis ulcers
  b. Confirm the presence of a DVT
  c. Assess the probability of a PE
  d. Stratify ankle-brachial index scores

167. Which of the following is a commonly used blood thinner that works by blocking the body's ability to adhere platelets together?
  a. Paroxetine
  b. Coumadin
  c. Heparin
  d. Aspirin

168. A WHNP is providing care to a postoperative patient with a urinary catheter. The WHNP knows that the most important contributing factor for the prevention of a catheter-associated urinary tract infection (CAUTI) is which of the following?
  a. Perineal care
  b. Frequent emptying of the drainage bag
  c. Hand washing
  d. Duration of catheterization

169. The WHNP is answering an HIV-positive patient's questions about the differences between the HIV-1 and HIV-2 viruses. Which information would the WHNP tell this patient?
  a. HIV-2 is highly transmissible.
  b. HIV-1 is the dominant strain worldwide.
  c. HIV-2 is well-studied and highly understood.
  d. HIV-1 is the weaker virus strain.

170. Which of the following traits was once diagnosed as a psychological disorder in the United States, but no longer is?
  a. Autism spectrum disorder
  b. HIV
  c. Homosexuality
  d. Seasonal affective disorder

171. Aminoglycosides such as gentamicin are absolutely contraindicated for the treatment of which condition?
  a. Multiple sclerosis
  b. Parkinson's disease
  c. Myasthenia gravis
  d. Amyloidosis

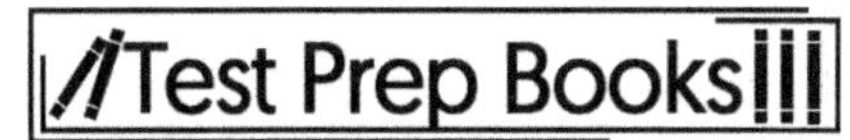

172. Which of the following statements about GINA is correct?
   a. Long-term care insurance companies are prohibited from using genetic information to set rates.
   b. Employers can use genetic information when making job assignments.
   c. Protection from GINA does not apply to conditions that were previously diagnosed.
   d. Health insurance companies can request specific genetic tests before quoting rates for coverage.

173. A postpartum patient notices swelling in their left calf. The WHNP assesses the leg and finds redness, heat, and a positive Homan's sign. After an ultrasound, a deep vein thrombosis (DVT) is identified. What intervention is likely to treat this problem and prevent new thrombi from forming?
   a. Sequential compression devices applied to bilateral lower extremities
   b. Anticoagulant medication, such as a low-molecular-weight heparin
   c. Placement of an inferior vena cava filter (IVC filter)
   d. Frequent walking and exercise

174. A small group of providers are choosing to improve an existing process related to patient discharge. They have identified that patients have a high re-admittance rate during the summer months. After mapping the current process, they note that patients leave the printout of discharge instructions that they are provided in their hospital room approximately 65% of the time. The providers set up a meeting to review potential solutions. In which part of the PDCA cycle is this performance improvement plan?
   a. Plan
   b. Do
   c. Check
   d. Act

175. The WHNP is caring for a patient after an emergency delivery in the ER. The newborn had an Apgar score of 8 at one minute and a score of 9 at five minutes after delivery. Which of the following statements is consistent with these scores?
   a. The scores are normal.
   b. The deficit is most likely due to decreased muscle tone.
   c. The newborn will require only short-term mechanical ventilatory support.
   d. The newborn is at risk for cardiac anomalies.

Answer Explanations #1

1. C: HRT has been linked to an increased risk of breast cancer in post-menopausal women, who are also more likely to be diagnosed with advanced disease. HRT has been linked to a slightly higher risk of ovarian cancer, making Choice *A* incorrect. Choice *B* is incorrect because long-term use of HRT has not been shown to increase the risk of lung cancer. Choice *D* is incorrect because estrogen may have a role in preventing colorectal cancer, but it has not been shown to have an impact on pancreatic cancer.

2. D: Chromosomal abnormalities of the fetus are the most common cause of early spontaneous abortions. Other factors that increase the risk include advanced maternal age, type 1 diabetes, renal disease, severe hypertension, thyroid dysfunction, anatomical defects of the uterus, illicit drug use, smoking, alcohol abuse, and non-ASA NSAID use; therefore, Choices *A* and *B* are not correct. Moderate exercise is not a risk factor for spontaneous abortion.

3. D: Low-grade cancer cells are malignant cells that look similar to healthy cells, which is a positive prognostic factor. Choice *A* is incorrect because tumors larger than 1 centimeter become associated with less favorable outcomes as they grow bigger. Choice *B* is incorrect because node-positive cancers have started spreading to surrounding lymph nodes and are associated with less favorable prognosis. Choice *C* is incorrect because hormone receptor-negative tumors have a less favorable initial prognosis than hormone receptor-positive tumors. However, hormone receptor-negative tumors do tend to have a lower recurrence rate than hormone receptor-positive tumors.

4. B: The most appropriate response is Choice *B*. This statement provides empathy to this patient and seeks to explore the extent of the patient's advance care planning. Ideally, advance care planning should begin at diagnosis and continue throughout treatment and beyond. However, WHNPs can encounter many challenging situations, particularly when family members and patients have differing wishes. The WHNP's job is to provide therapeutic communication, ensure the patient is well-educated on all potential options, and always advocate for the patient's wishes. Choice *A* is not the most appropriate choice because the WHNP is not acknowledging the patient's feelings or addressing their concerns. Although this is a pertinent assessment question, Choice *C* is not the most appropriate choice since it does not address what the patient is saying in their statement. Choice *D* is not the most appropriate answer choice because this statement does not advocate for or explore the patient's wishes.

5. A: The calcium-channel alpha to delta ligands potentiate the action of gabapentin in the treatment of chronic neuropathic pain. Gabapentin is the initial drug of choice for treatment of this type of pain. Opioids are seldom effective for neuropathic pain. Nonsteroidal anti-inflammatory drugs are not recommended due to the risk of bleeding. Nonopioid analgesics may be used, but they are less effective than gabapentin in treating the pain. Therefore, Choices *B, C*, and *D* are incorrect.

6. B: This scenario depicts a classic case of testicular torsion which is an emergent condition; therefore, the NP should call 911 first, Choice *B*. The NP could then order pain medications, Choice *D*. Choices *A* and *C* should be performed at the hospital.

7. C: Regular, routine testing is not generally necessary for asymptomatic men. Testing is recommended for high-risk groups, men who have new or multiple partners, and those who have been exposed to or are experiencing symptoms. While symptoms of the disease in men are more easily recognized, though many men experience no symptoms at all. Women are more commonly asymptomatic than men, which means that the disease is more advanced when diagnosed; therefore, Choice *A* is incorrect. Nucleic acid testing is more specific than antibody testing, but it is also more expensive, and in many cases neither of the tests is required for diagnosis because the patient's presenting symptoms are diagnostic. Therefore, Choice *B* is incorrect. Women with untreated chlamydia

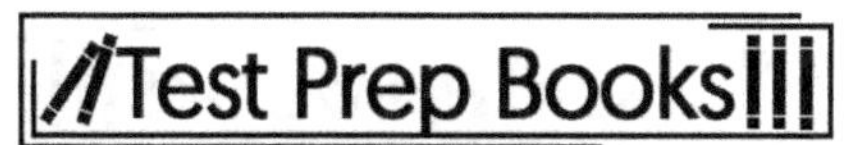

risk significant damage to the entire reproductive system, which may become systemic as in the case of pelvic inflammatory disease, so Choice *D* is incorrect.

8. C: Raloxifene is a selective estrogen receptor modulator (SERM) that may be used for reduction of fracture risk in women with osteoporosis or for reduction of breast cancer risk in postmenopausal women. A history of VTE is an absolute contraindication to this medication. Choice *A* is incorrect, as osteoporosis is a primary indication for this medication. Choices *B* and *D* are not contraindications to this medication, though type 2 diabetes mellitus may increase the long-term risk of VTE.

9. D: Massive urine production, or polyuria, is the result of a hyperglycemic state in the body and a hallmark sign of any diabetic condition. Urine is not concentrated, but rather diluted. Sodium, potassium, and other electrolyte imbalances may occur as a result of polyuria but are not a direct effect of hyperglycemia.

10. C: Vitamin K plays a role in the body's natural clotting process, and Warfarin works by inhibiting the synthesis of certain clotting factors dependent on vitamin K. Maintaining a consistent intake of vitamin K helps maintain the desired therapeutic effect of Warfarin without unnecessary restrictions. Choice *A* is incorrect because it suggests avoiding vitamin K–rich foods altogether, which is not necessary for most patients on Warfarin. Although Choice *B* recognizes the importance of a balanced diet, it does not highlight the important fact that vitamin K may alter Warfarin's effectiveness; therefore, it is incorrect. Choice *D* is not necessary and may lead to nutritional imbalances.

11. C: It is important to provide counseling on fertility preservation before the start of treatment, as it has a significant impact on quality of life during survivorship. The ability of a patient to have their own children is a central aspect of survivorship for all patients regardless of age, making Choice *A* incorrect. Fertility preservation counseling increases post-treatment quality of life by decreasing stress, depressive symptoms, and decisional regret, making Choice *B* incorrect. Oncofertility discussion is the standard of care and is recognized by ASCO even when emergent treatment is needed, making Choice *D* incorrect.

12. C: An atrial septal defect is not part of the tetralogy of Fallot. The tetralogy of Fallot includes a ventricular septal defect, an aorta arising from both ventricles (an atrial septal defect), and hypertrophy of the overworked right ventricle due to pulmonary valve stenosis.

13. D: A core needle biopsy entails using a needle to extract a small piece of tissue for examination by a pathologist to determine diagnosis. Choice *A* refers to an excisional biopsy, in which the goal is complete removal of the tumor for pathology. Choice *B* refers to a fine needle aspiration, while Choice *C* describes a bone marrow biopsy.

14. B: Inhibition of excretion of the medication results in increased plasma concentration of it, which may result in an overdose or ADR. Inhibition of excretion is more common than induction, which is an increase in the excretion rate of the drug. Induction can result in an inadequate systemic response to the drug that may also represent an ADR; therefore, Choice *A* is incorrect. Desensitization is the diminished body response to a drug that is administered over a long period of time. This predictable reaction is also the basis for reversing drug sensitivities in patients with allergies; therefore, Choice *C* is incorrect. Absorption is the first phase of pharmacodynamics and is defined as the presence of the drug in the bloodstream following administration; therefore, Choice *D* is incorrect.

15. C: In the female reproductive system, many different hormones work together to propagate the species. The function of each one is listed below.

Hormone	Source	Action
GnRH	Hypothalamus	Stimulates anterior pituitary to secrete FSH and LH
FSH	Anterior pituitary	Stimulates ovaries to develop mature follicles (with ova); follicles produce increasingly high levels of estrogen
LH	Anterior pituitary	Stimulates the release of the ovum by the follicle; the follicle is then converted into a corpus luteum that secretes progesterone
Estrogen	Ovary (follicle); placenta	Stimulates repair of endometrium of uterus; negative feedback effect inhibits hypothalamus production of GnRH
Progesterone	Ovary (corpus luteum); placenta	Stimulates thickening of, and maintains, endometrium; negative feedback inhibits pituitary production of LH
Prolactin	Anterior pituitary	Stimulates milk production after childbirth
Oxytocin	Posterior pituitary	Stimulates milk "letdown"
Androgens	Adrenal glands	Stimulates sexual drive
hCG	Embryo (if pregnant)	Stimulates production of progesterone

16. A: Iron deficiency anemia is a type of anemia typically caused by a low intake of iron in one's diet. Symptoms of iron-deficiency anemia include an inflamed and sore tongue, fatigue, brittle and spoon-shaped nails, dizziness, weakness, and cold hands or feet. Low iron levels cause the tongue to become reddened and painful because there is a lack of oxygen being received in the area. Choice *B* is incorrect as low iron levels would lead to increased fatigue and weakness due to the decreased oxygenation occurring in the body. Choice *C* is also incorrect as iron deficiency may cause increased heart rate, or tachycardia, due to the body attempting to compensate for low oxygen levels in the blood. Choice *D* is also incorrect because fingernail clubbing is a clinical manifestation of chronic obstructive pulmonary disorders. As mentioned above, iron-deficiency anemia leads to brittle and spoon-shaped nails due to malnutrition.

17. C: The WHNP should use the patient's chosen name and pronouns to respectfully address them. Choice *A* is incorrect as avoiding using pronouns can make the provider-patient interaction awkward and nontherapeutic, causing unnecessary stress for the patient. Choice *B* is also incorrect as this may be dismissive of the patient's gender identity. Choice *D* is also incorrect because this does not assist the current interaction with the patient.

18. D: Statistically, half of women who have annual mammograms will experience one false positive during a ten-year time period because mammograms have low specificity, which increases the incidence of false positives. False positives are associated with added expense, and in the case of mammograms increased stress for the patient. Choice *A* is incorrect because the item defines high sensitivity and high specificity, which is not common. Choice *B* is incorrect because mammograms cannot confirm the absence of disease. The mammogram report is worded in terms of high probability that the disease is not present. Choice *C* is incorrect because mammograms are affected by the patient's personal characteristics such as the tumor size, patient's age, and the patient's body size.

19. B: Levothyroxine can cause cardiac side effects, and the lowest dose should be started in the elderly and for people with a history of heart disease. The NP should evaluate for symptoms of angina, palpitations, and myocardial infarction. Therefore, Choice *B* is correct. The other answer choices are not true for the pharmacodynamics of levothyroxine.

20. C: Pregnant women with gestational diabetes need to exercise regularly, avoid excessive weight gain, and monitor food intake. They also need to seek regular prenatal care since gestational diabetes can affect fetal growth and increase the baby's risk of obesity. Therefore, Choices *A*, *B*, and *D* are not correct.

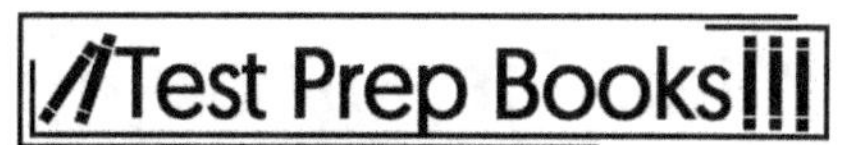

21. D: An ankle-brachial BP index is commonly used to diagnose peripheral arterial disease by comparing the blood pressures of the two sites, thus assessing blood flow. An echocardiogram is a sonographic test used to visualize the structures of the heart, such as in heart failure. A computed tomography (CT) scan would not be useful for visualizing arterial structures of the extremities, or at least it is not commonly used. An electrocardiogram is used to measure and track electrical activity of heart muscle.

22. B: The most effective method to educate families and facilitate learning is utilizing practice dolls and mannequins. This allows those who are learning to gain hands-on experience so they can be comfortable on their own. Although playing a pre-recorded video demonstration may be helpful, it is not the best choice because it does not allow the expectant parents to have hands-on practice, making Choice *A* incorrect. Providing written step-by-step instructions may be helpful as a reference, but it isn't the most effective way to facilitate learning, making Choice *C* incorrect. This is also true for Choice *D*, making it also incorrect.

23. A: Prehypertension is defined as systolic pressures ranging between 120 and 139 mmHg or diastolic pressures between 80 and 89 mmHg. Normal blood pressure is less than 120/80 mmHg. Stage 1 hypertension ranges from 140 to 159 mmHg systolic or 90 to 99 mmHg diastolic. Stage 2 hypertension is greater than or equal to 160 mmHg systolic or greater than or equal to 100 mmHg diastolic.

24. C: Choice *C* is correct because chest imaging is one of the diagnostic tests used to identify lung injury. All suspected transfusion-related acute lung injuries (TRALIs) will show pulmonary infiltrates on a chest x-ray. Choice *A* is incorrect because hypotension, not hypertension, is suspected in TRALI. Choice *B* is incorrect because sinus bradycardia is not a clinical finding used to diagnose TRALI. Choice *D* is incorrect because jugular venous distention is expected with fluid volume overload, seen in conditions such as transfusion-associated circulatory overload.

25. A: Patients who have received blood products (especially in the form of massive transfusion) are at increased risk of hypocalcemia due to the citrate concentration within blood products. Because of this, WHNPs caring for these patients should advocate for serum calcium level monitoring and calcium supplementation when needed, and assess for signs and symptoms of hypocalcemia. These signs and symptoms include muscle spasms, paresthesia, Chvostek's sign, Trousseau's sign, and, in some cases, increased confusion.

26. B: Ibuprofen is an NSAID, which is useful for dysmenorrhea since NSAIDs inhibit prostaglandins and thereby target one of the underlying causes of dysmenorrhea. Choice *A* is a corticosteroid and does not have a role in treating dysmenorrhea. Choices *C* and *D* are antidepressants, the former being a selective serotonin reuptake inhibitor (SSRI) and the latter a serotonin-norepinephrine reuptake inhibitor, which are useful in treating PMDD but not the actual pain of menses.

27. C: Schizophrenia and bipolar disorder are mental disorders in which hallucinations and delusion (key components of psychosis) are common. These characteristics can also result from mind-altering drugs, specifically methamphetamines, cocaine, and LSD. Antiviral medications used to treat HIV do not normally cause psychosis.

28. B: Given the patient's blood pressure is uncontrolled, the NP should increase the dosage of the medication he is already on. The prescriber should increase dosage of an existing medication to its maximum dose before adding additional therapies. Therefore, Choices *A* and *D* are incorrect. The NP should titrate up to the next dosage of 40 mg of Lisinopril and then reassess effectiveness at follow-up visits. Therefore, Choice *B* is correct. The prescriber should always use step therapy and not jump to higher doses as this can lead to symptoms of hypotension; therefore, Choice *C* is incorrect.

29. C: The epididymis stores sperm and is a coiled tube located near the testes. The immature sperm that enters the epididymis from the testes migrates through the 20-foot long epididymis tube in about two weeks, where viable sperm are concentrated at the end. The vas deferens is a tube that transports mature sperm from the epididymis to the urethra. Seminal vesicles are pouches attached that add fructose to the ejaculate to provide energy for sperm.

The prostate gland excretes fluid that makes up about a third of semen released during ejaculation. The fluid reduces semen viscosity and contains enzymes that aid in sperm functioning; both effects increase sperm motility and ultimate success.

30. D: Aseptic technique is the recommended technique to use when inserting a urinary catheter and will help in the prevention of catheter-associated urinary tract infections (CAUTIs). Sanitary and clean techniques are lower on the scale of techniques and therefore not adequate. Sterile technique is usually used in surgical procedures in which an environment without micro-organisms present is desirable.

31. A: The most common adverse effect associated with the Zika virus is microcephaly, which results in severe to fatal changes in the brain of the fetus. The remaining choices may or may not be present as a result of the microcephaly; however not one of them is the most significant effect. Therefore, Choices *B, C,* and *D* are incorrect.

32. B: Vena cava filters are also known as inferior vena cava (IVC) filters or Greenfield filters. They are used to prevent a pulmonary embolism (PE). Indications for the placement of a vena cava filter include:

- An absolute contraindication to anticoagulants
- Survival after a massive PE and a high probability that a recurrent PE will be fatal
- Documented recurrent PE

33. C: The split S_2 sound occurs because the pulmonic valve closes before the aortic valve during inspiration; this is more commonly observed in young adults. The sound is assessed with the diaphragm of the stethoscope at the sternal border of the left second intercostal space. In the elderly, it is often a normal sign as well unless the sound is also audible during expiration, which is defined as a wide splitting S_2. In patients without bundle branch block, S_1 is significantly less common than S_2. The use of additional diagnostic testing depends on the consideration of the patient's age and cardiac function because, most often, it is a normal sound. Therefore, Choices *A, B,* and *D* are incorrect.

34. D: This scenario is highly concerning for ovarian cancer, and the provider should waste no time seeking confirmation and specialist referral for treatment. Choices *A* and *B* are very unlikely to be the cause of this patient's drastic weight loss and constitutional symptoms. Choice *C* is certainly on the differential diagnosis list, but a unilateral adnexal mass favors an ovarian rather than endometrial origin.

35. D: The seminiferous tubules are responsible for sperm production. Had *testicles* been an answer choice, it would also have been correct since it houses the seminiferous tubules. The prostate gland (*A*) secretes enzymes that help nourish sperm after creation. The seminal vesicles (*B*) secrete some of the components of semen. The scrotum (*C)* is the pouch holding the testicles.

36. A: HELLP syndrome is characterized by hemolysis, elevated liver enzymes, and low platelet count. The presence of these laboratory findings, in combination with the patient's symptoms, is most consistent with a diagnosis of HELLP syndrome. The combination of lab values in Choices *B, C,* and *D* do not fit the diagnostic criteria of HELLP syndrome.

37. C: Lipid-soluble drugs move across the cellular membrane by passive diffusion, which means that the absorption rate is increased without the cellular expenditure of energy in the form of ATP. Drugs that are bound to plasma proteins are also capable of passive diffusion across the cellular membrane; therefore, Choice *A* is incorrect. Lipid solubility is one determinant of the absorption rate; however, the rate can also be affected by the remaining factors that are associated with the absorption rate; therefore, Choice *B* is incorrect. Choice *D* is incorrect because the first-pass effect is related to the route of administration rather than the solubility of the drug. All drugs administered orally are subjected to the first-pass effect because the drugs are absorbed in the stomach, and then they enter the GI vasculature and progress to the liver.

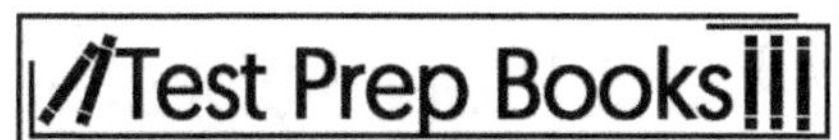

38. B: Choice *B* is the most appropriate response by the WHNP because it includes empathy and seeks to determine whether the patient has discussed this with another professional. The patient's statements could indicate they are experiencing depression, which is a very common experience amongst cancer patients. Choices *A* and *C* are not the most appropriate responses since these statements do not empathize or validate the patient's statement. Choice *D* is not the most appropriate response because responding with "I know how you feel," or responding with personal experiences would not be the most professional, therapeutic, or validating statement to make.

39. D: Choice *D* is the most concerning because acupuncture is an alternative therapy method that involves placing very small needles in the skin over different parts of the body to manage health conditions. This treatment is generally safe; however, there is a contraindication for use in individuals at risk for bleeding or infection. Chemotherapy treatments often inhibit the bone marrow production of blood cells (including red blood cells, platelets, and white blood cells). Therefore, any patient undergoing chemotherapy would be advised to work closely with their doctor to monitor blood levels before considering acupuncture. Choice *A* is incorrect because gentle activity, such as walking, is highly encouraged for chemotherapy patients because it can help with maintaining energy and mental wellness during treatment. Choice *B* is incorrect because taste changes are a very common and expected side effect of chemotherapy. This statement would warrant follow-up to determine if a patient is able to maintain dietary intake, but this is not the most concerning statement. Choice *C* is not the most concerning statement because nausea is another very common side effect of chemotherapy treatment, and ginger tea is a generally safe and effective complementary way to manage nausea. Although this symptom and treatment are generally not unexpected or concerning, the CMA would still record any symptom reported by the patient as well as any home remedies used to manage symptoms.

40. C: The Emergency Medical Treatment and Labor Act of 1986 (EMTALA) was a direct response to healthcare facilities turning away patients that were unable to pay for treatment, even in life-or-death situations. However, facilities are not reimbursed for losses by this law, and this has had an effect on overall healthcare costs.

41. D: Sequential compression devices are used to help prevent the formation of deep vein thrombosis in patients with decreased mobility. However, if the patient is already suspected of or diagnosed with deep vein thrombosis, the sequential compression devices can potentially dislodge the thrombus, causing it to travel within the patient's circulation. In the worst cases, this can lead to a clot lodging in the vasculature of the heart, lungs, or brain. The other choices listed are less likely to cause further complications from the deep vein thrombosis and more likely to decrease the risk of worsening deep vein thrombosis.

42. D: The Tennessee Classification System designates complete HELLP syndrome as having a platelet count of less than 10×10^9/L, AST greater than or equal to 70 units/L, and LDH greater than 600 units/L, which account for the alterations in liver function. Additional manifestations include red cell hemolysis, elevated liver enzymes, and coagulation defects. The syndrome is associated with abnormal blood clotting that commonly creates a hematoma in the liver tissue, not in the liver vasculature; therefore, Choice *A* is incorrect. The liver function is related to the degree of severity of the syndrome; however, the liver damage may or may not improve in a liver that has been previously damaged by systemic disease, prior trauma, or infection. Irreversible damage to the liver, including rupture of hematomas and liver capsule destroying a significant part of the liver, are commonly associated with this condition; therefore, Choice *B* is incorrect. Cerebral edema and hemorrhagic stroke are among the most common complications of the HELLP syndrome due to altered coagulopathy; therefore, Choice *C* is incorrect.

43. C: The uterus and ovaries aren't part of the birth canal, so Choices *A* and *D* are false. The cervix is the uppermost portion of the birth canal, so Choice *B* is incorrect, making Choice *C* the correct answer. The vagina is the muscular tube on the lowermost portion of the birth canal that connects the exterior environment to the cervix.

44. A: The most effective intervention to prevent a surgical site infection (SSI) in a patient is to administer prophylactic antibiotics before surgery. Choices *B* and *C* are also appropriate interventions, but they are not the most effective. Choice *D*, drawing labs prior to surgery, may be necessary to determine patient stability, but this intervention does not directly prevent SSI.

45. C: Choice *C* would provide the least support for the patient's iron deficiency anemia. Choices *A*, *B*, and *D* are all supportive of improved nutritional status regarding iron and should be encouraged via dietary intake.

46. A: Bladder training helps reduce incontinence and includes routine voiding, practicing suppression of the urge to urinate, Kegel exercises, and decreasing fluid intake in the evening. Choice *B* is incorrect; wearing briefs or pads assists in preventing accidents or leaks but does not reduce the frequency of incontinence. Choice *C* is incorrect, as the patient should be advised to avoid caffeine and other bladder irritants. Choice *D* is also incorrect. Using a straight catheter should not be a routine practice for incontinence because it can lead to infection.

47. D: Squamous cell carcinoma accounts for the overwhelming majority of vulvar cancers, with melanoma (Choice *A*) comprising a much smaller percentage. Choice *B* is not a common subtype of vulvar cancer, while Choice *C* is the most common subtype of bladder cancer.

48. D: Hypokalemia is associated with a prolonged P-R interval, which represents the time from the SA node firing to contraction of the ventricles. The remaining manifestations are associated with hyperkalemia; therefore, Choices *A*, *B*, and *C* are incorrect.

49. A: Choice *A* is the correct answer. Breast self-examination is recommended to be performed at approximately the same point during the menstrual cycle because hormone levels lead to changes in the breast tissue throughout the month. The end of the menstrual cycle is when tissue is less sensitive and less prone to inflammation; therefore, this will provide consistency, increased patient comfort, and smoother breast tissue. Choice *B* is not the best recommendation because the middle of the menstrual cycle can be a more challenging point for many women to identify. Choice *C* is less recommended because breast tissue tends to be more sensitive and engorged; therefore, this would not be the most comfortable and reliable timing for breast self-examination. Choice *D* is not the most appropriate recommendation because menstrual cycle length varies considerably from patient to patient and from month to month. Recommending the same date each month can lead to self-examination at different points within the menstrual cycle, which will reduce the consistency of breast tissue and lead to less reliable results.

50. D: Choice *D* demonstrates a normal finding when auscultating the patient's lungs. Choice *A* is not a normal finding over the lungs, but it is a normal finding over the stomach. Choice *B* is not a normal finding, as it is indicative of air hyperinflation, such as with asthma. Choice *C* is not a normal finding over the lungs; it is normal over dense areas such as the liver.

51. D: Bacteria ascension into the urinary tract from poor insertion technique, backflow of urine, or inadequate catheter hygiene is the most common cause of CAUTI. Choice *A* is incorrect because urinary retention can exacerbate the risk of CAUTI but is not a primary cause. Choice *B* is incorrect because, while many hospitalized patients do have compromised immune systems that make them more vulnerable to a CAUTI, the bacterial infection itself is the cause of CAUTI. Choice *C* is incorrect because trauma to the urethra from catheter insertion is not itself infectious.

52. C: Somatic pain is triggered by pain receptors in the tissues, muscles, bones, and skin. Visceral pain is due to inflammation or injury of involuntary muscles in body organs such as the heart. Referred pain is defined as pain that is perceived at an anatomical point distant from the site of injury. Radicular pain occurs when the nerve root is damaged, which is commonly the cause of lower back pain. Therefore, Choices *A*, *B*, and *D* are incorrect.

53. B: Choice *B* is the most common complication after abruptio placentae. Disseminated intravascular coagulation is a serious complication characterized by internal and external bleeding. Choice *A* is a genetic autoimmune disorder that can result in postpartum hemorrhage. Choice *C* occurs after birth and is the inability of the uterine muscle to

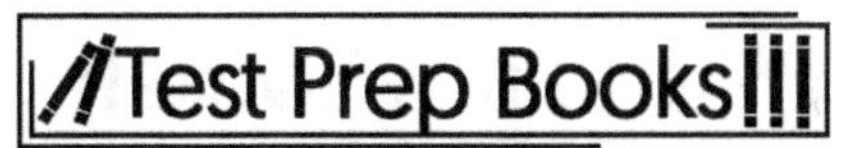

contract adequately. Choice *D* is a complication that can occur with any pregnancy. Pregnancy increases the risk of developing deep vein thrombosis with subsequent embolus.

54. B: Risk factors for ovarian cancer include hypothyroidism, a history of infertility treatment, tubal ligation, or the use of tamoxifen; therefore, Choice *B* is the correct answer, and Choices *A, C,* and *D* are incorrect.

55. C: Disseminated intravascular coagulation (DIC) is a disorder that causes abnormal coagulation. It can lead to organ damage by inappropriate development of clots and hemorrhage due to consumption of platelets and coagulation factors. Lab results will typically see decreased fibrinogen levels, decreased platelet counts, increased thrombin and prothrombin times, and increased D-dimer assay; therefore, Choices *A, B,* and *D* are incorrect.

56. D: Pain that continues or recurs longer than three months is considered chronic pain. Choice *A* is incorrect because the patient's pain has lasted longer than three months, but acute pain lasts less than three months. Choice *B* is incorrect because, while neuropathic pain can also be chronic, the patient's description of the pain does not have any hallmark features of neuropathic pain such as shooting, tingling, sharpness, or a pins-and-needles sensation. Based on their description, the patient's pain is unlikely to have a neuropathic origin. Choice *C* is incorrect because again, while visceral pain can also become chronic, the patient's pain clearly exists in the hip joint, while visceral pain can originate from the affected organ or be diffuse or referred. Based on the patient's description, the pain is unlikely to be visceral in origin.

57. B: Status asthmaticus is the Latin term for a severe asthma attack, characterized by wheezing and bronchoconstriction, that is unresponsive to the usual therapy of bronchodilators. Delirium tremens is the set of symptoms experienced by an alcoholic in withdrawal, making Choice *A* incorrect. Pulsus paradoxus is defined as a drop in the systolic blood pressure by ten points and a decrease in the amplitude of pulse waves during inspiration. This phenomenon can be observed during cardiac tamponade, making Choice *C* incorrect. Choice *D* is incorrect, as febre rubra is the Latin term for scarlet fever.

58. C: Of the four patients, the one described in Choice *C* has the greatest number of risk factors for SSI: advanced age, smoking, diabetes, and malnutrition. The patient in Choice *A* has the lowest risk of the four patients. Choice *B* is incorrect because, while their BMI is a risk factor, they are at lower risk than the patient described in Choice *C*. Choice *D* is incorrect because, while their BMI is also a risk factor, they too have fewer risk factors than the patient described in Choice *C*.

59. A: Using compression can move fluids toward the trunk of the body where they can be removed and processed. Choices *B*, *C*, and *D* are incorrect, as these interventions would only further increase the lymphedema.

60. A: *Streptococcus pneumoniae* is the most common cause of bacterial pneumonia. The other three organisms listed are also bacterial and may cause pneumonia but are not as common as *S. pneumoniae.*

61. B: Prenatal development occurs in three stages in order: germinal stage, embryonic stage, and the fetal stage. Therefore, Choice *B* is correct. Choice *A* is incorrect because it's the germinal stage that precedes the embryonic stage. Choice *C* is incorrect because it's the embryonic stage that precedes the fetal stage of development. Choice *D* is incorrect because the fetal stage doesn't precede the germinal stage, and the embryonic stage precedes the fetal stage.

62. D: Choice *D* is correct because one of the primary manifestations of malignant hyperthermia is hypercarbia. A carbon dioxide level of 47 mmHg is above normal. The normal CO_2 level is 35-45 mmHg. Choice *A* is not correct because a heart rate of 54 beats/min is not expected with hyperthermia. Tachycardia, or increased heart rate, is expected. Choice *B* is not correct because a temperature of 38.2 °C (100.7 °F) is on the higher end of normal. Choice *C* is not correct because a potassium level of 3.2 mEq/L is not expected in malignant hyperthermia. Hyperkalemia, an elevated potassium level, is consistent with the complication.

63. A: Choice *A* is a concerning response by the patient regarding their daily levothyroxine administration. This medication should be taken once daily on an empty stomach, at least 30 minutes before and four hours after meals. Choices *B*, *C*, and *D* all meet these administration guidelines and do not necessitate patient education at this time.

64. A: This patient has a Bartholin cyst, which forms when the ducts supplying the Bartholin gland become obstructed. She is largely asymptomatic; therefore, reassurance and monitoring are most appropriate at this time. Bartholin cysts typically resolve spontaneously, and mild symptoms may improve with over-the-counter analgesics and sitz baths. Symptomatic or persistent cysts may require drainage with Word catheter placement. Choice *B* would be appropriate for a Bartholin abscess, but this lesion has no fluctuance or purulence. Choice *C* would also be considered for an abscess but not a simple cyst. Choice *D* would indicate a suspicion for cancer, which is not the case in this patient.

65. A: Abnormal uterine bleeding in a postmenopausal woman is highly suspicious for endometrial cancer, and this should be considered the diagnosis until proven otherwise. Choice *B* is unlikely, as this patient has never had an abnormal Pap smear that would indicate risk for cervical cancer. Choices *C* and *D* often cause pelvic pain and a host of other symptoms, but painless vaginal bleeding would be an uncommon presentation, particularly in a postmenopausal patient.

66. D: A viral infection is considered an immunologic cause as the immune system is weakened by the viral infection and thrombocyte levels drop as a result. Nonimmunological causes arise from a source outside of the immune system, such as sepsis and acute respiratory distress syndrome. Folate deficiency, a cause for anemia, is a nutritional deficiency, not immunological.

67. B: In order, grieving people typically progress through the emotions of denying the event, anger at the event, bargaining to bring the loss back, depression when they realize the loss cannot come back, and finally acceptance of the loss. Depending on the individual and the context of the loss, this cycle can occur slowly or rapidly. People may also relapse into previous stages before finally arriving at acceptance.

68. D: Percussion and palpation of the abdomen can change the frequency of bowel sounds; therefore, auscultation beginning in the right lower quadrant and proceeding clockwise should be completed immediately after inspection. If the patient is reporting abdominal pain, the WHNP will palpate that area last; therefore, Choice *A* is incorrect. The assessment of the abdomen generally begins in the right lower quadrant and proceeds clockwise to the left lower quadrant before moving to the midline of the abdomen; therefore, Choice *B* is incorrect. Inspection of the surface of the skin is improved with a tangential view of the abdomen rather than a direct view. The WHNP should be seated at the patient's side to identify abnormal contours, pulsations, and peristaltic waves; therefore, Choice *C* is incorrect.

69. C: Placenta previa is the abnormal placement of the placenta over the internal cervical os or within 2 centimeters of the internal cervical os. The risk factors for placenta previa are previous C-section, maternal age greater than thirty-five years, and increased number of previous pregnancies. Other risk factors include infertility treatments, multiple births, previous abortions, and smoking or cocaine use.

70. B: Hyperglycemia occurs when the patient's blood sugar level is elevated, usually greater than 180-200 milligrams per deciliter. Common symptoms of hyperglycemia include polyuria (excessive urination), polydipsia (excessive thirst), nausea, abdominal pain, fruity-scented breath, and confusion. Choices *A*, *C*, and *D* describe symptoms of hypoglycemia.

71. C: Primary amenorrhea refers to the absence of menses either by age 15 when secondary sexual characteristics are present or by age 13 in the absence of secondary characteristics. Choice *A* is not correct, as thelarche typically precedes menarche by two to three years and is not a criterion for primary amenorrhea due to this variability.

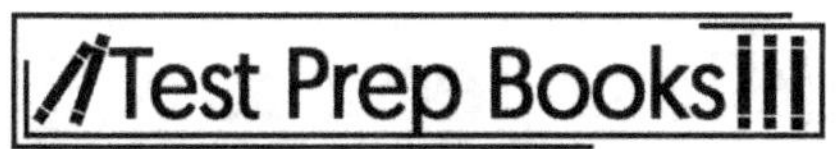

Choice *B* meets criteria for secondary amenorrhea, not primary. Choice *D* is almost correct, but the appropriate age for diagnosis is 13 as described above, not 14 years of age.

72. C: Polycystic kidney disease is an autosomal defect, which means that there has been a mutation in one of the first 22 non-sex genes. If both parents carry the gene without any symptoms of the disease, there are four possibilities for the offspring: There is a 25 percent chance that the child will inherit two normal genes, a 50 percent chance that the child will inherit one normal gene and one altered gene and will be a carrier without symptoms of the disease, and a 25 percent chance that the child will be born with two defective genes and will be at risk for developing the disease. Choice *A* is incorrect because hemophilia occurs when there is a recessive gene on the X chromosome. Choice *B* is incorrect because cystic fibrosis is an autosomal recessive disorder, which means that the offspring usually inherits one defective gene from each parent who is a carrier. Thalassemia is also an autosomal recessive defect; therefore, Choice *D* is incorrect as well.

73. C: During the course of a normal pregnancy, women typically receive the second pelvic exam during the third trimester to assess the development of the fetus and the status of the woman's reproductive system. Then, after birth, a postpartum pelvic exam is performed to assess the return of the reproductive organs to their nonpregnant state. Choices *A*, *B*, and *D* are incorrect because they give times that are either too early or too late for the second pelvic exam.

74. A: Choice *A* is the correct answer because light activity (e.g., walking) has been shown to improve cancer-related fatigue. Choice *B* is incorrect because eating with plastic utensils can help with treatment-related taste changes. Choice *C* is incorrect because eating small, frequent meals is advised for patients having trouble with appetite. Choice *D* is also incorrect, as application of lotion can assist patients who experience dry skin from cancer treatment.

75. D: The patient is describing tolerance, which means that changes made by the drug decrease some of the effects of the drug when given over an extended period of time. Addiction is a complex disease that may be due to genetic, environmental, or psychosocial factors. It is manifested by compulsive use of the drug without the control exhibited by individuals who are not addicted, so Choice *A* is incorrect. Habituation is not associated with the use of controlled substances and is defined as adjusting or adapting to something, so Choice *B* is incorrect. Physical dependence manifests with withdrawal syndrome if the substance is withdrawn abruptly or neutralized by an antagonist, so Choice *C* is incorrect.

76. D: This patient has interstitial cystitis, also known as bladder pain syndrome. It involves repetitive inflammation of the bladder's urothelium. While interstitial cystitis is a less common cause of pelvic pain, it substantially impacts quality of life. Patients often experience pelvic pain as well as urinary frequency and urgency; notably, patients often report improvement in symptoms with urination. Choice *A* is possible but less likely given the findings on cystoscopy. Choice *B* is not the best answer, as a UTI with negative leukocyte esterase and nitrites on urinalysis is possible but exceedingly rare. Bladder carcinoma, Choice *C*, is unlikely due to the patient's age and the absence of hematuria.

77. B: Choice *B* will best maintain organ perfusion. Elevating the lower extremities promotes venous return and shunts blood flow to vital organs. Choice *A* will help stop the bleeding but will not directly maintain organ perfusion. Choice *C* will help restore lost blood volume. However, this intervention does not immediately maintain organ perfusion. Choice *D* will facilitate the administration of multiple medications and fluid therapy. However, this intervention alone does not maintain organ perfusion.

78. D: Choice *D* should be omitted from the plan of care for a patient struggling with hemorrhoids because this patient would benefit from a high fiber diet. Choices *A*, *B*, and *C* all provide symptom relief and encourage the management or resolution of hemorrhoids; therefore, these measures should be included in the treatment plan.

79. A: Metformin (a biguanide) is the treatment of choice for prediabetes and type 2 diabetes because it promotes weight loss by decreasing the absorption of glucose, normalizing the hepatic production of glucose, and increasing the peripheral uptake and utilization of glucose. Metformin is the only oral hypoglycemic agent approved for children, and it can lower the HbA1c 1.5 percent to 2.0 percent. Choice *B* is incorrect because sulfonylureas are associated with weight gain and the risk for hypoglycemia that is increased if the patient is also taking clarithromycin, levofloxacin, sulfamethoxazole-trimethoprim, metronidazole, or ciprofloxacin. Choice *C* is incorrect because meglitinides are appropriate for postprandial hyperglycemia, but they require multiple doses. Choice *D* is incorrect because drugs in the alpha-glucosidase inhibitor class are used for type 2 diabetes, but they may be used if the patient is unable to tolerate metformin.

80. B: Research conducted over several years has found no evidence of any harmful effects occurring in a fetus as a result of being around computers during pregnancy, thus computers aren't considered a teratogenic agent. Therefore, Choice *B* is correct. Choice *A* is incorrect because saunas are another well-known teratogenic agent. Babies are unable to regulate their body temperature while in utero, which means they can't tolerate the severe heat of a sauna. Choice *C* is incorrect because potassium iodide readily crosses the placenta and can result in hypothyroidism if it enters a mother's system during pregnancy. Choice *D* is incorrect because maternal stress is actually another type of teratogenic agent. Maternal stress during pregnancy has been known to cause poor outcomes such as low birthweight, preterm births, and even infant mortality.

81. C: Patients with thrombocytopenia should always wear shoes to avoid injury to the feet. Choices *A*, *B*, and *D* are all incorrect. Bleeding precautions include using a soft toothbrush, implementing a bowel regimen to avoid constipation, only using electric razors, preparing the environment to reduce fall risk, and avoiding activity that can result in bleeding.

82. A: Tamoxifen is effective in reducing the risk of breast cancer in at-risk postmenopausal women. It is not effective in pre-menopausal women due to the added estrogen burden. Tamoxifen is commonly used in advanced disease and is only effective against estrogen-positive tumors.

83. B: In the event of major trauma, there is an increased incidence of fetal-to-maternal hemorrhage, which can alter the amount of Rho(D) immune globulin (RhoGAM) that is required to protect the fetus. The Kleihauer-Betke test can be used to quantify the concentration of fetal hemoglobin in the maternal blood, which then is used to calculate the appropriate dose of Rho(D) immune globulin (RhoGAM) in Rh-negative mothers; therefore, Choice *B* is correct. Although some authors recommend the use of the test in all patients as an indicator of preterm labor, the research indicates that this test is not specific for, or sensitive to, the occurrence of preterm labor and is not a reliable indicator for preterm labor; therefore, Choice *A* is incorrect. The transfer of fetal hemoglobin to the maternal circulation must be addressed with the first pregnancy to avoid the formation of anti-D antibodies; therefore, Choice *C* is incorrect. The test can only measure the concentration of fetal hemoglobin in the maternal circulation. It is not sensitive or specific to the degree of the precipitating trauma; therefore, Choice *D* is incorrect.

84. A: Spinal cord compression symptoms include changes in urinary function, weakness, and changes in sensation of the lower extremities. Choices *B*, *C*, and *D* are not represented by the scenario.

85. C: Urinary retention occurs when a patient has cessation of urination or incomplete emptying of the bladder. This may lead to overflow incontinence as the bladder becomes overfilled with urine, which then is involuntarily released from the overfull bladder. Therefore, *A*, *B*, and *D* are not correct.

86. B: Levothyroxine doses are calculated based on weight and then adjusted depending on follow-up TSH levels. Since this patient was recently started on the medication, they should have a close follow-up of six to eight weeks, Choice *B*. The TSH should not be redrawn before six weeks as the levothyroxine will not have reached its steady state yet; therefore, Choice *A* is incorrect. A six-month follow-up would be too long and could leave the patient on an inadequate dose for longer than needed; therefore, Choice *C* is incorrect. A twelve-month follow-up is

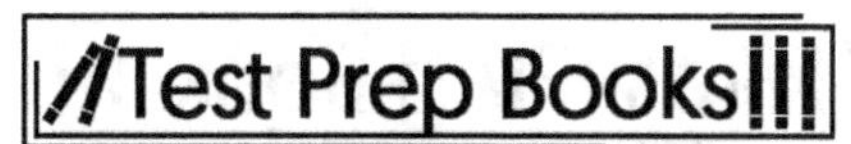

appropriate for a patient who has been determined to be on the correct dose of levothyroxine through repeat laboratory testing; therefore, Choice *D* is incorrect.

87. C: First-generation antipsychotics, such as haloperidol, can cause extrapyramidal symptoms like tardive dyskinesia, involuntary movements of the face and mouth. Therefore, Choice *C* is correct. Serotonin syndrome, Choice *A*, is caused by too much serotonin typically from antidepressants. First-generation antipsychotics can cause muscle rigidity and sexual dysfunction; therefore, Choices *B* and *D* are incorrect.

88. C: Barrett esophagus is associated with the development of esophageal adenocarcinoma; therefore, continued PPI therapy is recommended. Adverse effects of proton pump inhibitors (PPI) include non-traumatic fractures, *Clostridium Difficile* diarrhea, and acute interstitial nephritis. With consideration of these adverse effects and the success of the treatments for peptic ulcer disease, *H. pylori* infection, and gastro-esophageal reflux disease (GERD), PPI therapy is not recommended for the remaining conditions. Therefore, Choices *A*, *B*, and *D* are incorrect.

89. A: Pills is not one of the five P's of the sexual history. The missing pieces are partners and sexual practices; therefore, the five P's of the sexual history are partners, sexual practices, prevention of pregnancy, prevention of STIs, and a past history of STIs. Therefore, Choices *B, C*, and *D* are incorrect.

90. D: Seizures in the absence of a pre-existing seizure disorder indicate that the patient's condition has progressed from preeclampsia to eclampsia. Eclampsia is a severe and potentially life-threatening complication of preeclampsia that requires immediate medical intervention. While the symptoms in Choices *A*, *B*, and *C* are all characteristic of preeclampsia, they do not indicate a progression to eclampsia.

91. A: A woman may have flulike symptoms, anxiety, or jaw or back pain days to weeks before the actual cardiac event. These symptoms may be overlooked, and the correct diagnosis may be missed if the clinician is unaware of gender differences. The other three symptoms listed are classic, well-known symptoms of a myocardial infarction.

92. A: The concurrent use of spironolactone with simvastatin is contraindicated because the interaction between the two drugs causes a significant increase in the simvastatin levels. There are no reported interactions among spironolactone and KCl, Clorazepate, or metronidazole. Therefore, Choices *B*, *C*, and *D* are incorrect.

93. A: This patient is in need of emergency contraception. Currently, the two options for this are either the copper IUD or particular oral progesterone-only contraceptives, including levonorgestrel or ulipristal acetate. Choice *B* is highly effective for primary contraception but not for emergency contraception after unprotected intercourse. Choice *C* is incorrect, as the only approved emergency contraceptives do not contain estrogen. Choice *D* is not correct, as spermicide gel is neither an emergency contraceptive nor one of the most effective modes of primary contraception.

94. C: Occupational therapy is a type of rehabilitation that supports individuals in returning to a specific type of movement, often for their occupation or routine activities. Sierra is excited to return to her specific job role, and an occupational therapist can provide emotional and mental support, along with physical exercises to strengthen specific areas and build range of motion, that can help her on the job. Blood thinners, Choice *A*, are not necessary in this situation. Since Sierra wants to return to her original position, switching her to a new role or new shift (Choices *B* and *D*) are not the best options for her mental or emotional state; these are prohibitive to returning to "normalcy."

95. B: These hormones are produced by the adrenal glands and influence specific sexual and reproductive functions, such as building estrogen and testosterone.

96. D: This response best respects and addresses the patient's concern (pain) while also educating the patient about the risks of leaving the catheter in. Choice *A* is incorrect because the catheter should not remain in place longer than necessary. Choice *B* is incorrect because removal of the catheter is already part of postoperative order sets, and the timing of removal is firmly within the WHNP's scope of practice. Choice *C* is incorrect because, while it may be correct, this response does not acknowledge the patient's valid concerns about pain, nor does it explain the importance of removing the catheter.

97. C: Choice *C* is the appropriate intervention for this patient. During pregnancy, the enlarged uterus applies pressure to the vena cava when in the supine position and causes decreased venous return. Turning the patient to the left lateral position will relieve compression. Choice *A* should occur after non-pharmacological interventions have been attempted. Choice *B* is not indicated. The patient's airway has already been cleared and the symptoms are not indicative of respiratory complications. Choice *D* is indicated only if the patient's symptoms persist after performing initial interventions.

98. B: The onset of insulin aspart is five minutes after injection, which means that the patient's meal should be immediately available to prevent hypoglycemia. Choice *A* is incorrect because the onset of insulin aspart is five minutes. Choice *C* is incorrect because insulin aspart is one of the insulins that can be used with an insulin pump or pen. Choice *D* is incorrect because the peak action of insulin aspart is one to three hours, not five to six hours.

99. A: A lower GI bleed is typically caused by hemorrhoids or anal fissures, diverticulosis, colon polyps, and even cancers of the colon or anus. Because the bleeding is in the lower portion of the GI tract, the blood typically presents as frank red blood with the passage of stools, known as hematochezia. Choices *B* and *C* are incorrect because they are associated with an upper GI bleed. Hematemesis is the vomiting of blood, especially vomit that appears "coffee ground-like." Melena is dark and tarry stools that may appear black in color. Choice *D* is also incorrect as diarrhea can have several causes and does not directly indicate the potential for a lower GI bleed.

100. D: The three categories of notifiable diseases are outbreak, infectious, and noninfectious; therefore, Choices *A, B,* and *C* are incorrect.

101. B: The use of urinary catheters greatly increases the risk of urinary tract infections, which can have incredibly negative effects on patients' overall health outcomes. Because of this, urinary catheters should only be used when they are deemed necessary and when the risk of not having one outweighs the risk of potential infection. Choice *B* is not an example of an indication for urinary catheter placement. While mobility is limited initially, these patients can still use bed pans and external catheters to prevent risk of infection. Further, patients should be encouraged to increase their mobility early on to improve their rehabilitation. Choice *A* is an indication for a urinary catheter, as urinary incontinence will likely worsen the patient's wounds and increase the patient's chances of infection through the broken skin barrier. Choice *C* is an indication for a urinary catheter, as urinary retention in the best cases can lead to urinary tract infections and in the worst cases can lead to severe medical emergencies. Choice *D* is an indication for a urinary catheter because in critical patients, strict monitoring of intake and output can assist in early assessment of changes in condition. This benefit outweighs the risk of infection.

102. D: The correct answer is Choice *D*, status epilepticus. Status epilepticus is a state in which seizures recur before the patient has a return to baseline mentation. Choices *A* and *C* are incorrect. Tonic-clonic seizures were previously known as grand-mal seizures. These terms do not describe recurrent seizures.

103. A: The *T* in TNM refers to the size of the primary tumor. A tumor graded as *TX* indicates that there is a primary tumor that cannot be assessed, making Choice *A* correct. Choice *D* is incorrect because no evidence of a primary tumor would be graded as *T0*. Choices *B* and *C* are incorrect because these criteria are not part of the TNM model of tumor grading.

104. C: Patients with neuropathy often have limited sensation to their hands and feet, making them more prone to injury that can lead to infection. Patients should be counseled on regular examinations and care of hands and feet to prevent infection. Choices *A* and *B* are incorrect, as there is little data that exists to recommend routine vitamin E

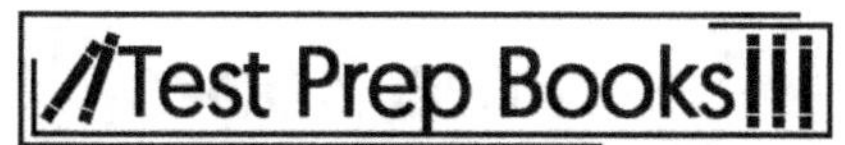

for the prevention of chemotherapy-induced peripheral neuropathy or lidocaine cream for the treatment of pain. For physical and emotional wellbeing, patients with neuropathy should continue to exercise as they are able, making Choice *D* incorrect. This may require a referral to physical therapy for an optimal program.

105. C: A Type III immune-mediated adverse drug reaction is the immune complex hypersensitivity reaction. An example of this reaction is the Arthus reaction to the tetanus vaccine. Examples of the type I reaction that is defined as IgE-mediated, immediate-type hypersensitivity are anaphylaxis and angioedema. Examples of the type II antibody-dependent cytotoxicity reaction is heparin-induced thrombocytopenia. Example of the type IV reaction—cell-mediated or delayed hypersensitivity—are drug rash and eosinophilia. Therefore, Choices *A, B* and *D* are incorrect.

106. C: Chlamydia and gonorrhea, sexually transmitted infections, are associated with the development of pelvic inflammatory disease (PID). When bacteria from these infections travel upward to the reproductive organs from the vagina or cervix, pelvic inflammatory disease may develop. The disorders and diseases represented by Choices *A, B,* and *D* are not associated with PID.

107. D: The CAGE assessment questionnaire is a four-question, provider-administered tool that is specific to alcohol abuse. The "C" refers to cutting down on drinking. The "A" asks if the patient has been annoyed by others questioning their drinking habits. The "G" asks if the patient has experienced guilt, and the "E" asks if the patient has ever found it necessary to drink in the morning. There is a form of this assessment that addresses drug abuse in addition to alcohol abuse. The DAST-20 tool is the Drug Abuse Screening Test for adolescents. TAPS is the Tobacco, Alcohol, Prescription medication and other Substance use scale that is either self-administered or provider-administered. The CRAFFT (car, relax, alone, forget, friends, and trouble) tool is used to assess the risk for substance use in adolescents. Therefore, Choices *A, B,* and *C* are incorrect.

108. C: Under the Patient Protection and Affordable Care Act (PPACA) in the FLSA, employers that have fifty or more employees are required to take extra precautions for their employees. This requirement mandates that employers provide a non-bathroom private location for expressing milk and provide breaks as much as needed. Compensation for breaks occurs the same as it would for other employees, but the breaks must be provided when needed. Choices *A, B,* and *D* fail to meet this criterion.

109. C: This patient most likely has uterine leiomyomata, or fibroids. The physical findings of an enlarged, tender, and irregular uterus are highly suggestive of this condition. TVUS is the preferred initial imaging study for confirmation. Choice *A* may be considered if TVUS is negative or inconclusive, but it is not first-line. Choice *B* is unlikely, as the patient and her husband have been struggling with infertility, and her last menstrual cycle began ten days ago. Also, TVUS would reveal pregnancy if it were the case. Choice *D* is not indicated for first-line workup in this patient.

110. A: Polycystic ovarian syndrome (PCOS) can be associated with Type 2 diabetes and metabolic syndrome given its ties with obesity and insulin resistance. Therefore, Choice *A* is correct. Endometriosis is a condition where endometrial cells migrate to places other than the uterus and cause pain during the menstrual cycle. It is not associated with PCOS and therefore Choice *B* is incorrect. There is no increased risk of cervical cancer with PCOS; therefore, Choice *C* is incorrect. While obesity can increase a patient's risk of developing hypertension, Choice *D*, it is not directly caused by PCOS and is therefore incorrect. Other risk factors such as diet, exercise, smoking, and age are more highly associated with hypertension.

111. C: It is possible that cancerous cells had spread before the mass from Paula's cervix was removed. Therefore, she will need to be monitored to ensure cancerous cells are not found or growing larger in other parts of her body. Choices *A, B,* and *D* make assumptions that the case facts do not support.

112. D: The lithotomy position (patient lying on back with legs in stirrups) is a common position used to perform general female pelvic examinations because it provides visualization of the vaginal and perianal areas and facilitates the insertion of speculum for exam. Choice *A* is incorrect because the supine position (patient lying on their back) does not provide visualization or access to the vagina for pelvic examinations. Choice *B* is incorrect because the Fowler's position (lying with upper body partially elevated) would limit visibility and access to the vaginal area. Choice *C* is incorrect because, although the Sims position can be useful for rectal examinations as well as for evaluation of vaginal prolapse, this left-lying position with knee bent is not regularly used for general pelvic exams.

113. C: The TWIST score was devised by urologists for use in establishing the diagnosis and treatment protocol for testicular torsion. The points assigned to the individual assessments include testis swelling (2 points), hard testis (2 points), absent cremasteric reflex (1 point), nausea/vomiting (1 point), and high-riding testis (1 point). The scoring system has also been validated for use by prehospital providers. In the presence of scrotal pain, a TWIST score of 0 is an indication that there is an alternative cause for the patient's manifestations. A TWIST score between 1 and 5 requires immediate ultrasonography to confirm the diagnosis. Immediate surgical intervention, without any delay to obtain ultrasonography, is the recommended intervention for a TWIST score of 6; therefore, Choice *C* is correct. The possibility of an alternative condition is associated with a TWIST score of 0; therefore, Choice *A* is incorrect. Ultrasonography is only recommended for patients with a TWIST score of 5 or less; therefore, Choice *B* is incorrect. Ultrasonography to confirm the diagnosis is recommended for a TWIST score of 5. However, immediate surgery is required for a TWIST score of 6; therefore, the scores have different implications, and Choice *D* is incorrect.

114. D: Whenever a patient has increased swelling to a limb, paired with limited mobility and pain, the WHNP should be concerned with a possible clot formation or worsening/new heart failure. With that in mind, sudden increased shortness of breath could be a sign of emergent changes to the cardiopulmonary system, such as pulmonary edema, or a pulmonary or cardiac embolism that may have traveled from the limb. Therefore, the attending physician and possibly other resources should be notified of the patient's condition immediately to prevent worsening outcomes. Choice *A* points to signs of venous insufficiency and possible heart failure. Choice *B* points to a possible infection in the limb causing the swelling and redness. Choice *C* points to a possible decreased pulse in the foot, which would require further monitoring in case of deep vein thrombosis formation. All of these choices may require physician notification and further assessment, but Choice *D* takes priority as it could indicate signs of emergent patient decompensation.

115. A: IV magnesium sulfate will be given to the pregnant woman experiencing eclampsia to prevent seizures. The other three IV medications listed are all used to correct fluid and electrolyte imbalances and may be used, but not specifically for the purpose of preventing seizures in a pregnant woman in hypertensive crisis.

116. D: An ABG result of pH 7.51, PaCO2 72 mmHg, and HCO3 41 mEq/L would indicate that the patient is in partially compensated metabolic alkalosis, making Choice D the correct answer. The patient is not in an acidotic state, making Choice A incorrect. A fully compensated metabolic alkalosis would have the pH returned to a normal level of 7.35-7.45, making Choice B incorrect. Lastly, the patient's PaCO2 is in the acidotic, not alkalotic, state to compensate for the metabolic alkalosis.

117. A: The antiemetic drug metoclopramide is a dopamine receptor antagonist that can increase the manifestations associated with Parkinson's disease by antagonizing the metabolism of dopamine and its derivatives. According to the 2019 BEERS report, the antiemetic should be avoided in all patients with Parkinson's disease. The remaining choices, Choices *B*, *C*, and *D*, have no known effect on dopamine function.

118. C: Under the Pregnancy Discrimination Act of 1978, an employer must give a woman a comparable position to the one that she held prior to her maternity leave (if the company does so with employees on short-term disability). An employer may not refuse accommodations, ask about pregnancy status, or in any way discriminate against an employee for reasons related to pregnancy, making Choices *A*, *B*, and *D* incorrect.

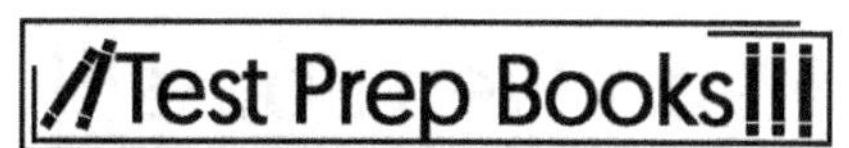

119. B: Noreen gave birth to her son ten months ago, but postpartum anxiety can manifest anytime from birth to one year after. It occurs in newer mothers and is characterized by an inability to sleep or relax. Panicked or worried thoughts typically relate directly to the baby. Generalized anxiety and social anxiety disorders can affect people of both genders in various life phases, so Choices *A* and *C* can be eliminated. Although Noreen is having trouble sleeping, she does not appear to have circadian rhythm sleep disorder, which is a disorder influenced by a person's hormones and environment. A person's internal circadian rhythms do not follow natural patterns, so the person may end up awake at night or asleep all day. This disorder tends to affect shift workers. Therefore, Choice *D* is incorrect.

120. C: The GAD7 is a screening tool used to assess anxiety symptoms over time; therefore, Choice *C* is correct. It should be given before treatment and then at each follow-up. If anxiety symptoms have decreased after treatment, the NP can conclude that the treatment is working. A PHQ9, Choice *A*, is used to assess depression. The MOCA screening, Choice *B*, is used to assess mild cognitive impairment. The CAGE screening, Choice *D*, is used to assess substance abuse.

121. D: HPV has been linked to multiple cancers, including anal, bladder, cervical, head and neck, penile, vaginal, and vulvar cancers. Choice *A* refers to cancers linked to the hepatitis virus. Choice *B* refers to cancers linked to *Helicobacter pylori* infections. Choice *C* refers to cancers associated with human immunodeficiency virus (HIV) infections.

122. A: This path correctly describes where blood flows after leaving the lungs in order to reach the tissues of the body. The other paths listed are incorrect, out of order, and list fictitious structures.

123. A: Loop diuretics, such as Lasix, are not appropriate for the initial treatment of HTN. Thiazide diuretics are used initially to minimize the effects of the drug on the kidneys and to avoid an electrolyte imbalance. Medications from the remaining categories are often used in the initial treatment of HTN; therefore, Choices *B, C,* and *D* are incorrect.

124. B: The pelvic cavity is the area formed by the bones of the hip. Housed in that space are the urinary bladder, urethra, ureters, anus, and rectum. This hollow space also contains the uterus in females. The other body cavities listed contain other organs not specified in the question.

125. B: Betamethasone therapy can improve the maturity of the fetal lungs by increasing the amount of available surfactant, which allows adaptation of the respiratory system immediately after birth. However, prolonged gestation, which permits additional time for the lungs to mature naturally is more effective than administration of additional corticosteroids; therefore, Choice *B* is correct. Research indicates that the administration of steroids such as betamethasone in the presence of the premature rupture of membranes (PROM) increases the incidence of infection; therefore, Choice *A* is incorrect. Successful treatment with betamethasone may reduce the incidence of respiratory distress syndrome in the newborn. However, there is no evidence that the risk is eliminated by betamethasone; therefore, Choice *C* is incorrect. Betamethasone is only used to mature the fetal lungs by increasing the amount of surfactant that is available to facilitate the expansion of the newborn lungs. It is not a tocolytic agent (an agent that decreases uterine contractions in preterm labor), and, in addition, tocolytic agents cannot be used for longer than 48 hours; therefore, Choice *D* is incorrect.

126. B: Increased arterial blood flow is not a factor that contributes to development of a venous thrombosis. Increased blood flow and perfusion may help decrease the likelihood of venous thrombosis. Choices *A, C,* and *D* are incorrect because endothelial injury, blood stasis, and hypercoagulability are all part of Virchow's Triad describing the three factors that can lead to venous thrombus formation.

127. A: Choice *A* is correct because pleuritic pain is one of the most common symptoms associated with a pulmonary embolism. Pleuritic pain is characterized by severe pain in the chest that worsens upon inspiration and expiration. Choice *B* is incorrect because a temperature of 99.8 °F (37.6 °C) is slightly above normal range. Low grade fever is a *non-specific* sign associated with pulmonary embolism. Choice *C* is incorrect because right calf erythema is an expected finding for deep vein thrombosis. This finding does not directly support a diagnosis of pulmonary embolism. Choice *D* is incorrect because a heart rate of 102 beats/min is slightly above normal. Tachycardia is associated with pulmonary embolism. However, it is not as specific to the respiratory system as pleuritic pain.

128. A: There is no chance that an offspring will have O blood or AB blood (see Punnett square).

	I^A	I^B
i	I^Ai	I^Bi
i	I^Ai	I^Bi

129. C: Patient and family-centered care (PFCC) is an approach to healthcare that involves collaboration among healthcare providers, patients, and their families to meet the patient's physical, emotional, and psychological needs. It recognizes the importance of involving patients and their families in the care and decision-making process. Choices *A*, *B*, and *D* do not demonstrate PFCC.

130. C: Women who are diagnosed with GDM should be tested for persistent diabetes or prediabetes at 6 to 12 weeks postpartum and then at least every three years. If the patient is diagnosed with prediabetes, the WHNP will consider metformin therapy and will provide counseling for lifestyle changes. Testing is positive for prediabetes if the HbA1c is 5.7-6.5 percent. Choice *A* is incorrect because the 1-hour OGTT is positive for GDM when the glucose level is ≥ 180 mg/dL. Choice *B* is incorrect because women with a history of GDM should be tested at least every three years. Choice *D* is incorrect because pregnant women with no history of diabetes should be tested at 24 to 26 weeks of gestation.

131. A: Choice *A* is the best action by the WHNP because encouraging the patient to discuss future reconstructive surgery will provide options for sexual activity. A total pelvic exenteration removes all organs within the pelvic cavity, including the vagina. Choice *B* is not the best action because the WHNP cannot predict the patient's recovery or promote false reassurance. Choice *C* is not the best intervention by the WHNP because the action does not address the patient's concerns regarding intimacy. Choice *D* is not the best action by the WHNP because the intervention ignores the patient's main concern regarding intimacy.

132. B: This patient's significantly elevated blood pressure in combination with their signs/symptoms suggests a hypertensive emergency, which requires immediate blood pressure reduction. Hypertensive urgency, Choice *A*, is characterized by significantly elevated blood pressure without signs of organ damage. Acute heart failure, Choice *C*, and acute stroke, Choice *D*, could be potential complications of a hypertensive emergency but do not fully explain this patient's symptoms and findings.

133. B: Hyperglycemia occurs when the patient's blood sugar level is greater than 200 milligrams per deciliter. Common symptoms of hyperglycemia include polyuria (excessive urination), polydipsia (excessive thirst), nausea, abdominal pain, fruity-scented breath, and confusion. Choices *A*, *C*, and *D* describe symptoms of hypoglycemia.

134. B: Asian populations have an increased incidence of lactose intolerance, which means that the WHNP will consider appropriate alterations to the nutritional plan of care.

135. B: This patient should undergo a screening mammogram. Every major guideline, including the USPSTF, recommends screening for breast cancer via mammography at least every two years after age 40 or 45. Some guidelines recommend annual screening. Choice *A* is not necessary, as the patient's last Pap smear was last year,

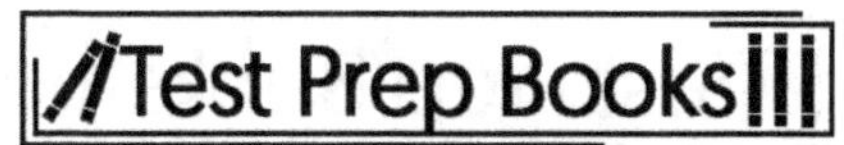

and current guidelines recommend this test every three years. Choice *C* is unnecessary because her last colonoscopy was only two years ago, but it would be prudent to seek the specialist's recommendation for when she should follow up. Choice *D* is not indicated but will be due soon; DEXA scans are recommended starting at age 65 for osteoporosis screening.

136. C: Coumadin, also known as warfarin, is an anticoagulant medication that prevents blood clots. Its mechanism of action is through interference with the synthesis of vitamin K-dependent clotting factors, which are important factors needed for blood to clot. Coumadin can be prescribed to prevent or even treat conditions including deep vein thrombosis or pulmonary embolism. Prothrombin time (PT) is the laboratory test used to measure how long it takes for blood to clot. Even though platelets are important in the clotting process, it does not indicate the effectiveness of Coumadin therapy. Instead, it is better at assessing the risk or possibility of bleeding or clotting disorders, making Choice *A* incorrect. Choice *B* is also incorrect because Coumadin does not have any effect on hemoglobin, or red blood cell count. Activated partial thromboplastin time (aPTT) is a test that can monitor the effectiveness of heparin therapy, another type of anticoagulant medication, making Choice *D* incorrect.

137. D: With medical therapy, many people with HIV are able to live normal, healthy lives. The patient should not wait until symptoms are present to seek medical care, since the earlier HIV is treated, the better the viral load can be managed; therefore, Choice *A* is not correct. Choice *B* is also incorrect since early medical care can enable a person with HIV to lead a normal life. Choice *C* is not correct, because not all treatment leads to undetectable viral loads.

138. A: This patient has PID, for which cervical motion tenderness (a positive chandelier sign) is a highly specific finding. Choice *B* is unlikely, as the urinalysis was negative for leukocyte esterase and nitrites, and the patient did not have costovertebral angle tenderness. Choice *C* should be on the differential diagnosis list for lower abdominal pain, but a positive chandelier sign makes PID much more likely. Choice *D* is incorrect given the above urinalysis findings. Also, the presence of a fever would automatically mean complicated cystitis rather than uncomplicated.

139. A: Spinal cord compression occurs when there is an impact to the spinal cord or cauda equina by the tumor, resulting in direct pressure, vertebral collapse, or both. Patients with breast, lung, prostate, renal, and melanoma are at high risk due to the affinity of the tumor to metastasize to the bone. Patients with metastatic disease at presentation are at higher risk than those with localized disease. Choice *A* is at highest risk due to having breast cancer that is widely metastatic. Choice *B* is low risk, as the patient has a locally advanced colon cancer. Choice *C* is incorrect, as the patient has localized bladder cancer. Choice *D* is incorrect, as the patient has a locally advanced prostate cancer.

140. D: In type 2 diabetes, the pancreas produces insulin, but the body does not use it effectively. This type of diabetes may be treated with oral anti-diabetic medications and, in some cases, insulin. However, many people can control their type 2 diabetes through lifestyle changes, such as losing weight and eating less carbohydrate-rich and sugar-laden foods, making Choices *A*, *B*, and *C* incorrect.

141. A: A grade 2 murmur is softly audible with the stethoscope, and it is NOT accompanied by a palpable thrill. Grade 3 murmurs are generally not accompanied by a palpable thrill; therefore, Choice *B* is incorrect. A grade 4 murmur is audible even with only partial contact between the stethoscope and the skin; therefore, Choice *C* is incorrect. A 5/6 murmur is audible with only minimal contact between the skin and the stethoscope; however, there is most often an audible thrill present as well; therefore, Choice *D* is incorrect.

142. B: Cigarette smoking is a major cause of atherosclerosis, the most common cause of aortic aneurysms. Following a low-fat diet would help with dyslipidemia, which may be a contributor to atherosclerosis, but it is not as important as stopping smoking, which causes the inflammatory, toxic effects that produce atherosclerosis. Exercise is helpful in coping with stress effectively, as is meditation, but not specific to atherosclerosis that causes aortic aneurysms.

143. C: Choice *C* is the best response by the WHNP because the question encourages the patient to talk openly about their feelings and promotes therapeutic communication. Choice *A* is not the best response by the WHNP because stating a fact of therapy does not address the patient's concern. Choice *B* is not the best response by the WHNP because the question encourages the patient to think about ending necessary medical treatment before other interventions are explored. Choice *D* is not the best response by the WHNP because the statement speaks negatively about the patient's partner.

144. B: Unfortunately, endometriosis cannot be definitively diagnosed with noninvasive testing.

Thus, exploratory laparotomy represents the gold standard for definitive diagnosis. Choice *A* would certainly be important to rule out other causes of pelvic pain and abnormal uterine bleeding; however, it would not itself rule in endometriosis. Choices *C* and *D* face similar challenges, and additionally, they are not as commonly utilized as ultrasound given their higher cost and demand.

145. A: DVT is the most common cause of edema caused by venous insufficiency. The other three factors are also causes, but not as common as DVT.

146. D: An ectopic pregnancy results from the abnormal implantation of the fertilized ovum at a site other than the uterus. The fallopian tube is the implantation site in 94 percent of ectopic pregnancies, which means that there is some impedance to the normal eight- to ten-day passage of the fertilized ovum from the fallopian tube to the uterus. The fallopian tube is lined by hair-like extensions, or cilia, which provide the motility that propels the ovum from the point of fertilization to the appropriate implantation site in the uterus. There is clear research evidence that one of the effects of smoking is the blunting or destruction of the cilia, which decreases the efficiency of this process, thereby contributing to the likelihood of faulty implantation.

The process of implantation and initial development of the placenta is a hypoxic environment in the initial weeks of the first trimester due to "plugging" alterations in the vasculature of the endometrium that prevent maternal hemorrhage. Hypoxia from smoking is associated with fetal intrauterine growth delay later in the pregnancy. However, it does not directly affect implantation; therefore, Choice *A* is incorrect. Smoking affects the lining of the fallopian tube but has no identified effect on progesterone levels; therefore, Choice *B* is incorrect. Smoking directly affects the lining of the fallopian tubes. However, there is no evidence of any similar effect on the endometrium; therefore, Choice *C* is incorrect.

147. C: Bone health depends on Vitamin D, Vitamin C, and sufficient calcium. The remaining choices are important to other processes; therefore, Choices *A, B,* and *D* are incorrect.

148. C: Warfarin has a long half-life, and it requires "bridging" from parenteral anticoagulants and frequent monitoring. In addition, there are multiple drug–drug and drug–food reactions associated with warfarin use. When compared to warfarin, the newer drugs have shorter half-lives that do not require bridging or frequent monitoring for safe administration. Therefore, Choices *A* and *B* are incorrect. Choice *D* is incorrect because warfarin has multiple interactions.

149. D: Unless facility policy describes otherwise, nurses are not to re-suture incisions. The surgeon or first-assist usually takes charge of such duties, as they are specially trained to do so. The nurse will monitor the wound, assess for signs of infection, maintain a clean dressing daily or as prescribed, and apply prescribed medications.

150. A: Fetuses are vulnerable to developmental delays during the first trimester of pregnancy; no links have been shown during the other two trimesters. This may be due to the robust amount of brain growth that takes place

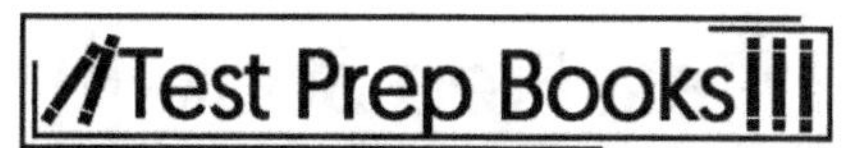

specifically during the first trimester. Any teratogenic agents may inhibit new neural pathways or brain matter from forming.

151. A: Fitz-Hugh–Curtis perihepatitis presents with characteristic "violin string" adhesions that are due to an inflammation of the surface of Glisson's capsule, which is a layer of connective tissue that surrounds the liver and encloses the hepatic artery, the portal vein, and the bile ducts within the liver. The condition is most often secondary to pelvic inflammatory disease caused by chlamydia or gonorrhea. Therefore, Choice *A* is correct. The hepatitis is the result of the infection by the pathogen that causes PID; it is not an autoimmune response. The pathogen is thought to migrate to the abdomen and liver from the fallopian tubes, causing the inflammatory process that results in right upper quadrant pain and altered liver function; therefore, Choice *B* is incorrect. The inflammatory process is most often caused by chlamydia or gonorrhea and is not associated with the late stages of syphilis infection; therefore, Choice *C* is incorrect. The patient may report little or no pelvic pain with this syndrome; therefore, Choice *D* is incorrect.

152. D: Enoxaparin therapy is generally done to prevent the formation of embolism and deep vein thrombosis in patients who have limited mobility. While it may be indicated for a patient who just had surgery, it is not likely to reduce atelectasis. The other choices will assist the patient to breathe more deeply, opening up the lungs to prevent atelectasis.

153. D: Treatment-related secondary cancers tend to develop within several years of initial exposure. Chemotherapy and radiation increase the chances of developing a secondary malignancy.

154. B: Chemotherapy treatment for testicular cancer typically includes cisplatin and etoposide, which are linked to leukemia. The risk increases if the patient is also treated with radiation. Melanoma is an uncommon secondary malignancy in this scenario, making Choice *A* incorrect. Prostate and rectal cancers are linked to radiation treatment, not chemotherapy, making Choices *C* and *D* incorrect.

155. D: This patient most likely has a prolactinoma. This is a benign pituitary tumor that secretes prolactin, the hormone that promotes expression of breast milk. MRI of the brain is the most sensitive imaging study for this condition. Choice *A* would be more appropriate if the patient's pregnancy test were positive. Choice *B* would not likely reveal any significant findings and would be more appropriate for unilateral breast discharge. Choice *C* would not necessarily be harmful, but it would similarly be more useful for unilateral discharge.

156. A: An INR is a lab test that can show medication effectiveness of Warfarin (Coumadin), a blood thinner. It has a therapeutic range of 2.0-3.0. Since the lab result was 2.8 and within the therapeutic range, the NP can determine the dose adjustment was effective and can keep the dosage the same, Choice *A*. Choice *B* is incorrect because the treatment was effective since she is now in the therapeutic range. Choice *C* is incorrect because the management is within the scope of practice of a nurse practitioner. Choice *D* is incorrect because the results are conclusive and within the normal range.

157. B: Hemolysis is the underlying defect of sickle cell disease, due to the abnormally shaped or sickled red blood cells, and hemolysis results in an increased concentration of free hemoglobin. Under normal circumstances, nitric oxide is responsible for triggering vasodilation and relaxation of the smooth muscle of the penis, resulting in tumescence. However, nitric oxide is scavenged by free hemoglobin, which means that the elevated levels of free hemoglobin due to hemolysis in sickle cell disease results in a deficit of nitric oxide and sustained venous outflow inhibition and failure of the tumescent process, causing priapism. Choice *B* is the correct answer. As noted, hemoglobin is released by hemolysis, which leads to *increased* free hemoglobin and continued venous outflow inhibition and sustained priapism; therefore, Choice *A* is incorrect.

Sickle cell disease is an inherited autosomal genetic defect that affects the structure of the red blood cell. It is associated with specific genes and does not involve alterations in the immune response. Sickle cell disease affects vasodilation by the release of free hemoglobin. The disease does not directly affect vasodilation; therefore, Choice *C* is incorrect. There is little research evidence for the efficacy of the prophylactic use of medications used to treat erectile dysfunction, and their use is not commonly recommended; therefore, Choice *D* is incorrect.

158. C: Reduced practice requires physician oversight only for prescriptive practice. Restricted practice requires physician oversight for all aspects of NP practice. Unrestricted practice places no restrictions on NP practice. Therefore, Choices *A* and *D* are incorrect. Choice *B* does not define a specific practice model; therefore, it is incorrect.

159. A: Anti-viral therapy will be started immediately after exposure, without waiting for further specialty consultation if the exposed person is pregnant due to the risk of the unborn fetus. HIV testing will be conducted at frequent intervals to monitor for the presence of evidence of infection; therefore, Choice *B* is incorrect. The precautions listed in Choice *C* are necessary to prevent possible contamination in the event that the exposure has resulted in infection of the exposed individual by the HIV virus; therefore, Choice *C* is incorrect. Renal, hepatic, and hematology studies are monitored to assess any effects of the HIV virus and/or the effects of anti-viral medications if ordered; therefore, Choice *D* is incorrect.

160. C: HbA1c levels from 4.5-5.6 are normal, from 5.7-6.4 indicates prediabetes, and 6.5 or higher indicates diabetes. This patient's HbA1c has lowered into the normal range due to her lifestyle modifications and therefore the dose of Metformin can be decreased, Choice *C*. Choice *A* is incorrect because the dose of Metformin should not be increased and is at its maximum dose. Choice *B* is incorrect because step-down therapy should be tried. The nurse practitioner should re-evaluate the HbA1c in three months and assess the need for dosage changes again. Choice *D* is incorrect because the dose should be slowly stepped down and not stopped abruptly.

161. B: Choice *B* is correct because it states that maintaining a healthy birth weight while carrying an embryo reduces the prospect of negative risks, which is accurate. This process of carrying an embryo is called gestation and sustaining a healthy birth weight during pregnancy can decrease the possibility of associated negative risks. Choice *A* is incorrect because research has shown that prenatal nutrition is one of the most important factors in ensuring a fetus's well-being. Some examples of nutritious foods for infants during prenatal development consist of lean meats, fruits, low-fat dairy products, vegetables, and whole grains. Choice *C* is incorrect because research shows that abusing substances while pregnant can result in long-term problems for infants. A few examples of some of these problems include neonatal abstinence syndrome, fetal alcohol syndrome, and sudden infant death syndrome. Choice *D* is incorrect because the developmental stage of an infant can indeed affect their susceptibility to teratogens. For instance, an infant in their first trimester is most prone to damage from different teratogenic agents.

162. B: Placenta previa often presents in the third trimester of pregnancy as vaginal bleeding that is painless. In this condition, the cervical os is either partially or completely covered by the placenta, leading to bleeding as the cervix begins to dilate or efface. Choice *A* is incorrect because placental abruption typically presents with abdominal pain, uterine tenderness, and sometimes vaginal bleeding, which is inconsistent with this patient's presentation. Choice *C* would generally present with abdominal pain and regular contractions, rather than painless vaginal bleeding. Choice *D* is characterized by the deep implantation of the placenta into the uterine wall, which can lead to significant bleeding during delivery. However, it is not typically associated with painless vaginal bleeding during pregnancy, as described by the patient's symptoms.

163. B: BV is often diagnosed using the Amsel criteria, of which three out of four must be met. The Amsel criteria include thin, homogenous white or yellow discharge; clue cells on microscopy; vaginal fluid pH greater than 4.5; and a fishy amine odor after addition of potassium hydroxide to the fluid. Choice *A* is incorrect, as nitrites on urinalysis are associated with a UTI, not BV. While pH is included in the Amsel criteria, Choice *C* features a pH of less than 4.5 rather than over 4.5. Choice *D* may be present in BV, but it is not part of the Amsel criteria and is more likely in cervicitis or trichomoniasis.

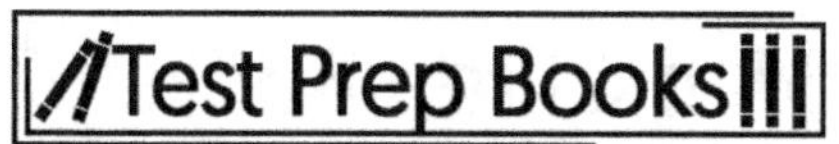

164. A: Virchow's triad identifies factors that contribute to the thrombotic process associated with deep venous thrombosis (DVT) and pulmonary embolism (PE). The triad consists of hypercoagulability, endothelial injury/dysfunction, and hemodynamic changes such as stasis and turbulence. Heart disease is a risk factor for DVT and PE, but it is not part of Virchow's triad.

165. C: Every patient seeking any nonbarrier method of contraception must be reminded that these methods do not protect against STIs. Thus, it is considered best practice to encourage patients to use condoms during intercourse regardless of their primary mode of contraception. Choice *A* is incorrect, as the Nexplanon® rod may remain in place for three years, not five years. It is indeed a highly effective method of contraception (Choice *B*) and may confer the added benefit of improved hormonal regulation, leading to reduction in symptoms such as breast pain or mood swings (Choice *D*).

166. C: The Wells score is a multi-step calculation that assesses the likelihood of a pulmonary embolism (PE). The assessment criteria include the presence of clinical signs and symptoms of DVT; a clinical decision that PE is the number one diagnosis or equally likely; a heart rate above 100; a history of immobilization for at least three days or surgery in the previous four weeks; a history of previous, objectively diagnosed PE or DVT; hemoptysis; and a history of malignancy with treatment within the last six months or palliative care. Each of these elements is scored as zero if the element is not present, or from one to three points if it is present. The Wells score cannot confirm the presence of a DVT, so Choice *B* is incorrect. Choices *A* and *D* are not associated with the Wells score and are therefore incorrect.

167. D: Aspirin works by inhibiting platelet aggregation to prevent clot formation. Paroxetine is used to treat anxiety and depression. Coumadin® (warfarin) works by blocking vitamin K-dependent clotting factors. Heparin enhances the effect of antithrombin III to inhibit thrombin activation.

168. D: Choice *D* is the most contributive risk factor for the development of catheter-associated urinary tract infections. The catheter should be removed as soon as possible to prevent bacteria from entering the urinary tract. Choice *A* is important. However, perineal care alone does not prevent bacterial colonization in other areas of the catheter, such as the drainage bag. Choice *B* helps prevent stagnant urine. However, this factor alone does not prevent CAUTIs. Choice *C* protects the healthcare providers from contamination but does not protect the patient from developing a CAUTI.

169. B: Of the two types of human immunodeficiency virus (HIV), HIV-1 is the dominant strain among global cases. HIV-2 is not highly transmissible, so Choice *A* is not correct. Since HIV-2 is poorly understood, Choice *C* is not correct. HIV-1 is the more severe strain.

170. C: Until the 1980s, homosexuality was classified as a psychological disorder in the DSM. Autism spectrum disorder is listed in the DSM-5, as is seasonal affective disorder (although listed as a subset of depression). Thus, Choice *A* and *D* are incorrect. Choice *B* is incorrect because HIV has never been listed as a discrete diagnosis in any edition of the DSM.

171. C: Aminoglycosides such as gentamicin alter neuromuscular transmission, which can cause muscle weakness. In patients with myasthenia gravis, muscle weakness results in respiratory depression. While there is a general caution for the use of aminoglycosides in the elderly, there is no contraindication for their use in the remaining diseases; therefore, Choices *A, B*, and *D* are incorrect.

172. C: One of the limitations of GINA is that the protections afforded by the law do not apply to manifested disease or previously diagnosed conditions, which may prevent patients from having the testing. Long-term care insurance providers are exempt from the provisions of GINA; therefore, Choice *A* is incorrect. Employers are not allowed to use genetic information for any employment decisions; therefore, Choice *B* is incorrect. Health insurance companies cannot use request genetic testing for any individual; therefore, Choice *D* is incorrect.

173. B: After a deep vein thrombosis is identified, the patient will begin receiving low molecular weight heparin subcutaneously. Unfractionated heparin may also be used in addition to aspirin or other anticoagulants. Choice *A* is incorrect; placing sequential compression devices on a leg with a DVT results in a risk of dislodging the clot, which can then travel through the body and cause a pulmonary embolism (PE). Choice *C* is incorrect. An IVC filter is placed for hypercoagulable patients in order to prevent a DVT from traveling to the lungs and causing a PE; it will not prevent new DVTs from forming. Choice *D* is incorrect. While walking and exercise are good interventions to prevent DVTs from forming, walking and frequent exercise can dislodge an existing DVT and could result in a PE.

174. A: The providers are in the planning stage. When they develop a change to implement, they'll be in the Do stage. Once the change has been implemented, they'll check the results and compare it to their baseline re-admittance and printout retention rates. Finally, they'll act to sustain any positive changes.

175. A: Apgar scores of 8 and 9 are normal scores for a healthy newborn with acrocyanosis, which is a benign condition manifested by peripheral cyanosis of the hands and feet that usually resolves within the first few hours after birth. Decreased muscle tone or flexion is most often associated with other deficits that would result in a lower Apgar score; therefore, Choice *B* is incorrect. If the newborn required ventilatory support, there would also be deficits of muscle tone and heart rate, resulting in lower Apgar scores; therefore, Choice *C* is incorrect. The Apgar score is not predictive of specific anomalies, and the indicated scores are considered as normal; therefore, Choice *D* is incorrect.

Practice Test #2

To keep the size of this book manageable, save paper, and provide a digital test-taking experience, the 2nd practice test can be found online. Scan the QR code or go to this link to access it:

testprepbooks.com/online387/npwh

SCAN ME

The first time you access the tests, you will need to register as a "new user" and verify your email address.

If you have any issues, please email support@testprepbooks.com.

Dear Future WHNP,

Thank you for purchasing this study guide for your NP Women's Health exam. We hope that we exceeded your expectations.

Our goal in creating this study guide was to cover all of the topics that you will see on the test. We also strove to make our practice questions as similar as possible to what you will encounter on test day. With that being said, if you found something that you feel was not up to your standards, please send us an email and let us know.

We would also like to let you know about other books in our catalog that may interest you.

PANCE

This can be found on Amazon: amazon.com/dp/1637758715

NP Family

amazon.com/dp/1637758006

We have study guides and flashcards in a wide variety of fields. If the one you are looking for isn't listed above, then try searching for it on Amazon or send us an email.

Thanks Again and Happy Testing!
Product Development Team
support@testprepbooks.com

Online Resources

Included with your purchase are multiple online resources. This includes the practice tests in an interactive format and a convenient study timer to help you manage your time.

Scan the QR code or go to this link to access this content:

testprepbooks.com/online387/npwh

SCAN ME

The first time you access the page, you will need to register as a "new user" and verify your email address.

If you have any issues, please email support@testprepbooks.com.
Thank you for letting us be a part of your studying journey!

www.ingramcontent.com/pod-product-compliance
Lightning Source LLC
LaVergne TN
LVHW061238100826
845148LV00008B/978
* 9 7 8 1 6 3 7 7 5 7 3 8 3 *